FIRST AID FAST for Babies and Children

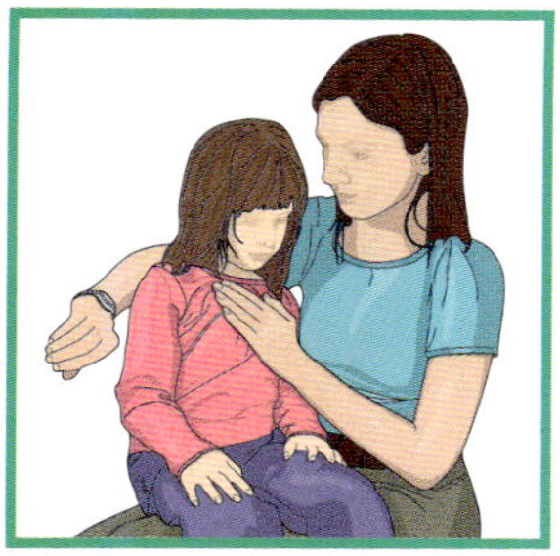
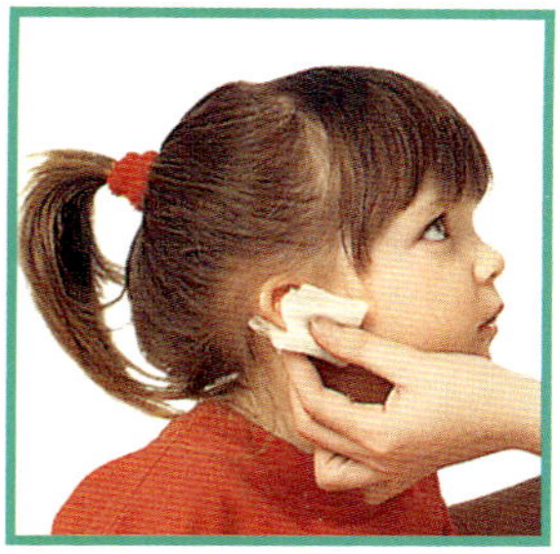
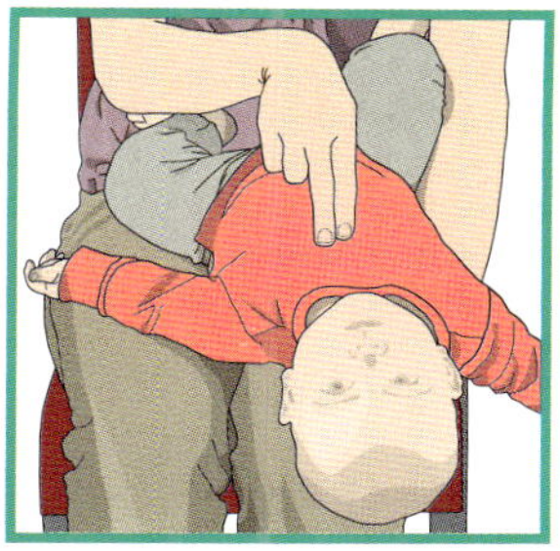
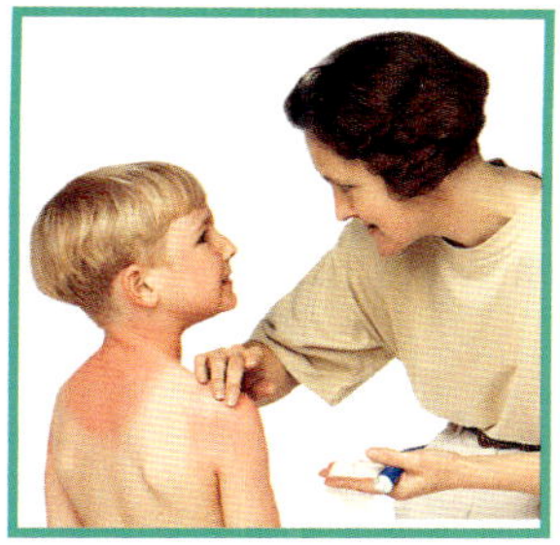

FIRST AID FAST for Babies and Children

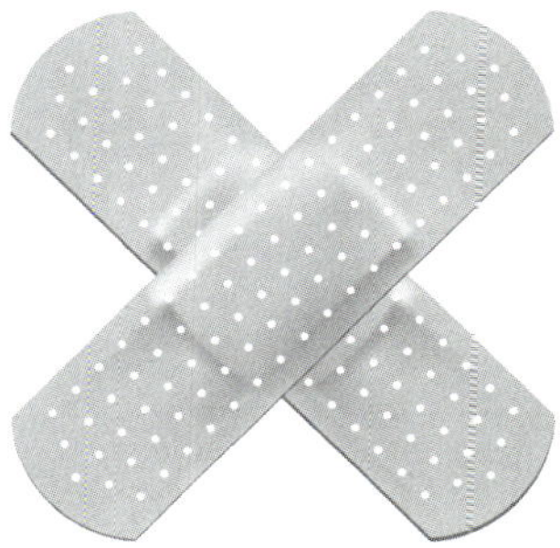

Emergency procedures for all parents and caregivers

2ND CANADIAN EDITION
Revised and Updated

Canadian Medical Consultant
DR. ANNA YVONNE KEMPINSKA, FRCPC

DK

DK Penguin Random House

DK LONDON

Consultant Editor Jemima Dunne
Senior Art Editor Sharon Spencer
Project Editor Miezan van Zyl
Jacket Designer Mark Cavanagh
Managing Editor Angeles Gavira
Managing Art Editor Michael Duffy
Pre-Production Producer Andy Hilliard
Producer Jude Crozier
Art Director Karen Self
Publisher Liz Wheeler
Publishing Director Jonathan Metcalf

DK INDIA

Art Editors Konica Juneja, Anjali Sachar
Senior DTP Designers Vishal Bhatia, Sachin Singh
Managing Editor Rohan Sinha
Deputy Managing Art Editor Anjana Nair
Pre-production Manager Balwant Singh
Production Manager Pankaj Sharma
Jacket Designer Dhirendra Singh
Managing Jackets Editor Sreshtha Bhattacharya

DK CANADA

Canadian Editors Barbara Campbell, Anna Kempinska

Second Canadian Edition, 2017
DK Canada 320 Front Street, Suite 1400, Toronto, ON M5V 3B6

17 18 19 20 21 10 9 8 7 6 5 4 3 2 1

001–308459–Oct/2017

Published in Great Britain by Dorling Kindersley Limited

Library and Archives Canada Cataloguing in Publication
First aid for children fast
First aid fast for babies and children / Canadian medical consultant, Dr. Anna Kempinska. -- 2nd Canadian edition.
Includes index.
Previous edition published under title: First aid for children fast.
Previous edition edited by Paul Munk.
ISBN 978-1-55363-287-0 (softcover)
1. Pediatric emergencies--Popular works. 2. First aid in illness and injury. I. Kempinska, Anna, editor II. Title.
RJ370.F58 2017 618.92'00252 C2017-901081-6

Printed and bound in China

Disclaimer:
First Aid Fast for Babies and Children provides information and guidance on initial care following an incident or if a child is unwell, but should not be regarded as a substitute for medical advice. The publisher and medical consultant do not accept responsibility for any claims arising from the use of this manual.

Foreword

As an emergency room pediatrician, I see many different types of ailments and injuries in children. Fortunately, serious accidents and illnesses rarely occur, but it is important to be prepared in case they do. Good and timely first aid care can not only save a life, but also help prevent further injury and speed recovery.

This updated edition of *First Aid Fast for Babies and Children* contains the latest Canadian guidelines for life-saving procedures as well as treatment of minor ailments and injuries. The informative text, user-friendly layout, and step-by-step photos will help parents and caregivers understand how to manage an injury or illness, know when to see a doctor, and identify more urgent situations when it is necessary to call 911 or go to the hospital.

The information contained in this book can help to reduce panic and increase confidence in your skills to handle an emergency. This book is an excellent resource, but I recommend also taking a first aid course from a reputable instructor such as St. John Ambulance or the Canadian Red Cross, particularly a course on Emergency Child Care and/or CPR.

The importance of injury prevention cannot be overstated. Most "accidents" are not accidents at all, but are preventable incidents. On each and every shift in the ER, I see children whose injuries could easily have been avoided had proper safety measures been in place. A child's curiosity and desire to explore are natural, but please take the time to read the Home Safety section in this book to make sure your child is having fun in a safe environment!

Warm wishes for safe play,

Anna Yvonne Kempinska, MD FRCPC

Contents

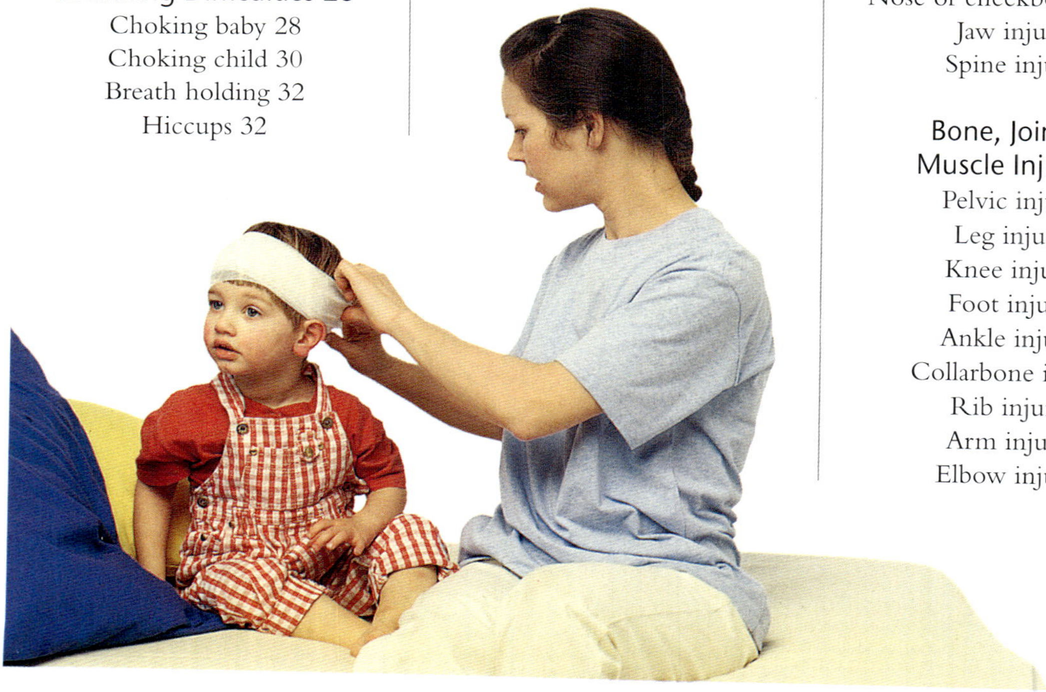

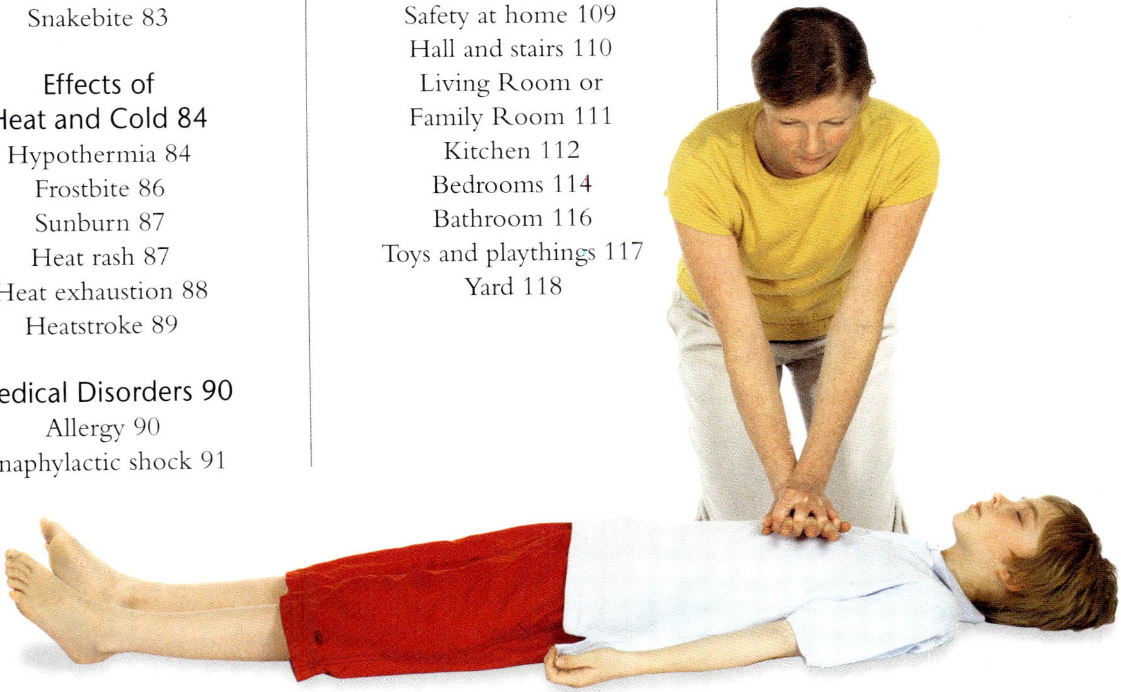

Introduction

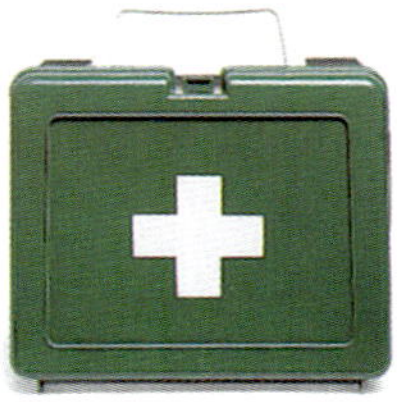

This book has been compiled primarily for parents but also for others—grandparents, teachers, playgroup leaders, and babysitters—who may regularly, or even just occasionally, find themselves in charge of babies and children. The content has been set out in a clear and logical way and the information is presented largely in pictorial form using simple words and captions to make it very easy to follow and to understand. The first aid advice given can be used to treat any age child and follows the most up-to-date clinical guidance at the time of publication.

Emergencies are, by their very nature, unexpected events and can be extremely frightening and stressful for anyone caring for a child. *First Aid Fast for Babies and Children* will help you learn various practical skills that will help you manage a wide range of first aid emergencies and everyday incidents, building your confidence and ensuring that you respond in the best way possible. The calmer you are, the more effective your help will be, and by listening and talking to the child you will be able to make the best decision for both of you, greatly improving the outcome.

In addition, there is reference information at the back of the book. A section on first aid kits and bandaging techniques also lists useful items to have at home and how to use them. The pages on Home Safety highlight potential danger areas around the home and how to fix them to minimize the risk of incidents in the first place.

How to use this book

This book covers first aid treatment for everything from minor cuts and abrasions to treating a child who is not responding. For every condition a series of photographs or illustrations shows you exactly what to do in an emergency. Key pieces of information are indicated on the photographs, and supplementary advice can be found alongside in the step-by-step text.

The injuries are organized by type, in coloured sections such as Breathing Difficulties or Wounds and Bleeding. However, in an emergency, the thumbnail index on the back cover will direct you straight to the relevant page. There are also sections, such as Action in an Emergency, Bandages and Dressings, and Home Safety, that contain information for general reference.

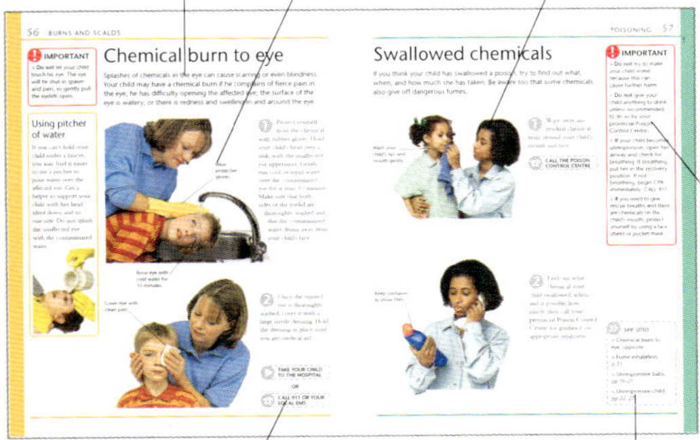

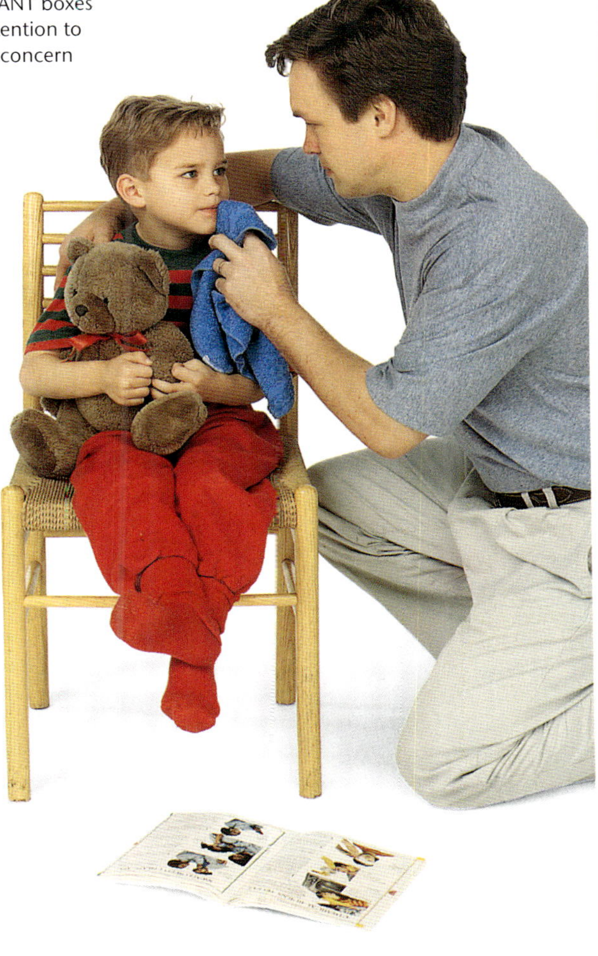

Guide to the symbols

The following symbols and instructions appear if your child needs further medical attention:

SEEK MEDICAL ADVICE

Depending on your area, call your doctor's office, nurse practitioner, or telehealth service for advice.

TAKE YOUR CHILD TO THE HOSPITAL

Take your child to the nearest hospital emergency department if you have help and transportation.

CALL 911 OR YOUR LOCAL EMS

Your child needs urgent medical attention and is best transported by trained medical experts to the hospital.

Action in an emergency

In any emergency, particularly one involving children, it is important to remain calm and act logically. Remember four steps:

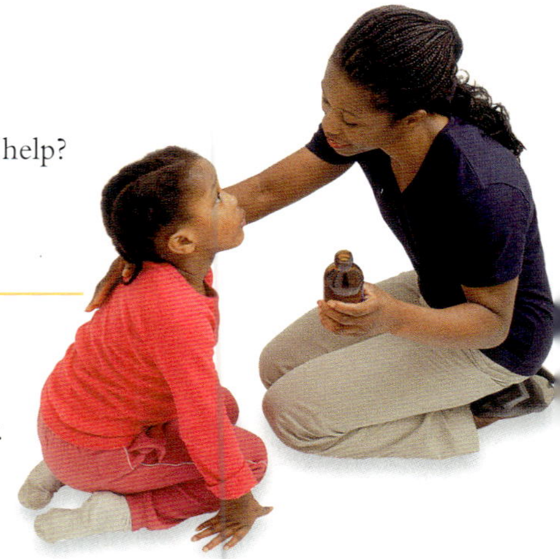

1 Assess the situation

- What happened and how did it happen?
- Is it safe for you to approach?
- Is there more than one injured child?
- Is there anyone who can help?
- Do you need emergency medical services?

2 Safety is important

- Do not risk injuring yourself—you cannot help if you become a casualty.
- Remove any source of danger from your child. Move your child only if it is safe for you and it's essential for her safety, and do so very carefully.

3 Treat serious injuries first

The primary considerations that immediately threaten life are:

- Serious bleeding, which can result in life-threatening shock (*see p.36*).
- Obstructed airway, which prevents breathing, can result in the heart stopping (*see p.16*).

IMPORTANT

- If more than one child is injured, go to the quiet one; she may be unresponsive and not breathing.

4 Get help

Shout for help early and ask others to:

- Make the area safe.
- Seek medical advice or call 911.
- Help with first aid.
- Move a child to safety, if necessary.

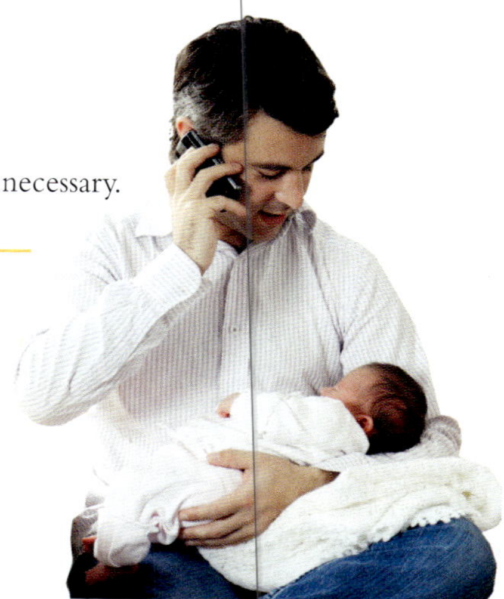

Telephoning for help

When you call 911 or your local EMS, use a hands-free phone so that you can treat the child at the same time. Provide the following:

- Your telephone number.
- The location of the incident.
- The type of incident.
- The number, sex, and ages of the casualties.
- Details of injuries.
- Information about hazards such as gas, power lines, or fog.

Fire

Write down an escape plan for your home and make sure everyone knows what to do.

- How would you get out of each room?
- How do you help babies and young children?
- Where will you meet when you've escaped?

Action for a frying pan fire

- Turn off heat source, then cover pan with lid, wet dishtowel, or fire blanket. Leave this on for half an hour—NEVER throw water over the flames.
- If fire is not under control, get out of the house, close doors behind you, and call 911.

Escaping from a fire

1. Feel the door. If the door is cool, leave the room.

OR

2. If the door is hot, don't open it. Go to the window.

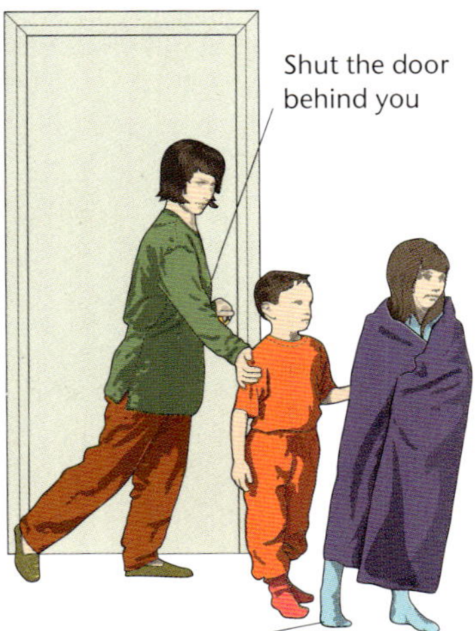
Shut the door behind you
Leave quickly
DO NOT GO BACK

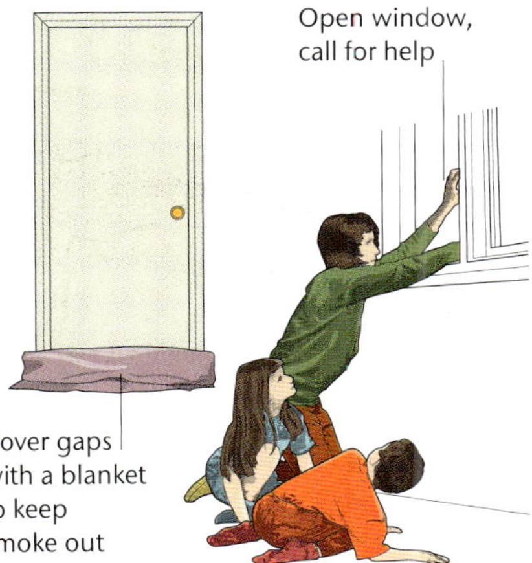
Open window, call for help
Cover gaps with a blanket to keep smoke out
Stay low down where air is clearest

IMPORTANT

- **Carry** babies and toddlers.
- **Don't** ask children to do anything other than look after themselves.
- **Close** all doors behind you.
- **Meet** outside your house.
- **Never** go back inside.
- **Phone** for help from elsewhere.

If you have to escape through a window:

- If you have to break the glass, put a blanket over the frame before you escape.
- **Slide** your child out, hang onto him, then ask him to drop down, if it is safe to do so.
- **Slide** out yourself, hang from the ledge, then drop.

Clothing on fire

If clothing is on fire:

Stop your child from moving; movement will fan the flames.

Drop him to the floor and wrap him in a coat or blanket, if available, to help smother the flames.

Roll him on the ground.

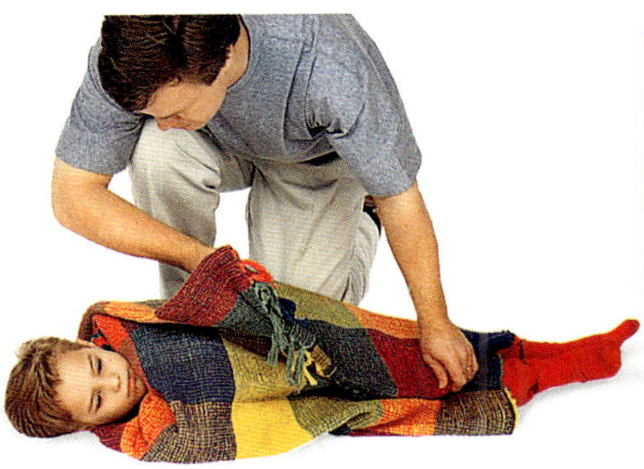

IMPORTANT

- **Do not** let your child run around; rapid movement will fan the flames.
- If water is available, lay him down, burning side uppermost, and douse him with water or a nonflammable liquid.

Electrical injury

Children are at risk of injury from domestic electricity if they play with electrical sockets or cords, or if cords are worn. Electrical current causes muscle spasms that keep a child from letting go of an electric cord and may cause burns both where the current enters and where it leaves the child's body. The current may also cause breathing and heart to stop.

! IMPORTANT

- **You** can safely approach the child if he is no longer in contact with the electric cable.
- **If** your child is no longer in contact with the electricity and is unresponsive and not breathing normally, begin CPR immediately with 30 compressions. If breathing, place in the recovery position. CALL 911 OR EMS.

CALL 911 OR YOUR LOCAL EMS

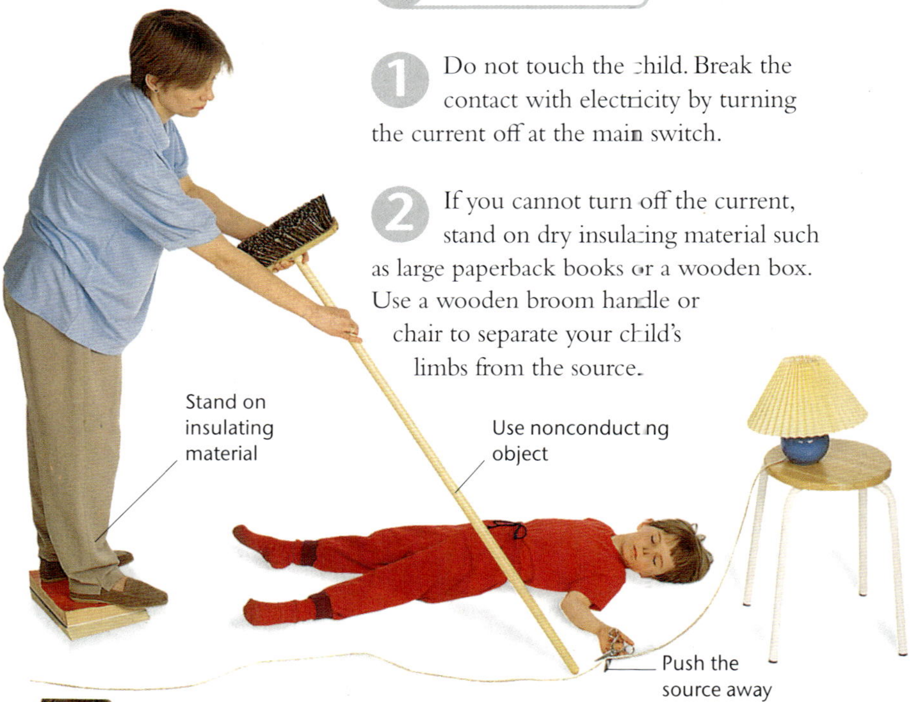

1. Do not touch the child. Break the contact with electricity by turning the current off at the main switch.

2. If you cannot turn off the current, stand on dry insulating material such as large paperback books or a wooden box. Use a wooden broom handle or chair to separate your child's limbs from the source.

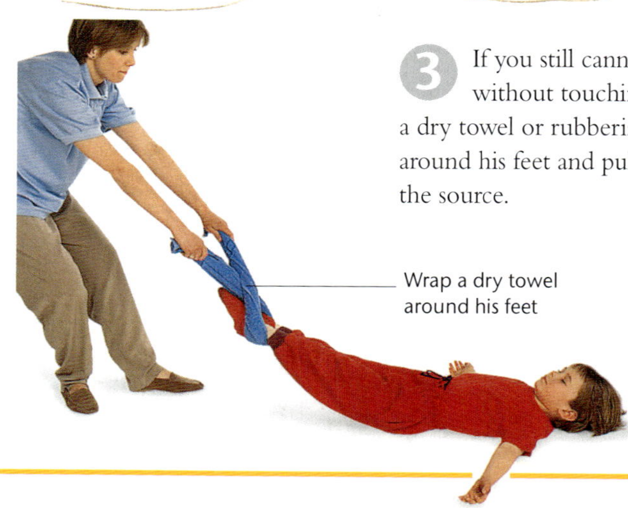

3. If you still cannot break the contact without touching your child, wrap a dry towel or rubberized exercise band around his feet and pull him away from the source.

4. Once the contact is broken, treat any injuries. If the child appears unharmed, monitor his breathing, pulse, and response while waiting for help.

High-voltage current

Contact with electricity from power lines and overhead cables is usually fatal. Severe burns result and the child may be thrown some distance from the point of contact. DO NOT approach the child unless you are officially informed that the power has been cut off.

see also

- Checking vital signs, *p.14*
- Electrical burn, *p.54*
- Unresponsive baby, *pp.19–21*
- Unresponsive child, *pp.22–27*

Water incident

Babies and young children can drown quickly if they slip into a pool or pond or are left unattended in a bath. Even 2.5 centimetres (1in) in a bath, or several centimetres in a bucket of water is enough to cover a baby's nose and mouth if he falls forward.

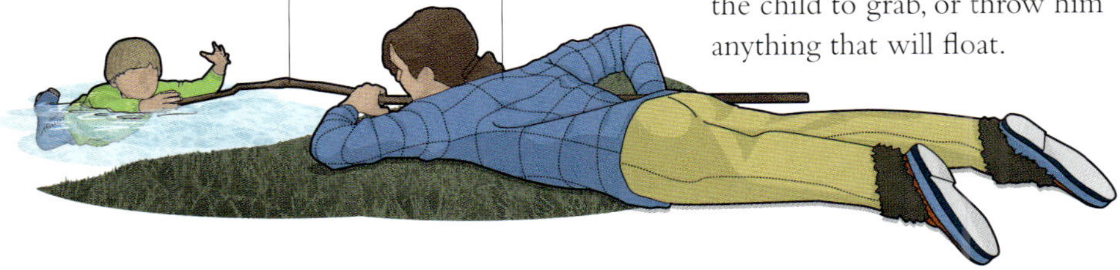

1 Get the child out of the water as quickly as possible. If the child is conscious and able to follow directions, hold out a branch or rope for the child to grab, or throw him anything that will float.

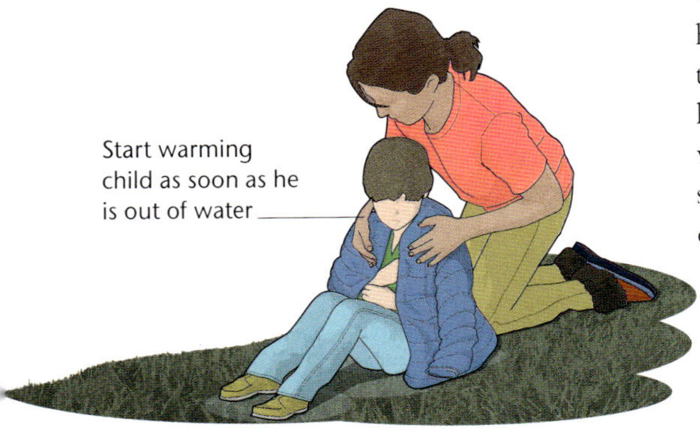
Start warming child as soon as he is out of water

2 Once the child is out of the water, protect him from cold and get him to a shelter. Treat him for hypothermia and replace any wet clothes with dry ones as soon as possible. Even if the child seems to have recovered,

TAKE YOUR CHILD TO THE HOSPITAL

OR

CALL 911 OR YOUR LOCAL EMS

IMPORTANT

- **Do not** put yourself in danger when attempting a rescue; don't enter the water unless you have to in order to save the child's life or you are a trained lifesaver.
- **If** the child is too small to follow commands, or unable, you may have to go in and rescue the child if possible.
- **Always** seek medical advice even if the child appears to have recovered because he may have inhaled some water, which can cause lung damage.
- **If** your child becomes unresponsive and is not breathing normally, begin CPR with 30 compressions immediately. CALL 911 OR YOUR LOCAL EMS.
- **Be** prepared to roll the child onto his side to clear airway because it is possible that he may regurgitate his stomach contents.

DROWNING CHAIN OF SURVIVAL FOR UNTRAINED RESCUER

Prevent drowning Stay safe and supervise your child in and around water.

Recognize distress Ask someone to call for help if the child is in distress.

Provide flotation Getting a float to a child can prevent submersion.

Remove from water Attempt this only if it is safe to do so.

Give first aid Treat as appropriate and seek medical advice.

see also
- Hypothermia, *p.84*
- Unresponsive baby, *pp.19–21*
- Unresponsive child, *pp.22–27*

IMPORTANT

- **Do not** move your child unnecessarily.
- **Stay calm** and reassure the child.
- **Write** down your findings each time you check the child.
- **If** you suspect serious illness or injury, TAKE YOUR CHILD TO THE HOSPITAL or CALL 911 OR YOUR LOCAL EMS.

Checking vital signs

When you are looking after a baby or child who is sick or injured, you need to check her vital signs—breathing, pulse, level of response, and fever—as part of assessing the severity of a condition. Then continue to monitor the signs while you are looking after your child or waiting for medical help to arrive, because the information can indicate whether a child's condition is changing (either improving or deteriorating). Note that here you are checking and monitoring for quality of pulse or breathing, not the presence or absence of them.

Breathing

When assessing breathing you are looking at how many times a child breathes in a minute, as well as the quality of the breaths—for example depth and ease. A baby may breathe as many as 40 breaths a minute; a toddler or child up to five years, 20–30 times; a child up to 12 years old, 12–25 times a minute; and an older child, about 12–18 breaths.

You can sit with the child and watch and listen for breaths, or for a baby or younger child it may be better to place your hand on the chest. Make a note of the breathing rate (the number of breaths in a minute) and as well as whether they are deep or shallow, easy or difficult, painful and/or quiet or noisy—and if the latter, what do they sound like?

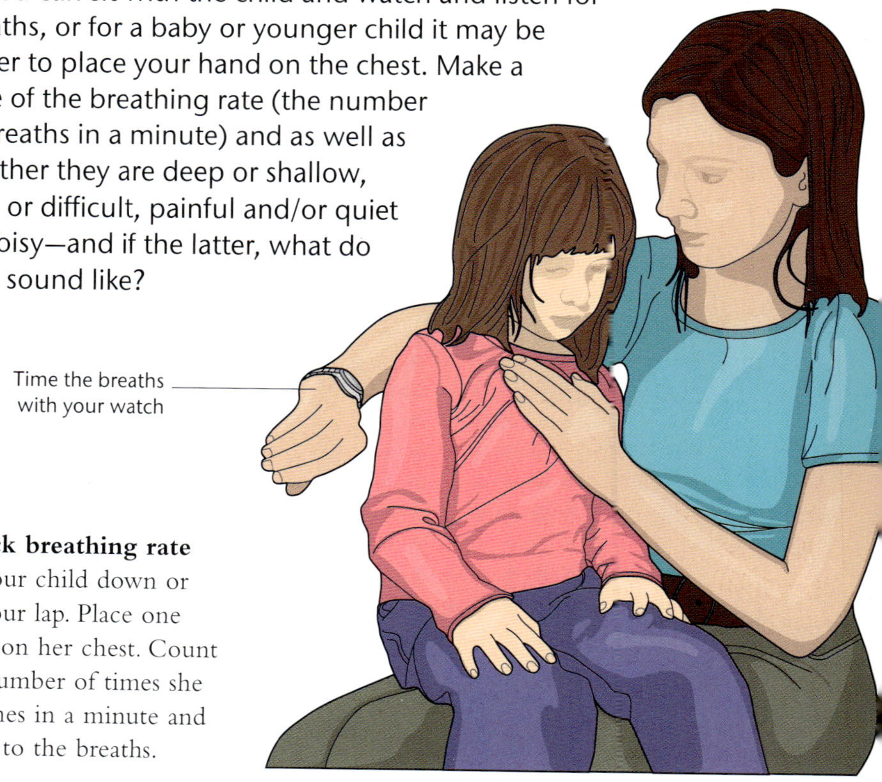

Check breathing rate
Sit your child down or on your lap. Place one hand on her chest. Count the number of times she breathes in a minute and listen to the breaths.

Pulse

Every time the heart beats, a wave of pressure passes along the blood vessels that carry blood from the heart to the body (arteries). This "wave" can be felt where the arteries lie close to the skin. For a baby check the pulse in the upper arm; for older children check it at the neck, groin, or wrist. The normal pulse rate for an infant is 100–160, but it decreases with age. A toddler has a heart rate of 85–130; at ages 2–5, 80–115; for 5–12-year-olds, 75–110; and over 12 years, 60–100. Count the rate (number of beats in a minute), and note whether it is strong or weak and regular or irregular.

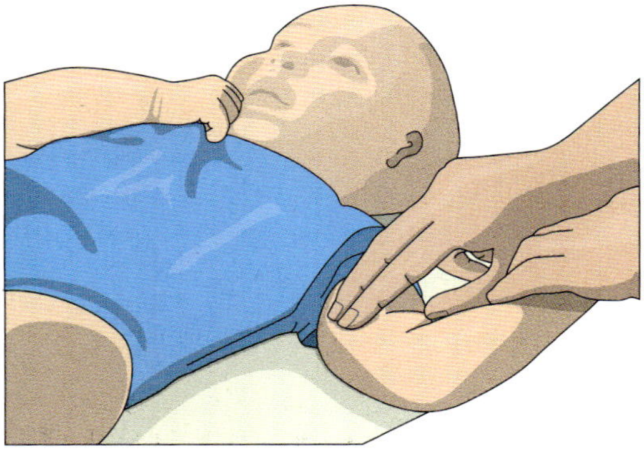

BRACHIAL PULSE

Place the pads of two fingers against the inner side of the baby's upper arm.

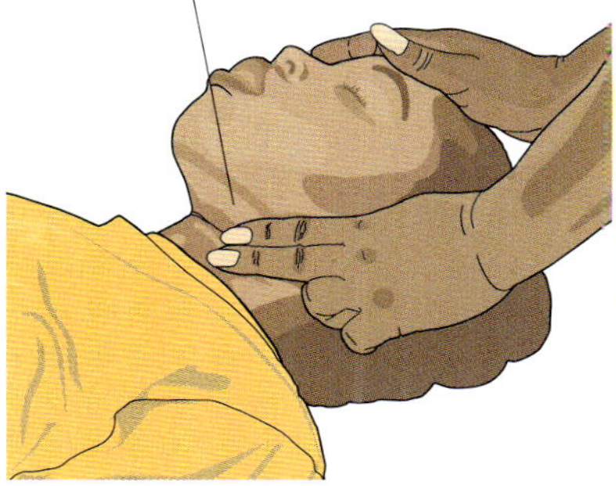

CAROTID PULSE

Place the pads of two fingers on the neck, just to the side of the windpipe.

Level of response

Some illnesses and injuries can affect your child's level of response and she may be fully alert or totally unresponsive or somewhere between. Assess your child right away and then again at regular intervals.

- *Child is fully alert* Her eyes will be open and she responds normally when you ask questions.
- *Responds only to voice* Does your child answer simple questions and obey instructions? Can she open her eyes?
- *Responds only to pain* Does your child open her eyes or move if you tap her shoulder or flick her foot?
- *Unresponsive* The child does not respond to any stimulus.

Body Temperature

- Viral and bacterial infections, including colds, flu, bronchitis, and gastrointestinal and urinary tract infections, are the most common causes of a raised body temperature.
- A body temperature below 35°C (95°F) indicates hypothermia.
- The temperature that should be checked by a doctor increases with age. For infants under three months of age, seek medical advice for a fever of 38°C (100.4°F), measured rectally. In toddlers, a rectal temperature over 39°C (102.2°F) should be checked. In older children, a temperature over 39.6°C (103.3°F) should be investigated by a doctor.

Unresponsiveness

A baby or child needs to inhale oxygen into his lungs. This oxygen passes into the bloodstream and is pumped around the body by the heart. If a baby or child is unresponsive, the air passage, or airway, to the lungs may be blocked, which means oxygen can't enter the body. Lack of oxygen slows down the heartbeat until it stops altogether (cardiac arrest) and no oxygen will reach the brain.

What you can do to help

Always make sure it is safe to approach the baby or child; you can't help him if you become a casualty too. If you are certain you are safe, first assess whether he is responsive. If he is unresponsive and his breathing is abnormal or absent, you need to help pump some blood by doing chest compressions. If circulation stops, blood cannot travel around the body and vital organs such as the brain and heart are deprived of oxygen. Start CPR immediately with 30 chest compressions, followed by opening the airway so that you can breathe into the lungs. The combination of rescue breaths and chest compressions is known as cardiopulmonary resuscitation (CPR). An AED can be used to restore a normal heartbeat (*see p.23*).

Chain of survival

An unresponsive baby or child's chances of survival are greater if:

- You call for expert help;
- CPR is given as soon as possible;
- An AED is used early;
- Advanced care by healthcare professionals is received as soon as possible.

For a baby (under 1 year)

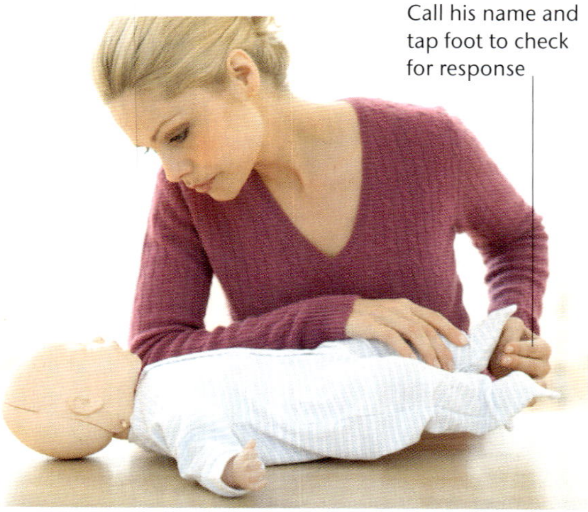

Call his name and tap foot to check for response

For a child (over 1 year)

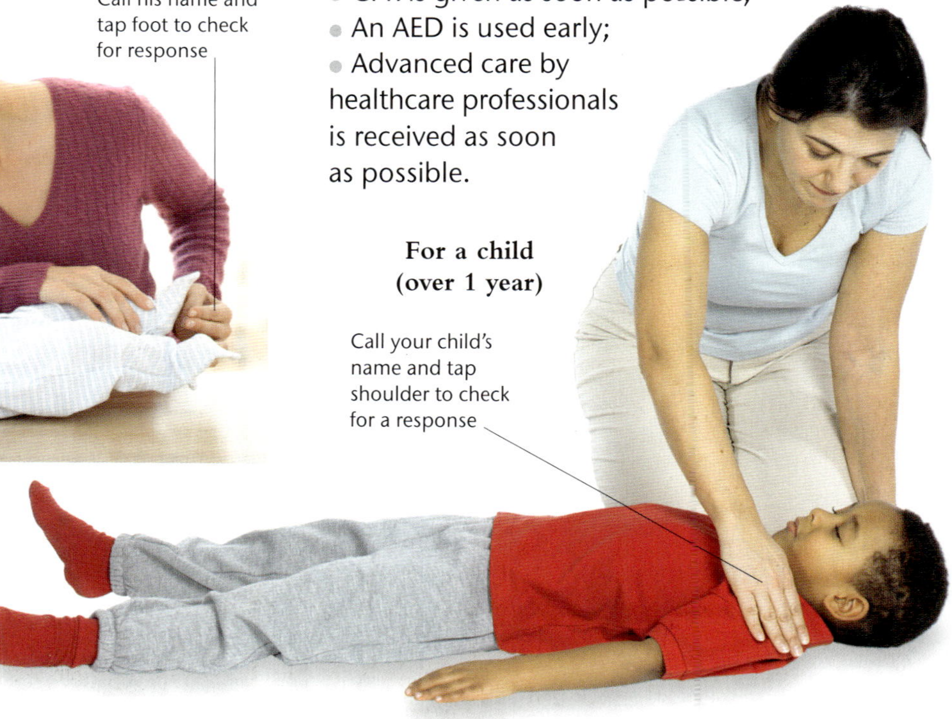

Call your child's name and tap shoulder to check for a response

When to call 911 or your local EMS

If there is somebody else present to help, always ask him or her to call 911 as soon as you realize that your child is not breathing. If you are on your own, give a combination of 30 chest compressions and 2 rescue breaths (CPR: baby *p.20*, child *p.24*) for two minutes before stopping to make the call. Then continue CPR until help arrives or the child recovers.

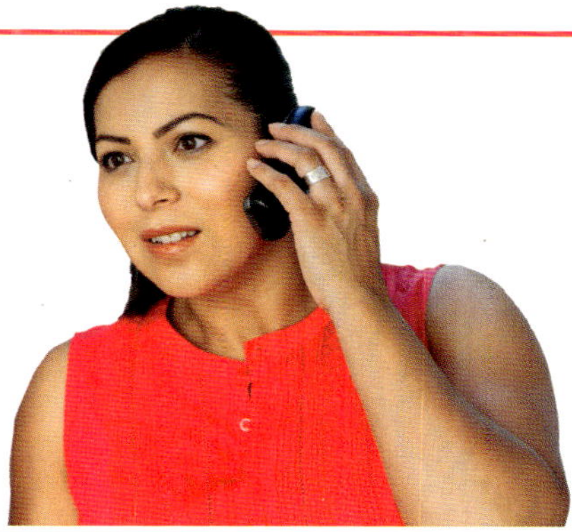

Maintain blood circulation

If your baby or child's heart has stopped beating, giving chest compressions will drive blood containing oxygen around the body. These will be more effective if alternated with rescue breaths. The combination of techniques is known as cardiopulmonary resuscitation (CPR).

For a baby (under 1 year)

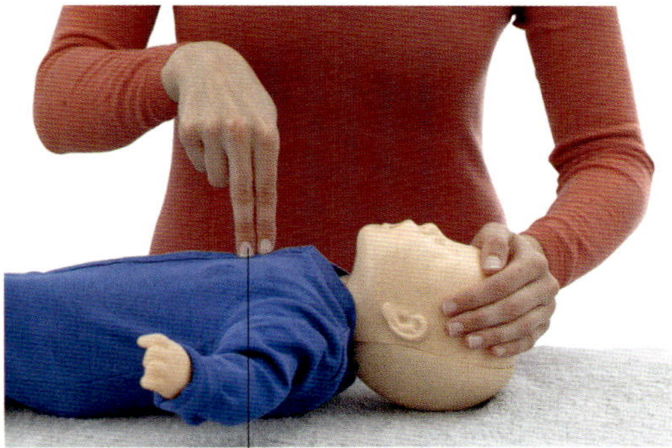

Press on centre of the chest with two fingers just below the nipple line

For a child (over 1 year)

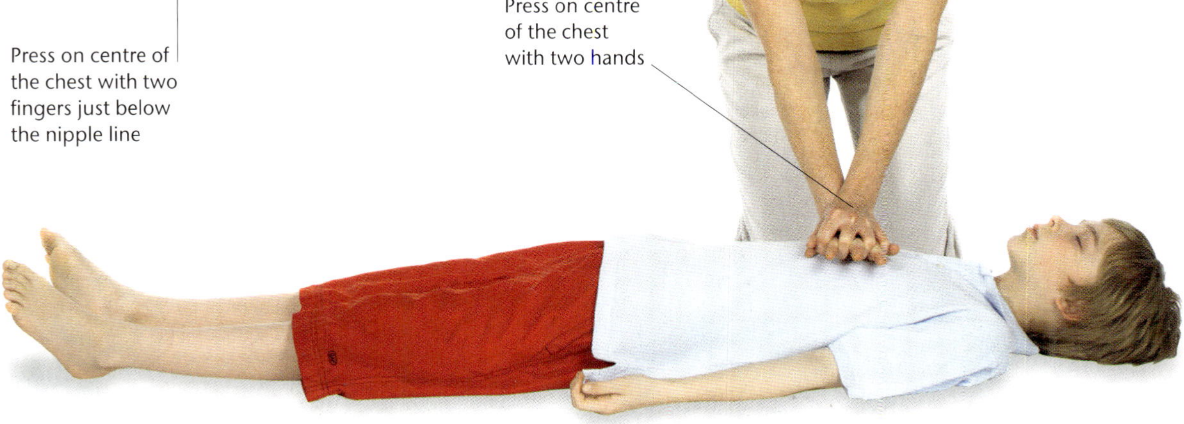

Press on centre of the chest with two hands

Open the airway

You need to open the airway before you can give breaths. Place one hand on the forehead and gently tilt the head to bring the tongue away from the back of the throat. Place one or two fingers of your other hand on the chin to lift. **If you suspect a neck injury, use the jaw thrust method to open the airway** (*see p.61*).

For a baby (under 1 year)

For a child (over 1 year)

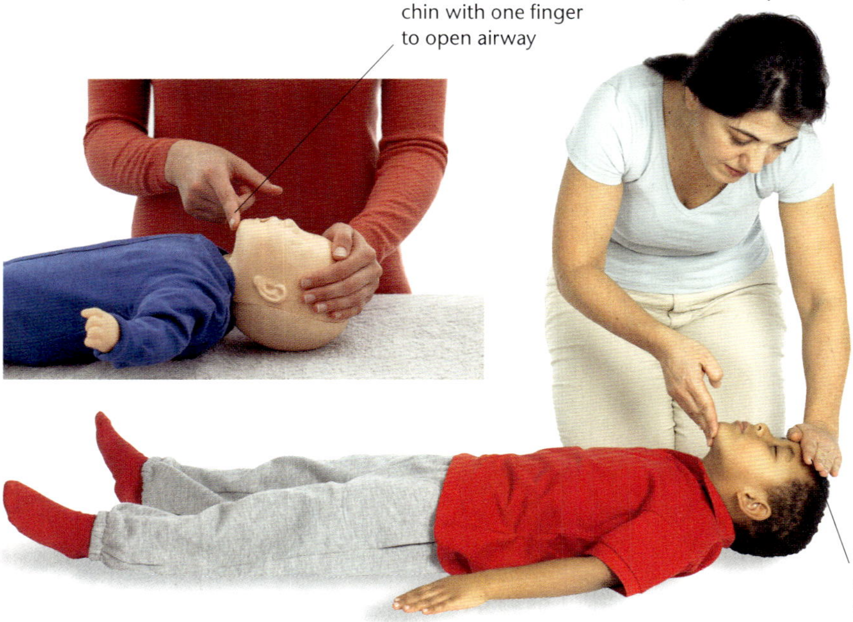

Airway

If a child is on his back the tongue may fall back and may block the airway.

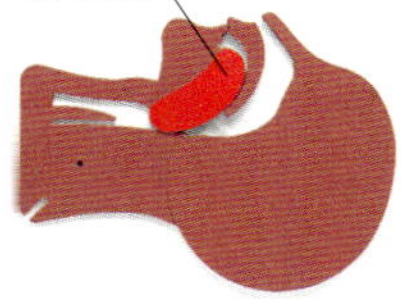

Head not tilted—airway blocked

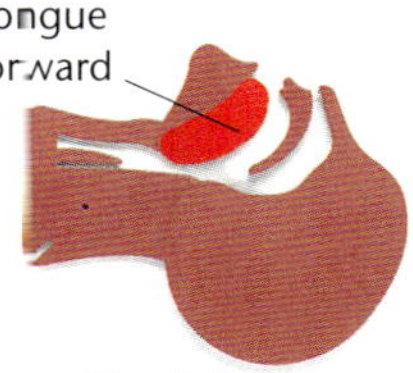

Head tilted—airway unblocked

Breathe for the baby or child

If your baby or child is not breathing, take a breath and blow oxygen into the child's lungs. This is known as rescue breathing. Blow just enough air in to see the chest rise.

For a baby (under 1 year)

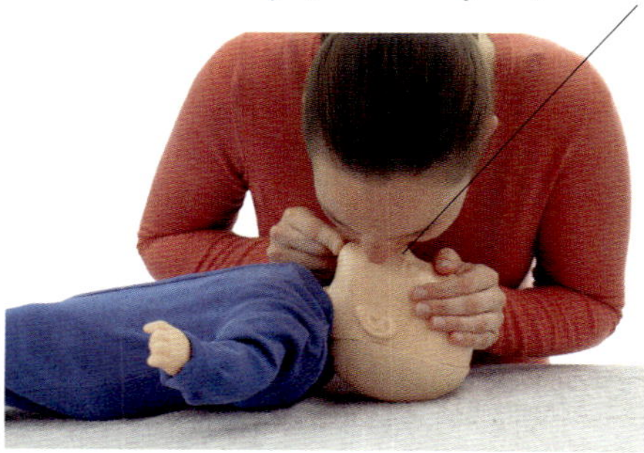

For a child (over 1 year)

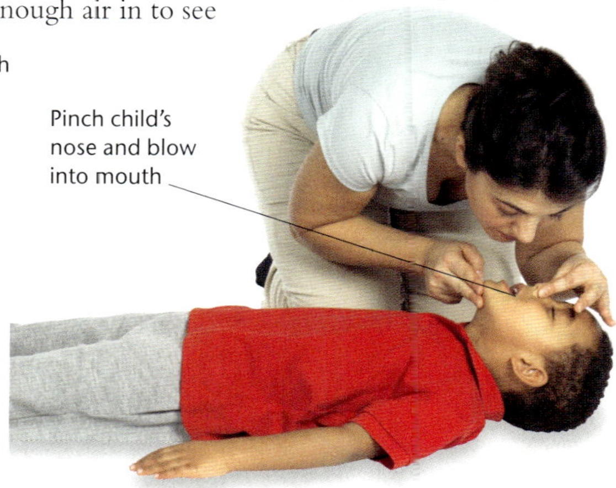

Unresponsive baby
(under 1 year)

Assess your baby before calling for help. If you are alone and the baby is not breathing, begin chest compressions and rescue breaths. For instructions on using an AED, *see p.23*.

1 Check for response

- Call her name and tap her foot gently. Never shake a baby.
- If there is no response,

CALL 911 OR YOUR LOCAL EMS

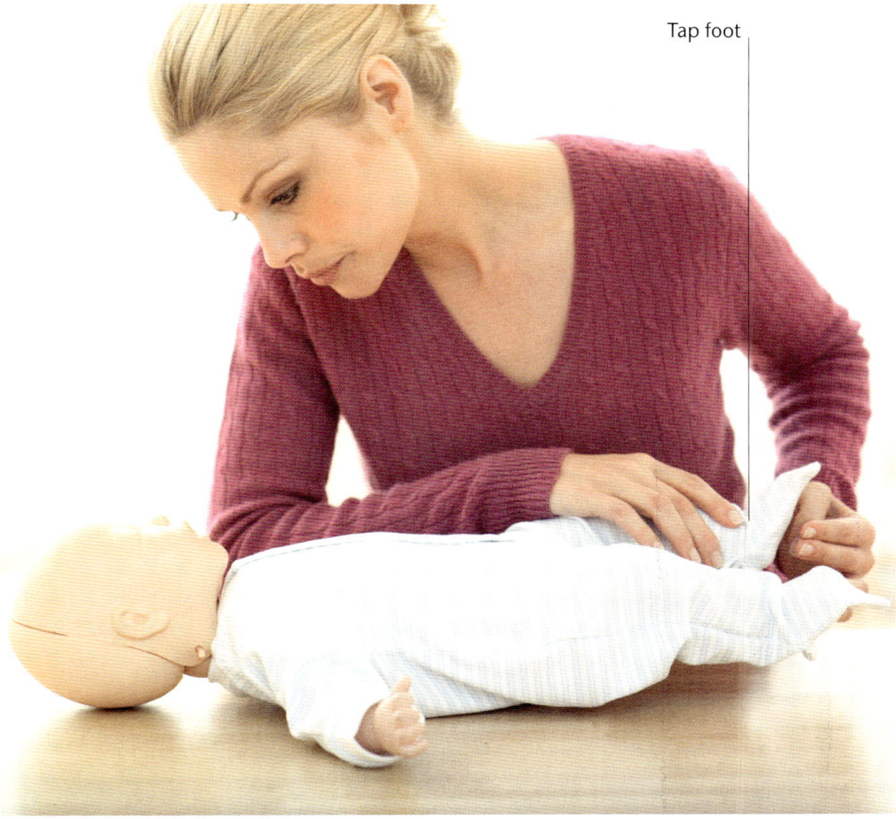

Tap foot

Resuscitation summary

Unresponsive baby

↓

No breathing or just gasping

↓

Send helper to

CALL 911 OR YOUR LOCAL EMS

↓

Start CPR: give 30 chest compressions

↓

Open airway and give 2 rescue breaths

↓

Repeat 30:2 for two minutes

↓

If not already done,

CALL 911 OR YOUR LOCAL EMS

↓

Continue CPR until help arrives

IMPORTANT

- If you are unable or unwilling to give rescue breaths, you can give chest compressions only.

Resuscitation summary

Unresponsive baby

↓

No breathing or just gasping

↓

Send helper to

CALL 911 OR YOUR LOCAL EMS

↓

Start CPR: give 30 chest compressions

↓

Open airway and give 2 rescue breaths

Repeat 30:2 for two minutes

↓

If not already done,

CALL 911 OR YOUR LOCAL EMS

↓

Continue CPR until help arrives

IMPORTANT

- **If** you are unable or unwilling to give rescue breaths, you can give chest compressions only.

CPR: baby (under 1 year)

This is to be used for an unresponsive baby who is not breathing. Always start with 30 chest compressions, followed by two breaths. If you are alone, continue sets of 30 compressions and two breaths for two minutes before calling 911 or your local EMS. **If your breaths aren't going in and you suspect choking, refer to Choking baby** (*see p.28*).

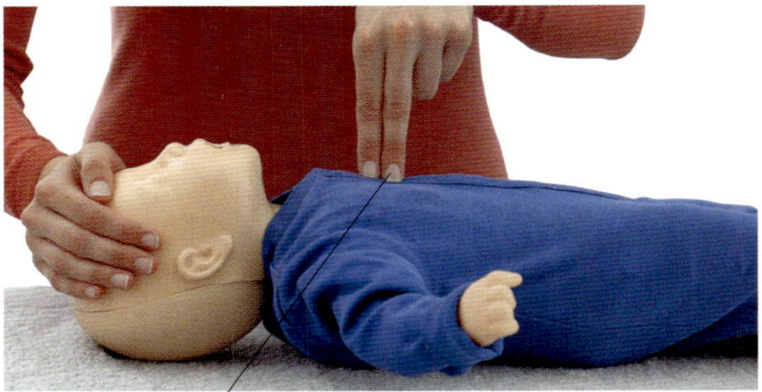

Press down by at least one-third of the depth of the chest

1 Begin chest compressions. Place two fingers of your lower hand on the centre of the baby's chest. Press down vertically on the breastbone to depress it by at least one third of its depth, or at least 4 cm (1.5 in). Release pressure, but don't move your fingers; allow the chest to come back up fully. Repeat to give 30 compressions at a rate of 100–120 per minute.

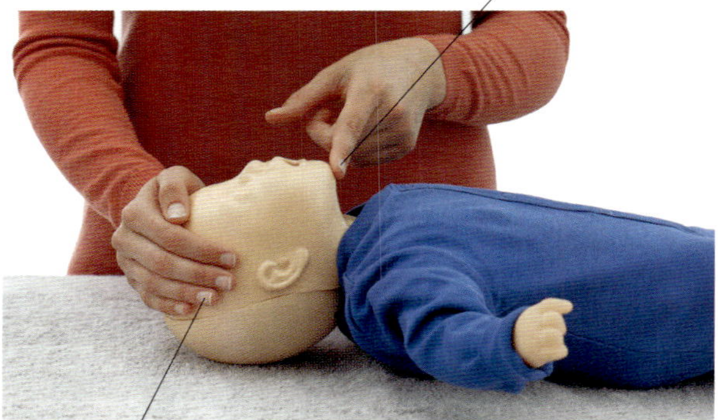

Lift point of chin with one finger

Tilt head back

2 Make sure that her airway is open. Put your finger on the point of the chin and lift it. Take care not to press on the soft part of the neck under the chin because that can block the airway.

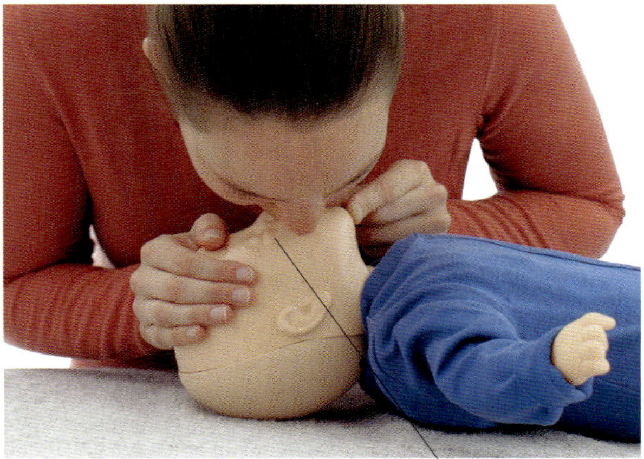

Blow into the baby's mouth and nose

3 Take a normal breath, then seal your lips tightly around your baby's mouth and nose. Blow gently until you see the baby's chest rise—Do NOT blow the whole adult human breath into the baby. Do NOT remove mouth from baby's for this stage; just watch chest fall out of the corner of your eye. If the chest does not rise, tilt the head and lift the chin a bit more.

Repeat 30 chest compressions

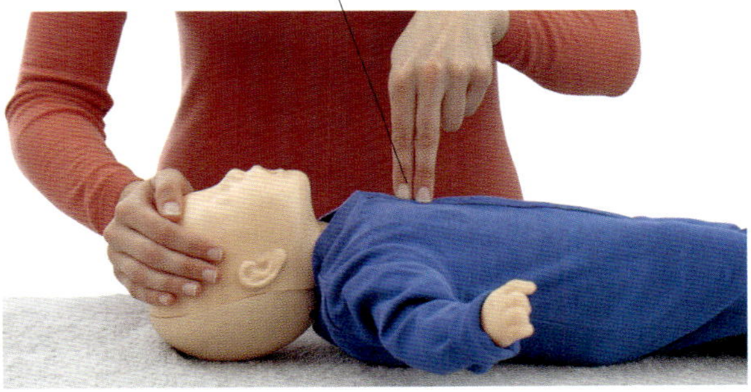

4 Continue CPR with 30 chest compressions.

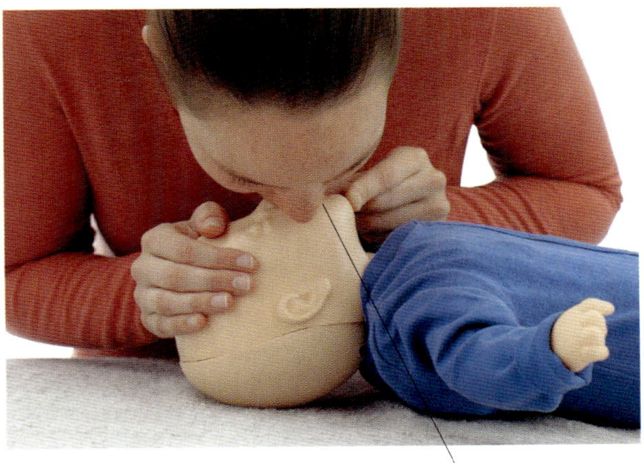

Follow with two rescue breaths

5 Return to the baby's head and give two rescue breaths, followed by another 30 chest compressions. Continue at a rate of 30:2 until the emergency services arrive; your baby shows signs of becoming responsive (coughing, opening her eyes, and moving) and she is breathing normally; or you are too exhausted to continue.

! IMPORTANT

- **Do not** sweep the mouth with your finger to search for an obstruction.
- **If** there is more than one rescuer, one gives 15 chest compressions followed by the other giving 2 breaths. There should be minimal pause between groups of compressions and breaths. You can switch positions if the person giving compressions becomes exhausted.
- **If** your baby shows signs of becoming responsive (*see below left*) and she is breathing normally, cradle her in your arms with head tilted down until the ambulance arrives (*below*). Monitor breathing, pulse, and level of response (*see p.14*) until the help arrives.

The recovery position

Hold the baby in your arms with her head tilted downward and supported. This keeps her airway open and clear and allows fluid to drain away.

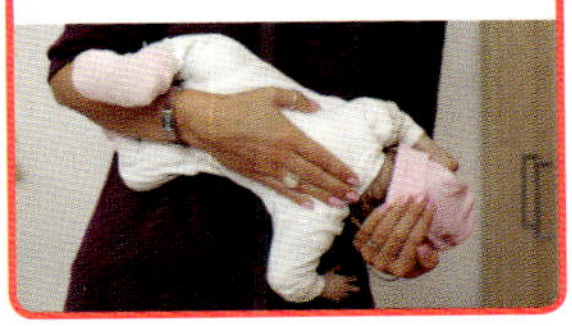

Resuscitation summary

Unresponsive child

↓

No breathing or just gasping

↓

Send helper to

CALL 911 OR YOUR LOCAL EMS

↓

Start CPR: give 30 chest compressions followed by two rescue breaths

↓

Repeat 30:2 for two minutes

↓

If not already done,

CALL 911 OR YOUR LOCAL EMS

↓

Continue CPR until help arrives

IMPORTANT

- If you are unable or unwilling to give rescue breaths, you can give chest compressions only.

Unresponsive child

(over 1 year)

Assess a child (aged one year to puberty) before you call for help. If you are on your own and the child is not breathing or just gasping, begin CPR.

1 Check for response

- Call his name, or tap his shoulder gently. Never shake a child.
- If there is no response,

CALL 911 OR YOUR LOCAL EMS

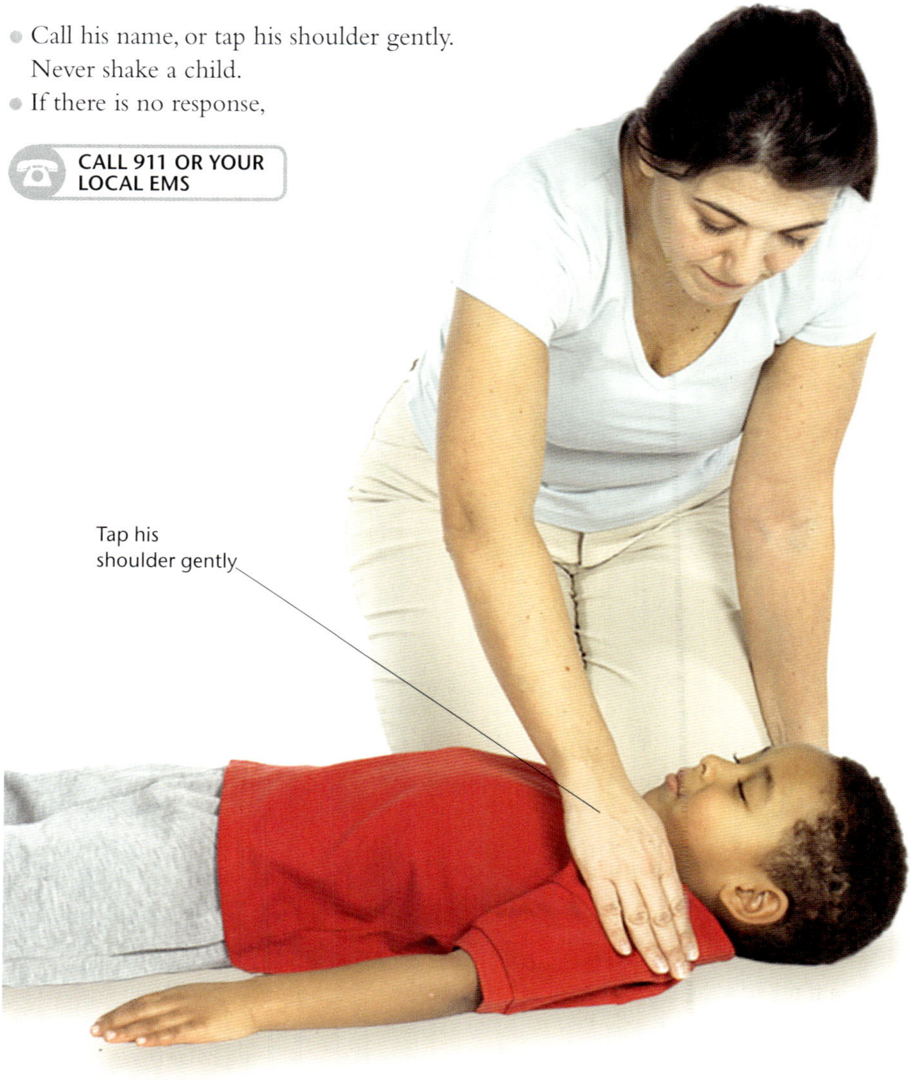

Using an AED (Automatic External Defibrillator) on a baby or child

Machines called AEDs can be used to analyze the heart rhythm and if necessary correct it by delivering an electric shock. If a baby or child is unresponsive and not breathing, start chest compressions, followed by rescue breaths (CPR, *see p.24*), and CALL 911 OR YOUR LOCAL EMS. Ask a helper to find an AED and use it as soon as it arrives—don't leave the child to look for one yourself. The machine will give you audible prompts to follow. If a shock is needed, the machine will deliver it; if not, it will not be given.

1. Turn on the machine. Pads may be connected to the machine (if not, the machine will tell you to connect them). If there are both adult and pediatric pads in the kit, use the right ones for the child's size. Remove any clothing or objects from the child that may come into contact with the pads.

2. Place the pads directly onto the child's chest. Peel off the backing paper and put one on the upper right side of the child's chest and the other on her lower left side.

3. Once the pads are attached, make sure no one is touching the child. The AED will analyze the heart rhythm and may recommend delivering a shock. Listen to the machine's instructions.

IF A SHOCK IS ADVISED

- The AED will start to charge up—make sure everyone is clear of the child, then follow the machine's prompts to deliver the shock.
- Continue CPR for 2 minutes or until the machine asks you to stop.
- The AED will reanalyze the child's heart rhythm at regular intervals; listen to the prompts.

IF A SHOCK IS NOT ADVISED

- Continue CPR. The AED will reanalyze the child's heart rhythm at regular intervals.

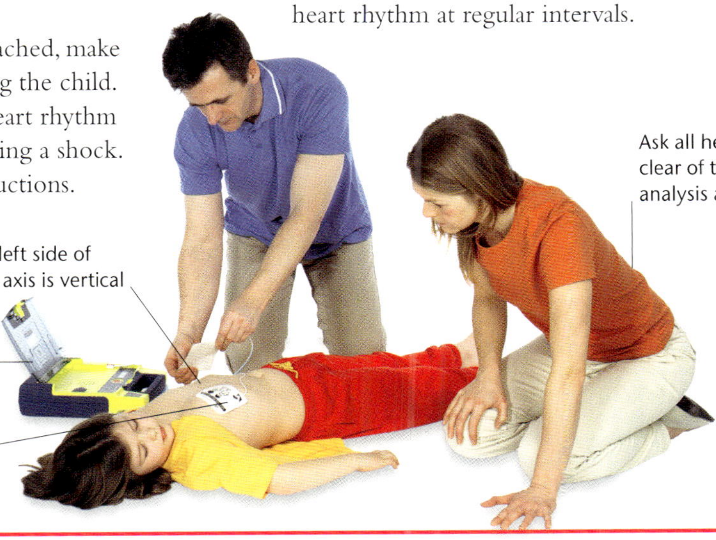

IMPORTANT

- **If** there are both adult and pediatric pads in the AED, use the pediatric ones, but adult pads can be used if pediatric pads are not available.
- **If** the child is very small, place one pad in the centre of her back and the other one in the centre of the chest. Both pads should be vertical.
- **If** she starts coughing, opening her eyes, speaking or moving purposefully, and is breathing normally, leave pads attached and put her in the recovery position.
- **If** the child is in water, remove the child from the water before using the AED.

Resuscitation summary

Unresponsive child

↓

No breathing or just gasping

↓

Send helper to

CALL 911 OR YOUR LOCAL EMS

↓

Start CPR: give 30 chest compressions, followed by two rescue breaths

↓

Repeat 30:2 for two minutes

↓

If not already done,

CALL 911 OR YOUR LOCAL EMS

↓

Continue CPR until help arrives

IMPORTANT

- If you are unable or unwilling to give rescue breaths, you can give chest compressions only.

CPR: child (over 1 year)

This is to be used for an unresponsive child who is not breathing. Always start with 30 chest compressions, followed by two breaths. If on your own, give CPR for two minutes before calling 911 or your local EMS. **If your breaths aren't going in and you suspect choking, refer to Choking child** (*see p.30*).

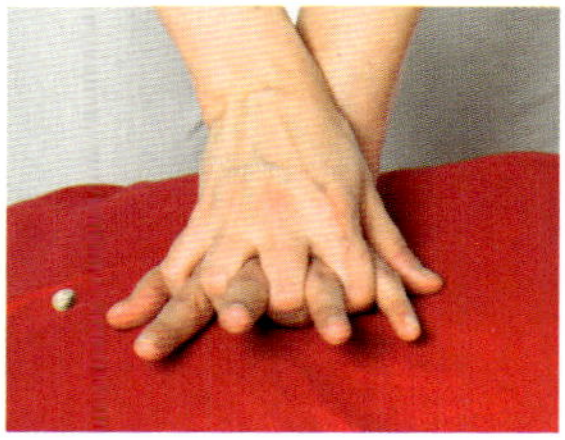

Interlock the fingers

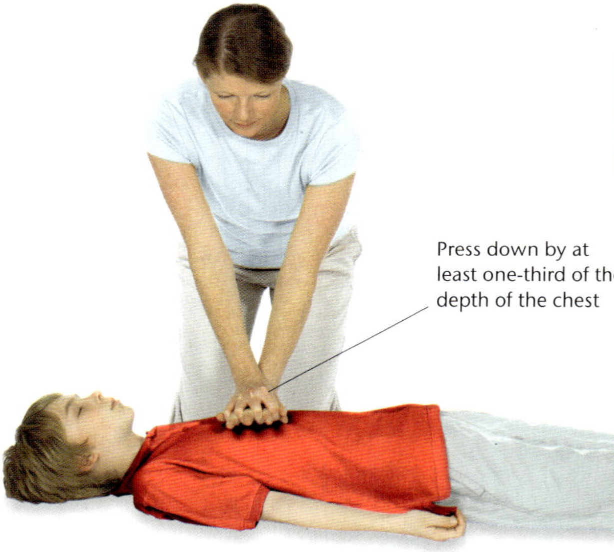

Press down by at least one-third of the depth of the chest

1 Begin chest compressions. Place the heel of one hand over the centre of the child's chest (on the breastbone). Place the heel of your other hand on top of the first hand and interlock your fingers. Lean forward over the child so that your shoulders are directly above your hands. Press down vertically to depress the breastbone by at least one-third of its depth, or about 5 cm (2in).

2 Release the pressure but don't move your hands; let the chest come back up. Repeat to give 30 compressions at a rate of 100–120 per minute.

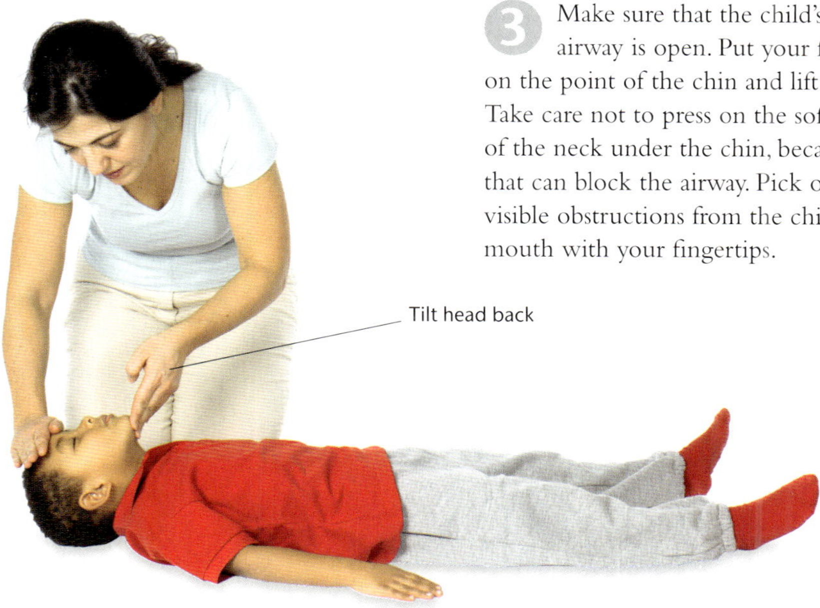

3 Make sure that the child's airway is open. Put your fingers on the point of the chin and lift it. Take care not to press on the soft part of the neck under the chin, because that can block the airway. Pick out any visible obstructions from the child's mouth with your fingertips.

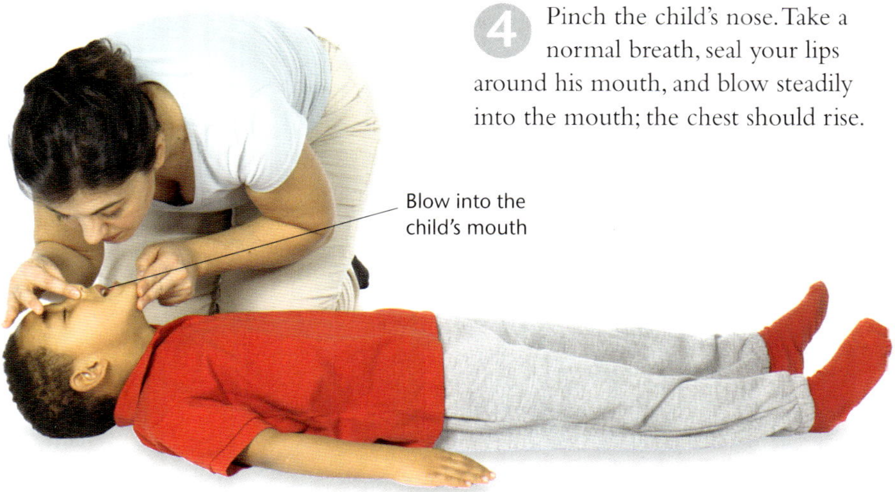

4 Pinch the child's nose. Take a normal breath, seal your lips around his mouth, and blow steadily into the mouth; the chest should rise.

5 Remove your mouth, but not your hands, and watch the chest fall—this is a rescue breath. Each complete rescue breath should take one second. If the chest does not rise, tilt the head and lift the chin a bit more.

6 Continue at a rate of 30:2 until the emergency services arrive; your child shows signs of becoming responsive (coughing, opening eyes, speaking, and moving purposefully) and is breathing normally; or you are too exhausted to continue.

! IMPORTANT

- **Do not** sweep mouth with your finger to search for an obstruction.
- **If** there is more than one rescuer, one gives 15 chest compressions followed by the other giving 2 breaths. There should be minimal pause between groups of compressions and breaths. You can switch positions if the person giving compressions becomes exhausted.
- **If** your child shows signs of becoming responsive (*see left*), and is breathing normally, place him in the recovery position (*see p.26*). Monitor breathing, pulse, and level of response (*see p.14*) until help arrives.

> **! IMPORTANT**
>
> - **If** you suspect a spinal or neck injury, do not move your child. Use the jaw thrust method to open the airway (*see p.61*).

Recovery position

Put your child in this position if she is unresponsive but breathing to prevent her tongue or vomit from blocking her airway. If the child is found lying on her side or front, not all the steps will be needed.

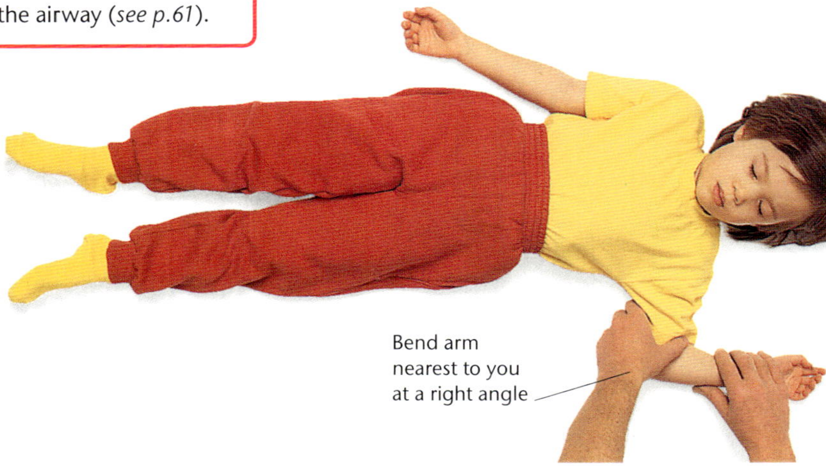

1 Kneel beside your child. Place the arm closest to you up alongside her head with the elbow bent and palm of hand uppermost.

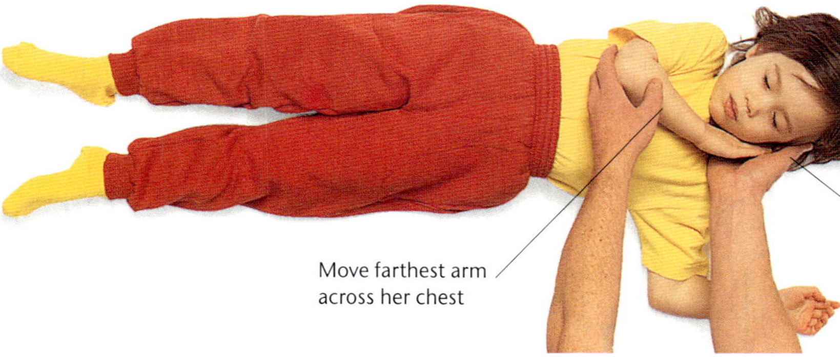

2 Bring her other arm across her chest and hold the back of her hand against her cheek.

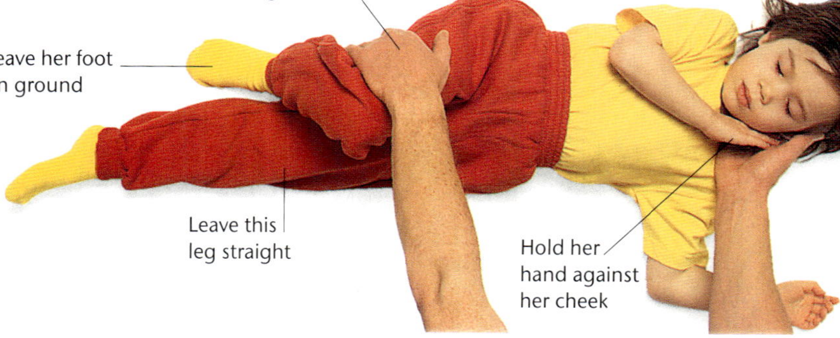

3 With your other hand, pull up the knee of the leg farthest from you to bend the leg, leaving the foot on the ground.

Eyeglasses

If the child is wearing eyeglasses, remove them and keep them safe.

4 Pull the bent leg toward you to roll your child onto her side. Keep your child's hand against her cheek to support her head.

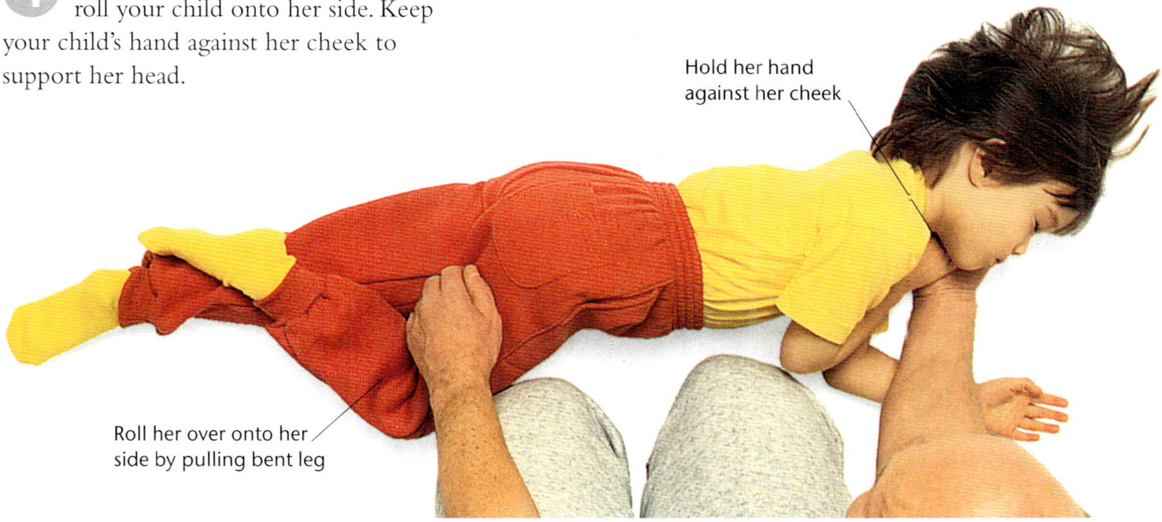

5 Adjust her uppermost leg so she cannot fall forward, and tilt her head back to make sure her airway is open.

CALL 911 OR YOUR LOCAL EMS

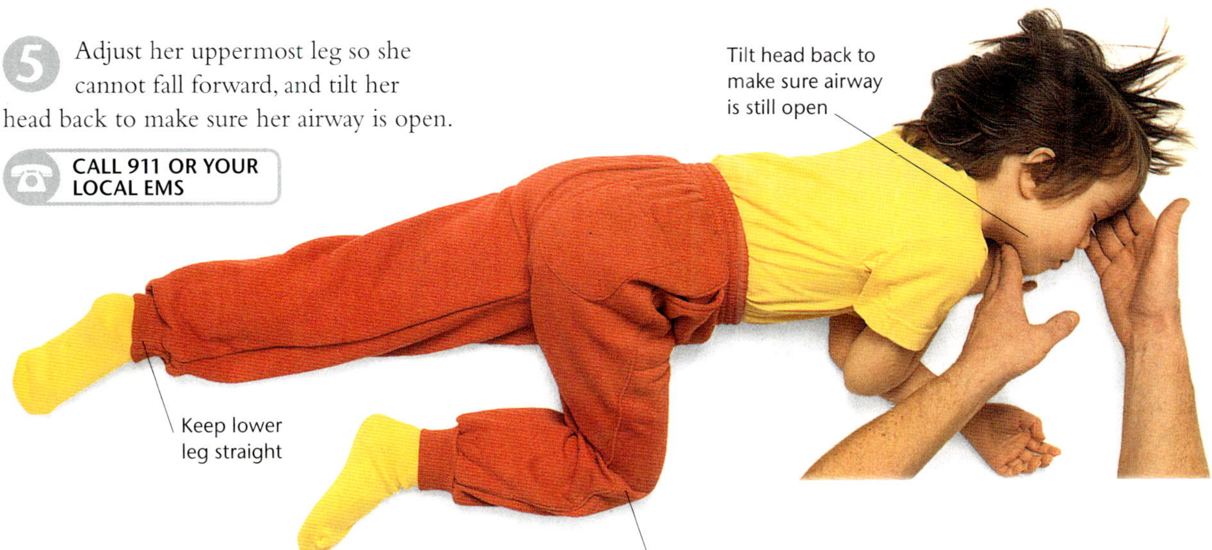

6 Check your child's breathing, pulse, and level of response while you are waiting for help to arrive.

see also
- Checking vital signs, *p.14*

IMPORTANT

- **Do not** shake a baby.
- **Do not** sweep the mouth with your finger to search for an obstruction.

Choking baby (under 1 year)

If the baby has an incomplete airway obstruction, he may be coughing, have noisy breathing, or be in distress. If he is choking, there will be no noise. Give chest thrusts then back blows to relieve a blockage. Send someone to CALL 911 OR YOUR LOCAL EMS.

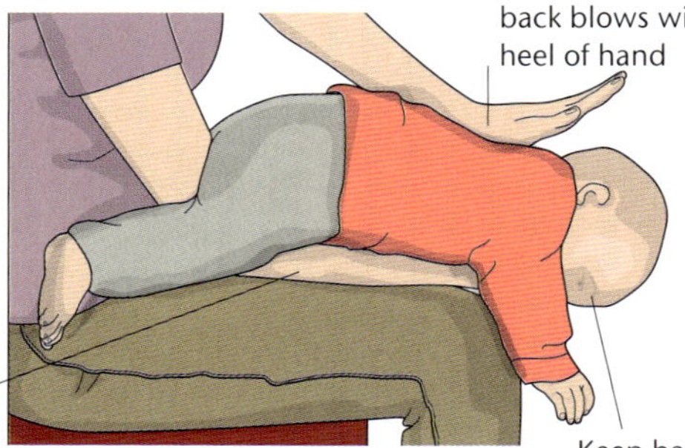

1 If your baby is unable to cough, cry, or breathe, lay him face down, head lower than his chest, along your forearm and rest your arm on your thigh. Support the baby's head with your hand. Give up to five back blows between his shoulder blades with the heel of your other hand.

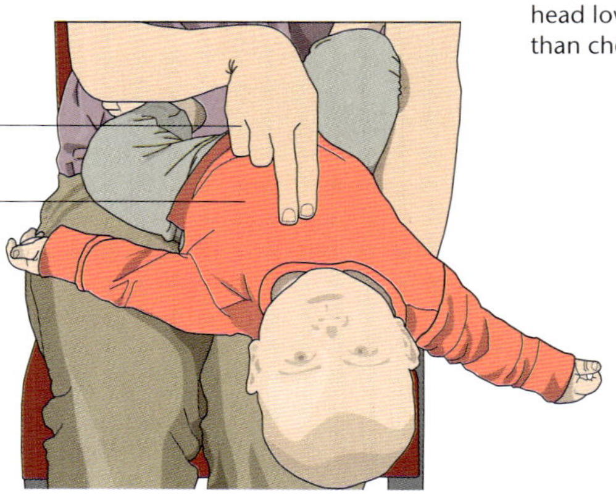

2 If the obstruction has not cleared, give chest thrusts. Turn him face up along your other arm. Place two fingers on the nipple line and push downward at least one third to one half of the depth of the chest. Repeat to give up to five thrusts; stop if the obstruction clears. If the obstruction has still not cleared,

CALL 911 OR YOUR LOCAL EMS

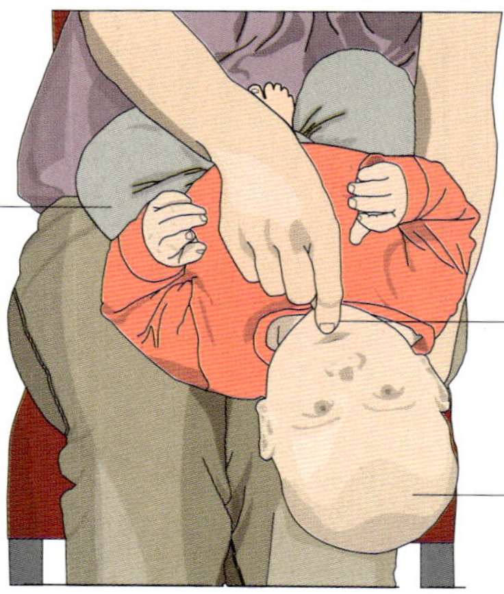

3 Check the mouth. Pick out any obvious obstruction from the mouth with your fingertips.

4 Continue back blows followed by chest thrusts until help arrives, the obstruction clears, or the baby becomes unresponsive.

If your baby becomes unresponsive

If your choking baby becomes unresponsive, begin CPR (*see p.20*). If he starts breathing at any stage, cradle him in your arms with his head down in the recovery position (*see p.21*). Send someone to CALL 911 OR YOUR LOCAL EMS.

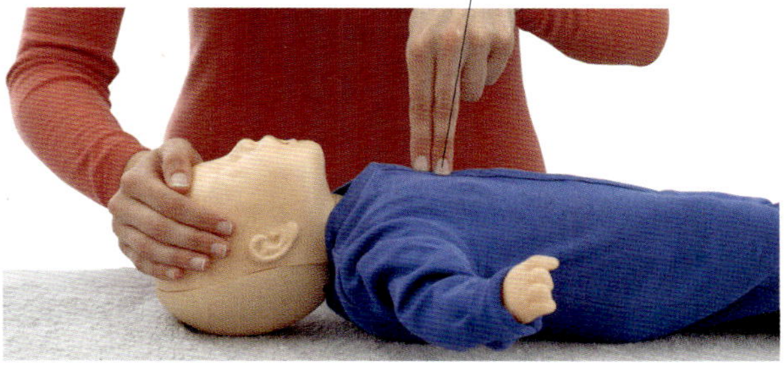

1. Give 30 chest compressions (this may dislodge obstruction).

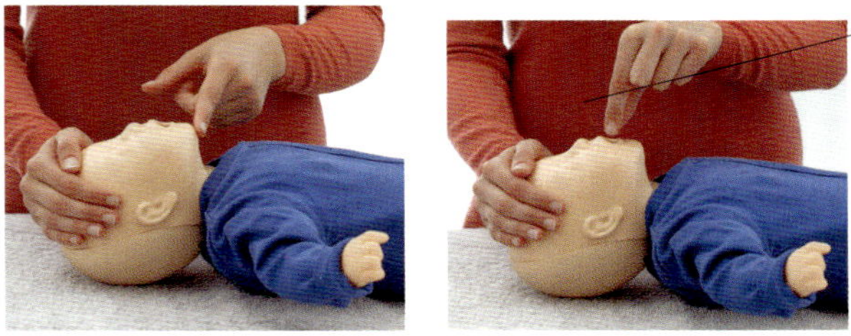

2. If your baby is not breathing, clear any visible obstruction from his mouth; do not do a fingersweep.

3. Begin rescue breaths. Give two rescue breaths by breathing into your baby's mouth and nose.

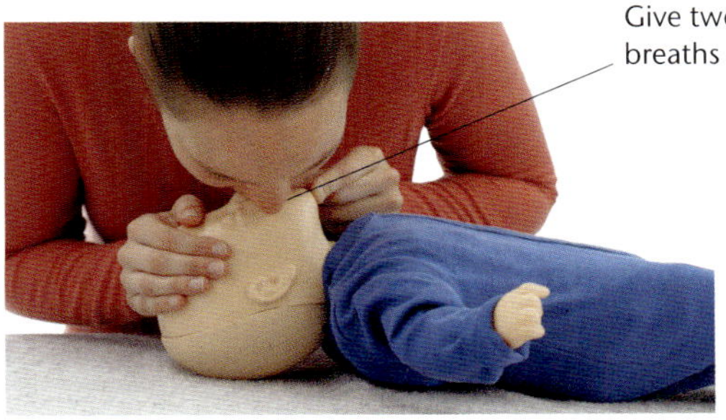

4. Repeat 30 chest compressions, then two rescue breaths. Continue to give 30 compressions followed by two rescue breaths for two minutes.

CALL 911 OR YOUR LOCAL EMS

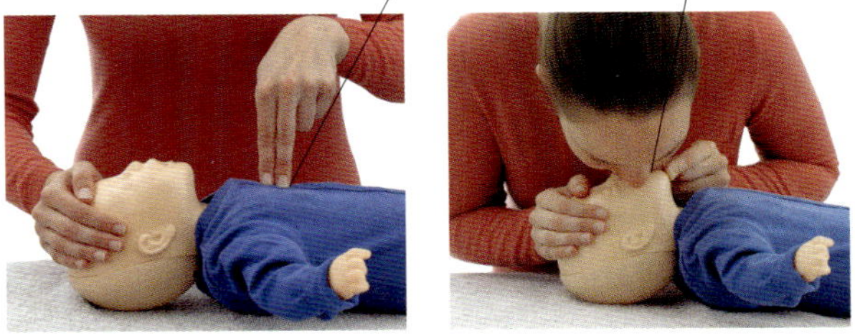

5. Continue alternating 30 chest compressions with two rescue breaths until help arrives, your baby shows signs of recovery (*see box, above right*), or you are too exhausted to continue.

IMPORTANT

- If you are alone, do 5 cycles of CPR (2 minutes), then stop to call 911. Return to performing CPR until help arrives, your baby shows signs of recovery, or you are too exhausted to continue.
- If your baby shows signs of recovery such as coughing, opening his eyes, and moving purposefully, and is breathing normally, CALL 911 OR YOUR LOCAL EMS if not already done. Cradle him in your arms with head tilted down (recovery position, *see p.21*) until emergency help arrives. Monitor breathing, pulse, and level of response until help arrives.

see also

- Checking vital signs, *p.14*
- Unresponsive baby, *pp.19–21*

IMPORTANT

- **Do not** put a finger blindly down the throat to search for the cause of choking.
- **Any child** who has been given abdominal thrusts must be seen by a doctor.

Choking child (over 1 year)

Start by asking your child if she is choking. If the blockage is mild, she will be able to speak, cough, and breathe. If it is severe, she will not be able to speak, cough, or breathe. Send someone to CALL 911 OR YOUR LOCAL EMS.

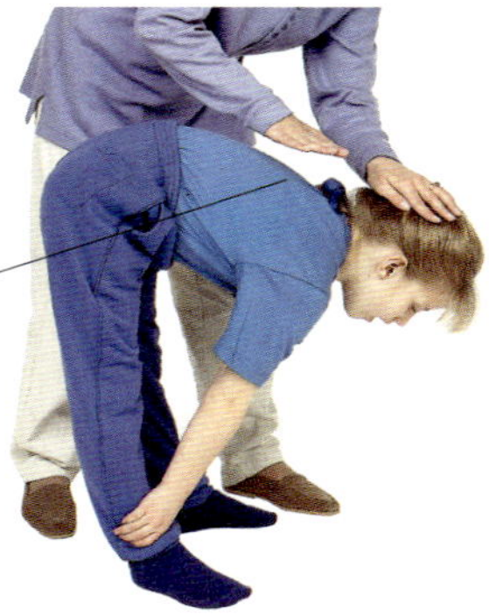

1 If your child can cough, encourage her to do so to remove the object.

2 **Back blows:** Stand or kneel behind her. Bend her forward until her upper airway is parallel to the ground. You may also wrap one arm diagonally across her chest. With the heel of your hand, give 5 firm back blows between the shoulder blades.

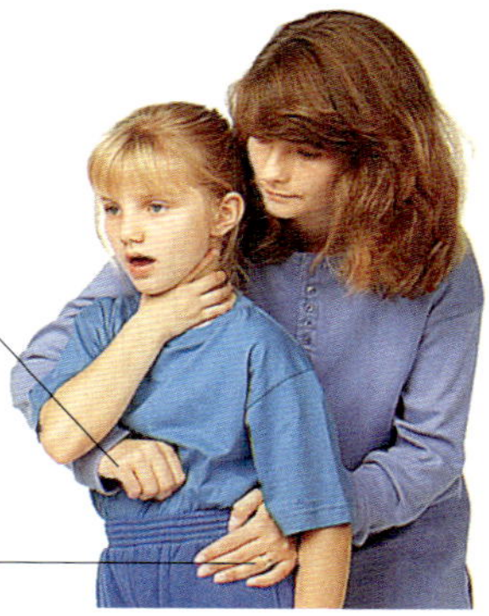

3 **Abdominal thrusts:** Wrap your arms around her waist. Make a fist with one hand. Place the thumb side of your fist against the middle of her abdomen, just above her navel.

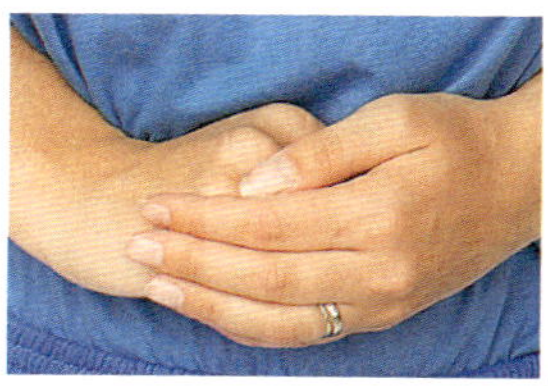

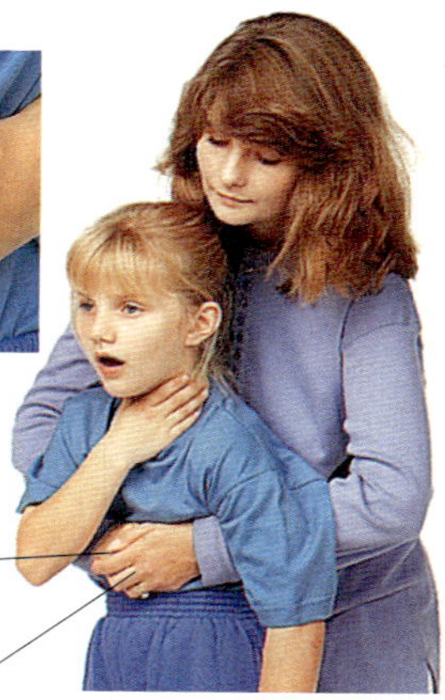

4 Grasp your fist with the other hand and press into her abdomen with a quick inward and upward thrust. Give up to 5 abdominal thrusts.

5 Continue the cycle of 5 back blows and 5 abdominal thrusts until the obstruction clears or the child becomes unresponsive.

CALL 911 OR YOUR LOCAL EMS

If your child becomes unresponsive

If your choking child becomes unresponsive, lower him to the floor, and treat as shown below. Send someone to CALL 911 OR YOUR LOCAL EMS.

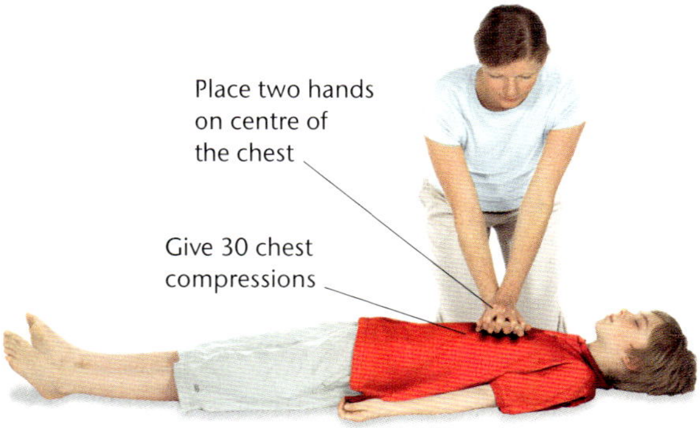

1 Begin CPR with 30 chest compressions (this may dislodge the obstruction).

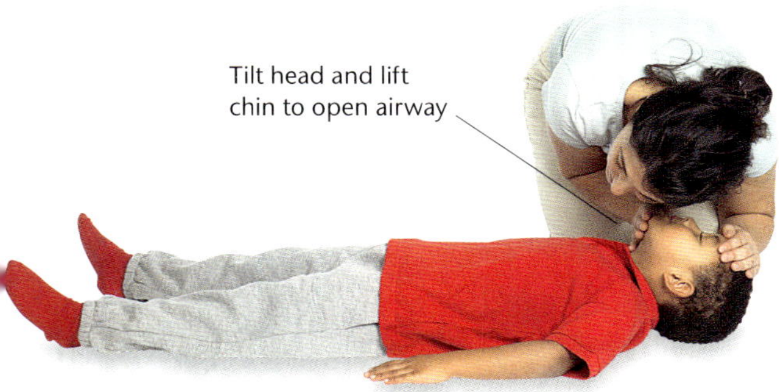

2 Open his airway. If your child is not breathing, clear any visible obstruction from his mouth. Do not do a blind finger sweep.

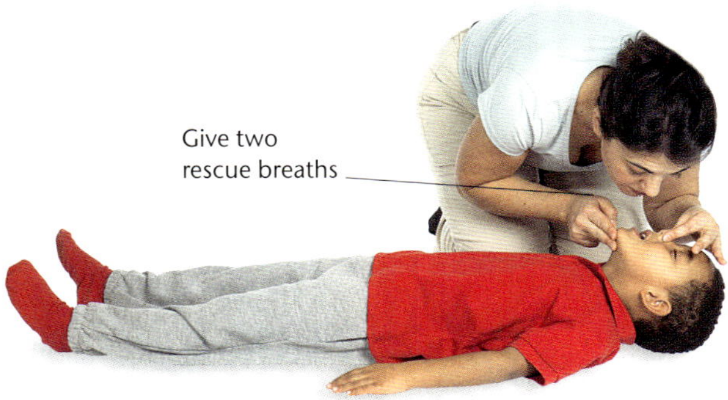

3 Attempt two rescue breaths into the nose. If his chest does not rise after the first breath, perform the head-tilt and chin-lift again before the second breath. Continue to give 30 compressions followed by two rescue breaths for 2 minutes.

CALL 911 OR YOUR LOCAL EMS

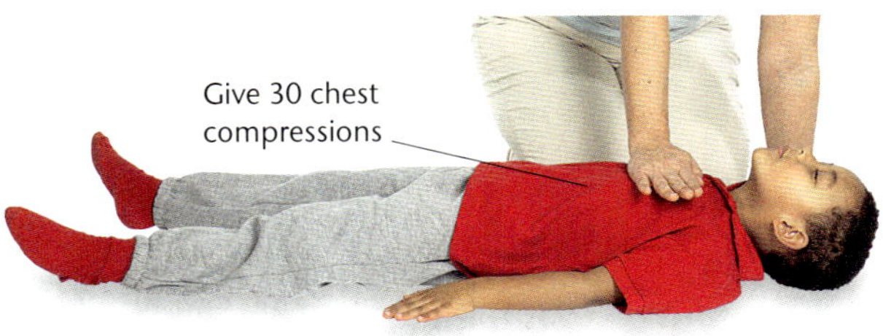

4 Continue cycles of 30 chest compressions followed by two rescue breaths until help arrives, your child resumes breathing, or you become too exhausted to continue.

IMPORTANT

- **If** you are alone, do 5 cycles of CPR (2 minutes), then stop to call 911. Return to performing CPR until help arrives, your child shows signs of recovery, or you are too exhausted to continue.

The recovery position

If the child starts breathing again but remains unresponsive, place him in the recovery position (*see p.26*) and CALL 911 OR YOUR LOCAL EMS.

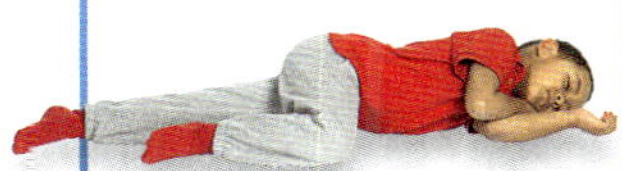

see also

- Unresponsive child, *pp.22–27*

IMPORTANT

- **Do not** shake a baby or young child.
- **If** he becomes unresponsive, open the airway and check breathing. If he is breathing, place him in the recovery position. CALL 911.

Breath holding

This is the result of rage and frustration. Your child is holding his breath if he cries, then breathes in but does not breathe out. He may go blue in the face and stiff and may even become unresponsive momentarily.

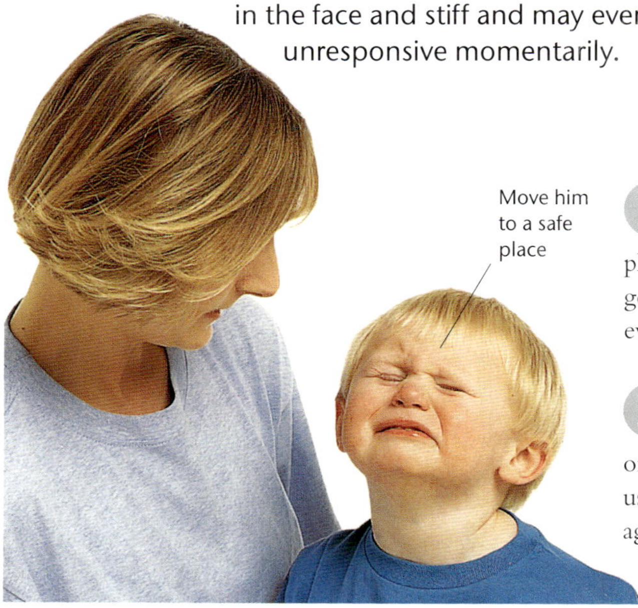

1. Make sure your child is in a safe place where he will not get hurt in the unlikely event that he falls.

2. Try to stay calm. Do not shake him or make a fuss. He will usually start breathing again spontaneously.

see also

- Unresponsive child, *pp.22–27*

IMPORTANT

- **If** the hiccups go on for longer than a few hours, SEEK MEDICAL ADVICE. A long attack can be worrying, tiring, and painful.

Hiccups

These are very common and usually only last for a few minutes, but often seem to go on for a long time. Children can become distressed.

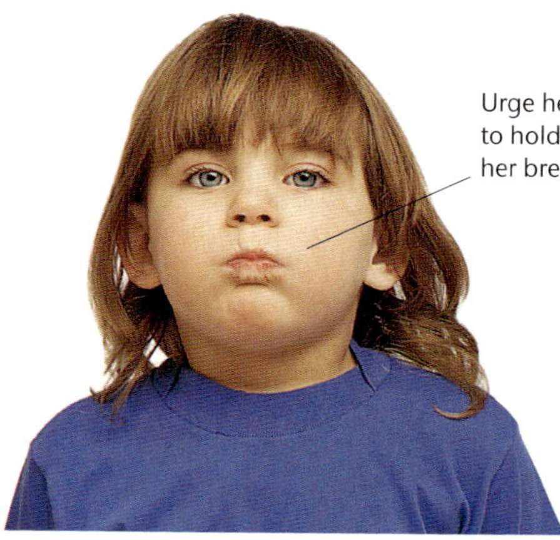

1. Tell your child to sit still and hold her breath for 5–10 seconds, then encourage her to breathe out slowly.

2. Get her to repeat this until hiccups have stopped.

Suffocation and strangulation

Strangulation results from a constriction around the child's neck that prevents breathing. Suffocation occurs when there is an obstruction over the mouth or nose, a weight on the child's chest or abdomen preventing normal breathing, or because the child is inhaling smoke- or fume-filled air, which prevents oxygen entering the lungs.

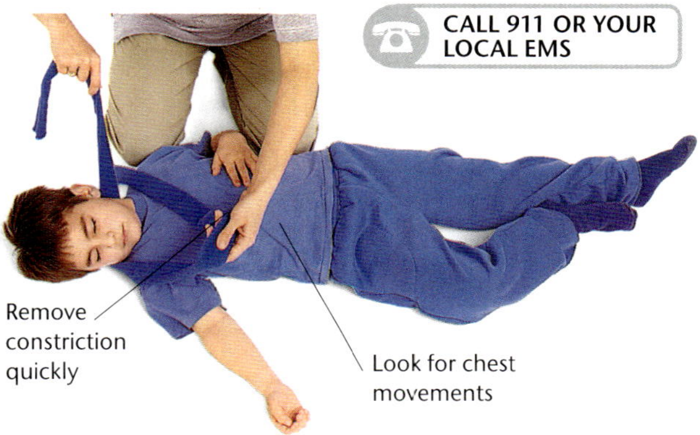

Remove constriction quickly

Look for chest movements

CALL 911 OR YOUR LOCAL EMS

1 Remove the obstruction quickly. Be very careful if you use scissors to cut the constriction if necessary. Breathing may restart.

2 Open your child's airway and check his breathing. If he is breathing, place him in the recovery position.

! IMPORTANT

- If your child is hanging, support his body while you remove or cut the rope or cord.
- Begin CPR immediately with 30 chest compressions

see also

- Unresponsive baby, *pp.19–21*
- Unresponsive child, *pp.22–27*

Fume inhalation

Fume, gas, and smoke inhalation requires urgent medical attention as the fumes prevent the child breathing in oxygen. Carbon monoxide prevents tissues taking up oxygen from air breathed in.

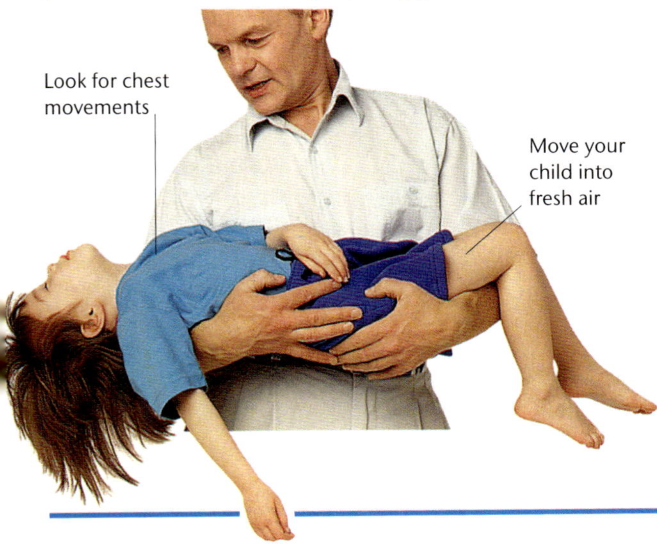

Look for chest movements

Move your child into fresh air

CALL 911 OR YOUR LOCAL EMS

1 Ensure that you do not put yourself at risk. Then carry your child away from danger area.

2 Open her airway and check her breathing. If breathing, place her in the recovery position, and treat any injuries found.

! IMPORTANT

- **Do not** enter the area if fumes, gas, carbon monoxide, or smoke are still present. CALL FIRE DEPARTMENT and 911.
- Begin CPR immediately with 30 chest compressions

see also

- Burns and scalds, *p.52*
- Unresponsive baby, *pp.19–21*
- Unresponsive child, *pp.22–27*

IMPORTANT

- **If** the attack is severe or prolonged, CALL 911 OR YOUR LOCAL EMS.
- **If** the attack is severe, there is a risk that he is suffering from a rare condition called epiglottitis. Suspect epiglottitis if your child has a high temperature and is obviously in distress, and has not had the Hib vaccination. CALL 911 OR YOUR LOCAL EMS.

Croup

This condition is caused by a viral infection. It can be alarming and often occurs at night, but usually passes quickly. Your child will have difficulty breathing, and a short, distinctve barking cough when he breathes out. He may be making a crowing or whistling noise. In a severe attack, he may use muscles around his nose, neck, and upper arms in his attempts to breathe. IF HE HAS blue-tinged skin or signs of a severe attack (*see box, left*), CALL 911 OR YOUR LOCAL EMS.

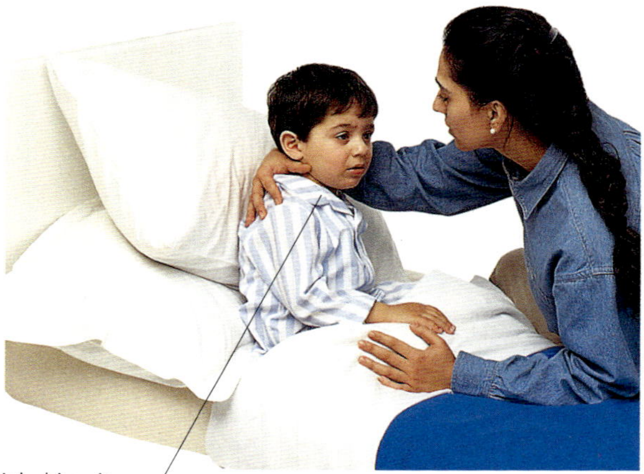

Help him sit up, supporting his back and head

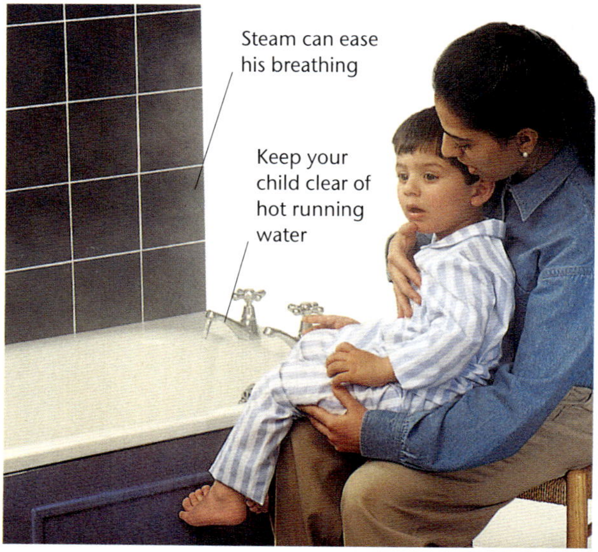

Steam can ease his breathing

Keep your child clear of hot running water

1. Help your child into a comfortable breathing position. Sit him up in bed, propped by pillows, or sit him on your lap supporting his back. Reassure him.
2. Stay calm—if you panic it could frighten the child, which can worsen the attack.
3. If it is safe to do so, create a steamy atmosphere. Take the child into the bathroom, and run a hot faucet or shower, or boil some water in the kitchen.
4. If he has not improved after 10 minutes, cool air can be helpful. Put him in front of a cool-mist humidifier, open the window in his bedrooom, or take him outside briefly to breathe in the air.

SEEK MEDICAL ADVICE

Asthma

If your child suffers from asthma, familiarize her with her medication so that she knows how to use it in an attack. You can recognize an attack if your child has difficulty breathing and is coughing; is wheezing, especially when breathing *out;* is distressed and anxious. She may also be tired by efforts to breathe and have a bluish tinge to face and lips.

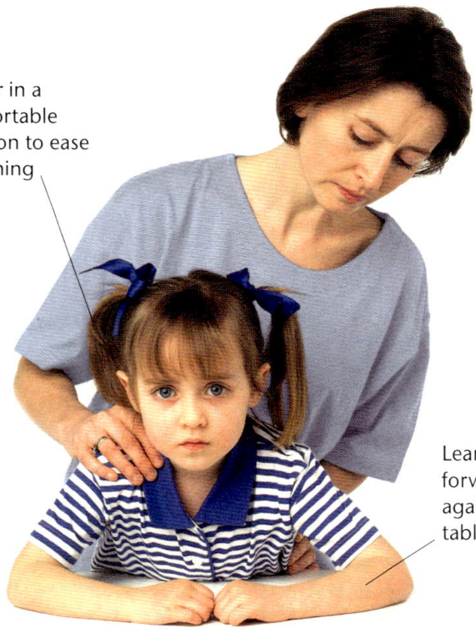

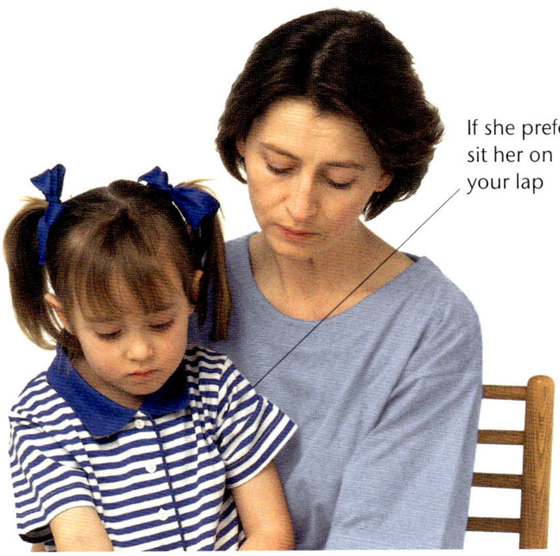

1. Give your child her usual dose of the medication as soon as an attack starts (see right). Stay calm and reassure her. Tell her to breathe slowly and deeply.

2. Help your child relax. Sit her down in a comfortable position for breathing. This could be leaning forward with her arms resting on a table, or if she prefers, sit her on your lap. Make sure the room is well ventilated and smoke free.

3. If the attack does not ease within a few minutes, give her the prescribed number of puffs of her medication (usually 4–8 puffs).

4. If the attack still does not ease,

CALL 911 OR YOUR LOCAL EMS

IMPORTANT

- **If** it is a first attack, CALL 911 OR YOUR LOCAL EMS.
- **If** the attack is severe, medication has no effect, child is exhausted, breathlessness makes talking difficult, and/or skin has a bluish tinge, CALL 911 OR EMS.

Using medication

Give your child her medication as soon as an attack starts. Usually if a child has an inhaler she will also have a spacer device to use with it, so use that as well because it's easier to take in the medication. Follow the instructions from your doctor carefully.

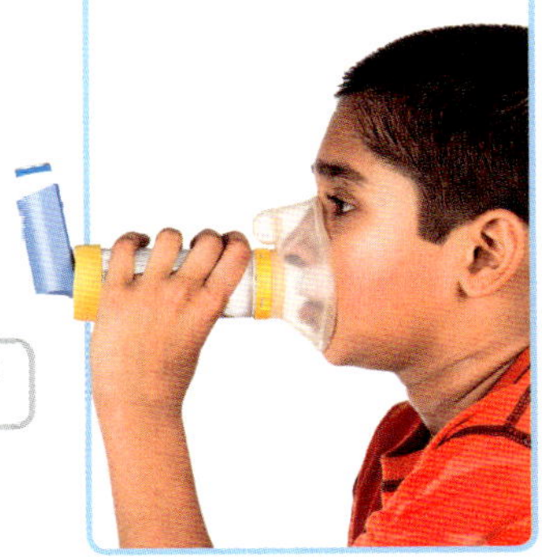

> **! IMPORTANT**
>
> - **Do not** move your child unnecessarily.
> - **Do not** give your child anything to drink or eat because he may need an anesthetic. If he is thirsty, moisten his lips with water.
> - **If** you suspect a broken leg, only raise the *un*injured leg.

Shock

The most likely cause is serious bleeding or a severe burn—injuries that must be treated without delay—dehydration, or a bacterial illness. There could be internal bleeding if shock develops with no visible injury. Early signs are increased respiratory rate and agitation; later signs include pale, cold, and sweaty skin with purplish blotching, bluish lips, rapid pulse, vomiting, confusion, becoming weaker, yawning, and thirst; eventually he will be unresponsive.

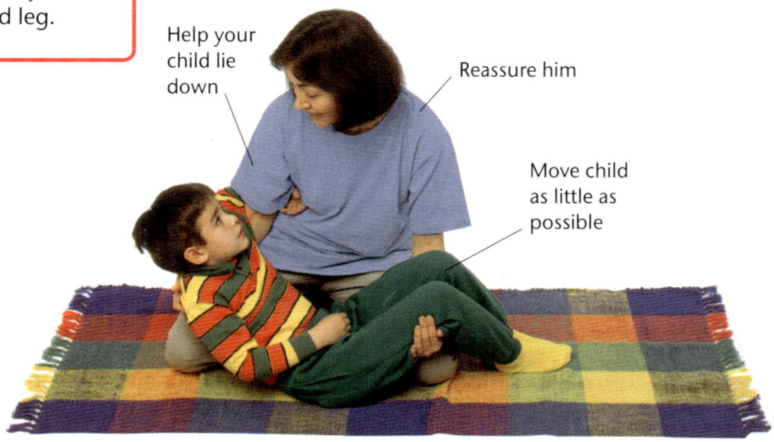
Help your child lie down
Reassure him
Move child as little as possible

1 Treat any obvious injury. Help your child lie down flat, on a blanket or rug if possible, to protect him from the cold. Stay calm and reassure him.

CALL 911 OR YOUR LOCAL EMS

2 Keep your child's head low; don't put a pillow under it. Carefully raise your child's legs above the level of his heart to help blood flow to the vital organs; support them on pillows, a chair, or a pile of books padded with a cushion.

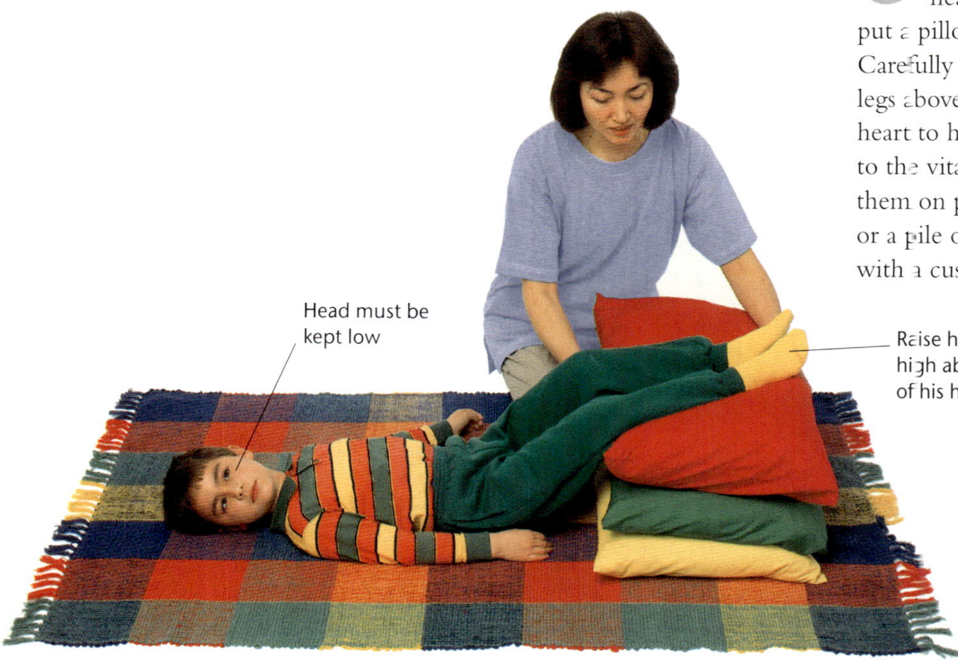

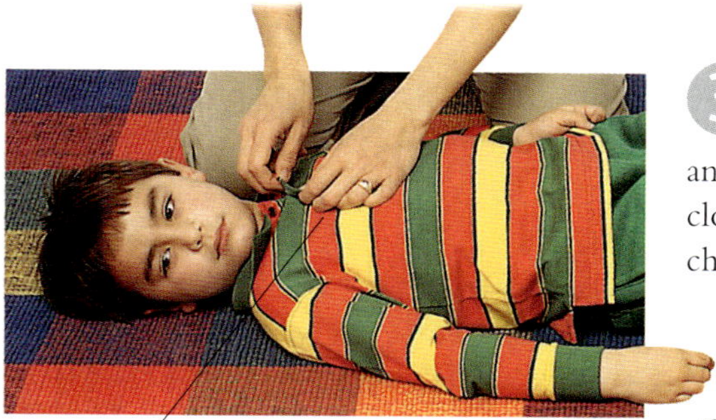

3 To make breathing easier, loosen any buttons or tight clothing at his neck, chest, and waist.

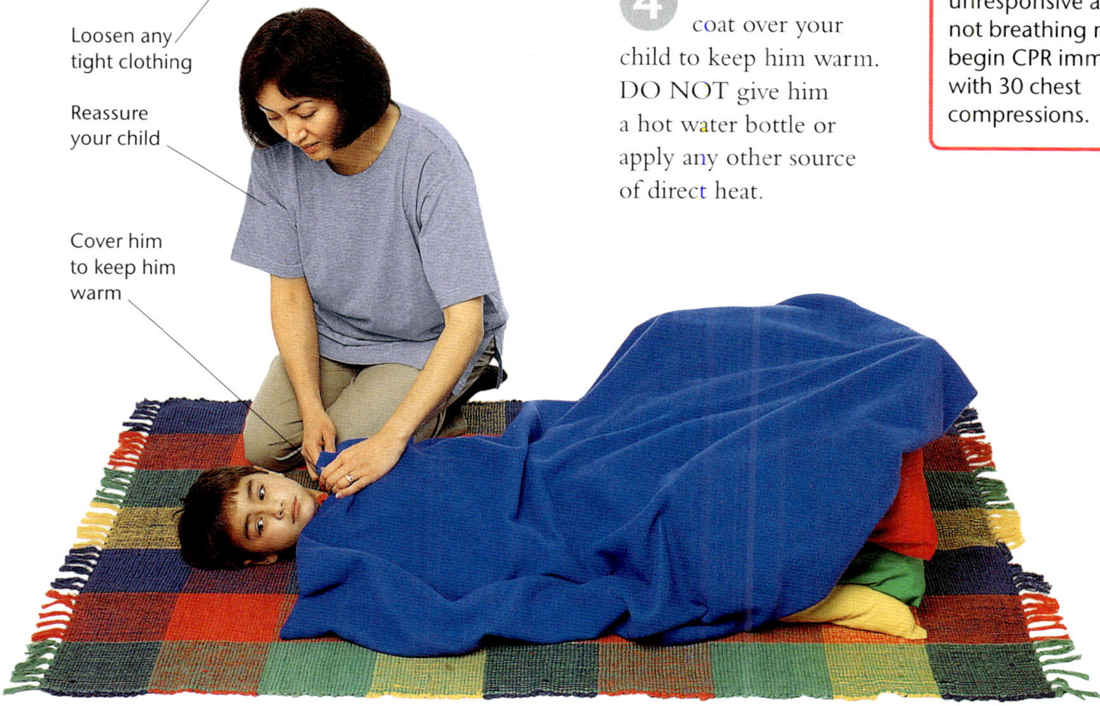

4 Put a blanket or coat over your child to keep him warm. DO NOT give him a hot water bottle or apply any other source of direct heat.

IMPORTANT

- **Do not** leave a child in shock alone, unless you absolutely have to get medical help. If you can, ask someone else to call 911 OR YOUR LOCAL EMS while you stay with him.
- **If** your child becomes unresponsive and is not breathing normally, begin CPR immediately with 30 chest compressions.

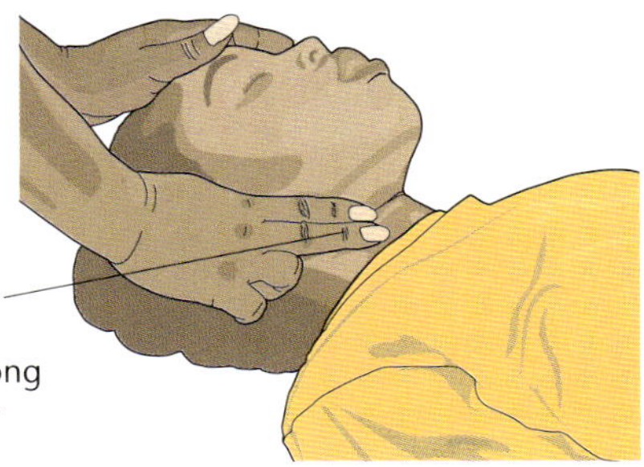

5 Monitor his breathing, pulse, and level of response while you wait for emergency help. Encourage him to talk or answer questions to help you assess any change in his condition. Make a note of any changes and tell the medical personnel.

see also

- Severe bleeding, *p.38*
- Burns and scalds, *p.52*
- Unresponsive baby, *pp.19–21*
- Unresponsive child, *pp.22–27*

Severe bleeding

Any incident that results in severe bleeding can be very distressing for you and your child. If it is not controlled quickly, a life-threatening condition known as shock could develop. Large wounds may also need stitches. Send someone to CALL 911 OR YOUR LOCAL EMS.

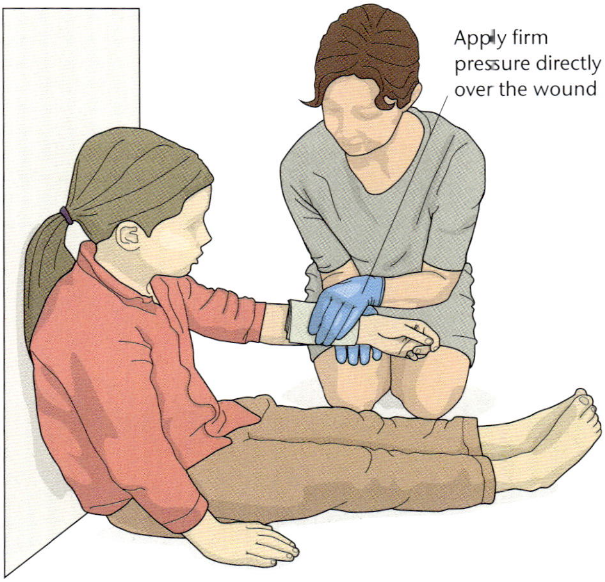

1 Apply direct pressure over the wound immediately, with a clean pad if available, but anything can be used, even a bare hand. Encourage the child to help with this.

2 While you maintain direct pressure, ask a helper to:

CALL 911 OR YOUR LOCAL EMS

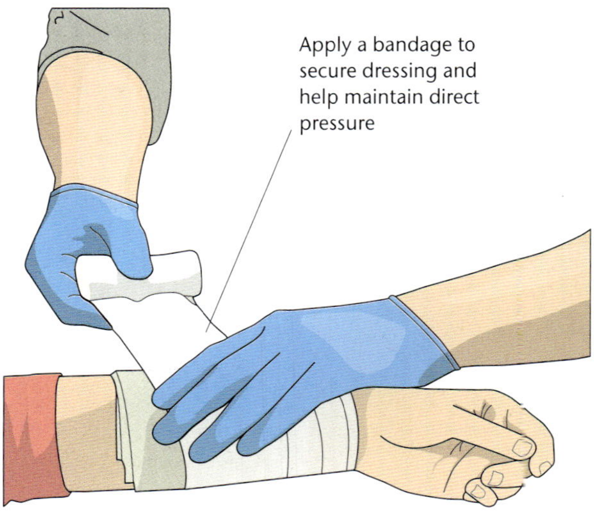

3 Secure the dressing with a bandage that is firm enough to maintain pressure, but not so tight that it affects the circulation beyond the bandage. Check the circulation in the hand or foot by pressing the nail. If colour does not return right away, the bandage is too tight; if bleeding has stopped, loosen it.

IMPORTANT

- **Do not** give anything to eat or drink in case anesthetic is needed.
- **Remove** or cut away clothing to expose a wound if necessary; don't remove anything that is stuck to the wound because it may worsen the bleeding.
- **Do not** apply direct pressure if there is an object embedded in the wound—press on either side of the object (do not remove it) to control bleeding (*see p.40*).
- **If** the bleeding follows a head injury, and there is thin watery fluid draining from the ears, nose, or an open skull wound, CALL 911 OR YOUR LOCAL EMS.
- **If** your child becomes unresponsive and is not breathing normally, begin CPR with 30 compressions immediately. CALL 911 OR YOUR LOCAL EMS.

see also

- Check circulation, *p.105*
- Dressings, *p.104*
- Embedded object, *p.40*
- Shock, *p.36*
- Unresponsive child, *pp.22–27*
- Triangular bandages, *p.106*

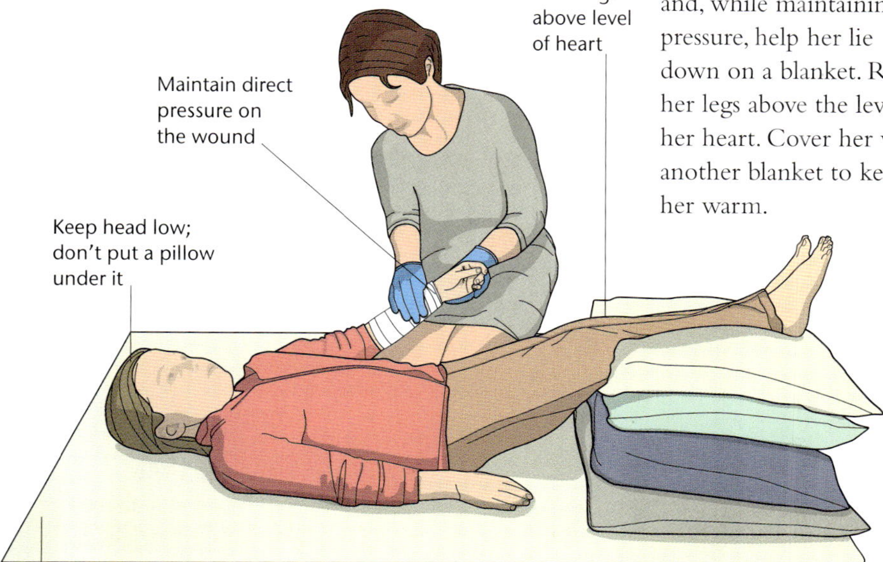

4 Shock is likely to develop if bleeding is severe. Support and elevate the injured part and, while maintaining pressure, help her lie down on a blanket. Raise her legs above the level of her heart. Cover her with another blanket to keep her warm.

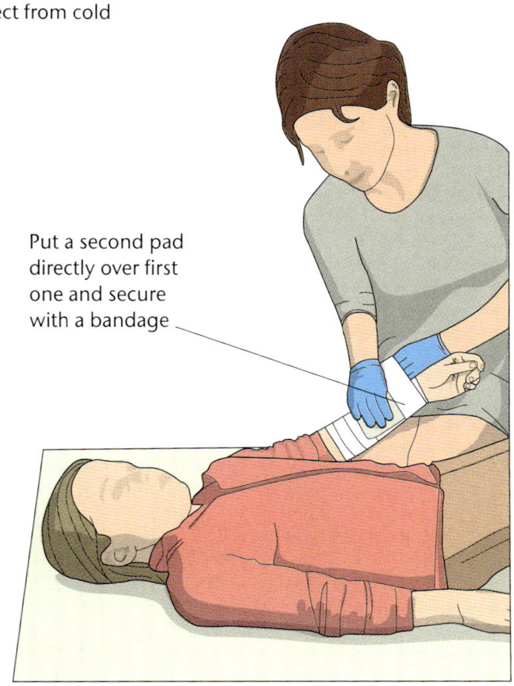

5 If bleeding shows through the first dressing, put another pad on top of the first and secure with a bandage. If bleeding continues, more items (such as dressings and gauze) may need to be added.

6 Monitor child's breathing, pulse, and level of response while waiting for emergency help to arrive.

When bleeding stops

If the bleeding has stopped and there is no risk of shock, help the child sit down and support an injured hand or arm in an elevation sling for extra comfort on the way to the hospital.

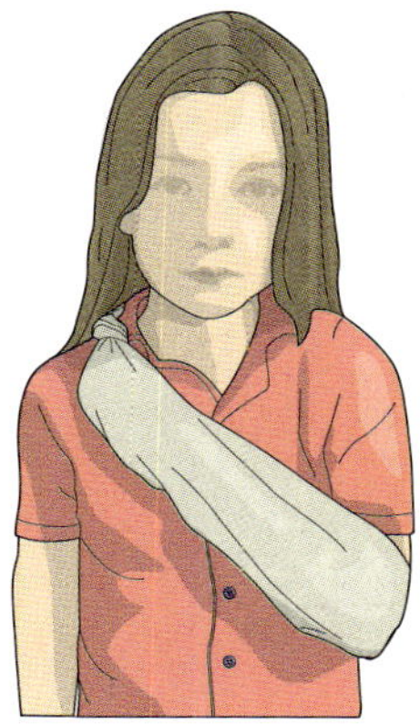

IMPORTANT

- **Do not** try to remove or dislodge objects that are embedded in a wound because you may cause further damage and bleeding.

Bandaging around larger objects

If the object is very big, build up padding on either side, then bandage above and below the object instead of over the top.

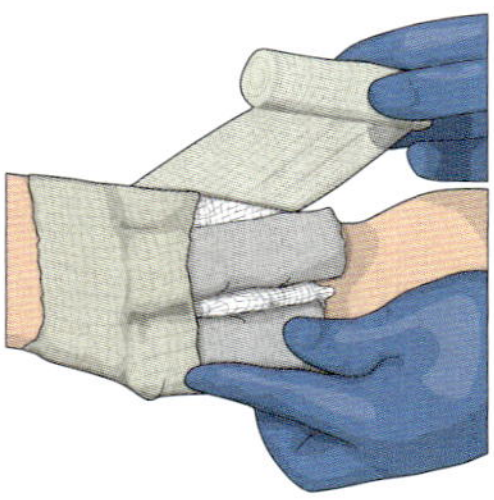

Embedded object

An object such as a piece of glass that becomes stuck in a wound is serious because it may be plugging the wound, preventing bleeding. Do not remove it. Protect it with padding and bandages and get medical help.

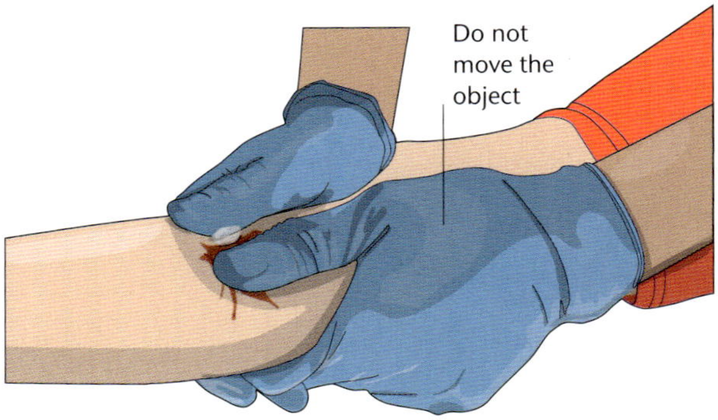

1. Help your child lie down and keep him calm. If pressure is necessary to slow bleeding, take care not to move the object and cause further damage. Apply pressure around the object.

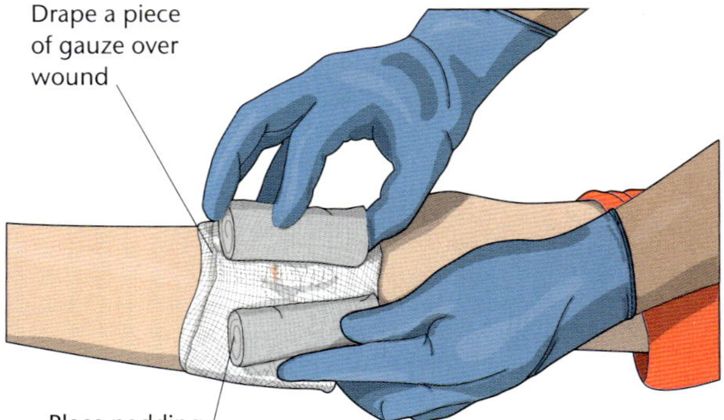

2. Loosely drape some gauze over the wound and object to minimize the risk of infection. If the object is small, build up padding so that it is slightly higher than the embedded object; spare roller bandages are ideal for this. If the object is large, *see box left*.

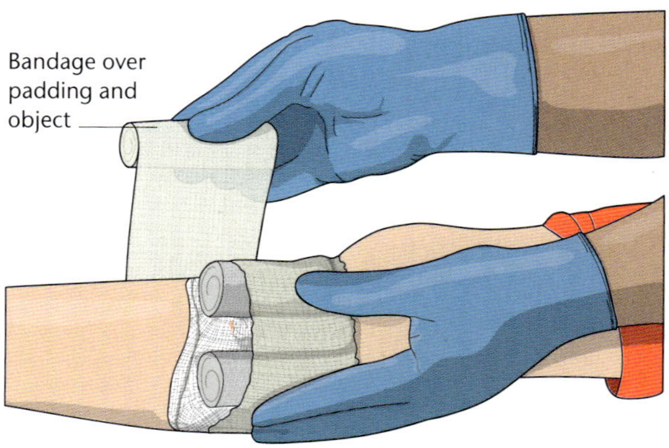

3. Secure padding in place by bandaging over it, being careful not to press down on the embedded object.

TAKE YOUR CHILD TO THE HOSPITAL

OR

CALL 911 OR YOUR LOCAL EMS

see also

- Severe bleeding, *p.38*

Cuts and abrasions

Children can be very upset by the tiniest abrasion. Reassure your child and wash the wound. Covering the wound with an adhesive bandage keeps it clean and often makes the child feel better.

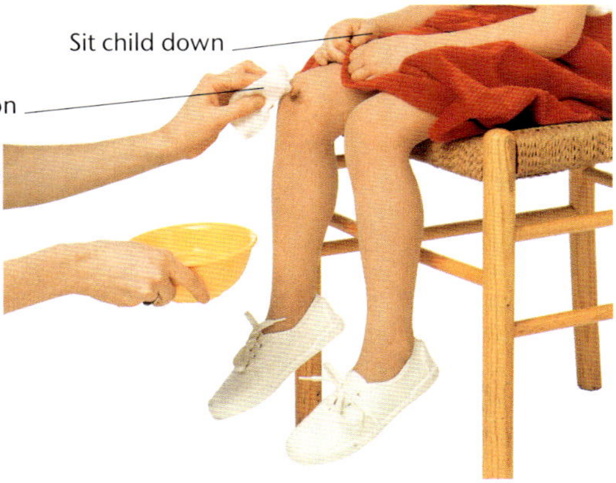

1 Help your child sit down and reassure her. Gently wash the abrasion with soap and water using a gauze pad or washcloth. If the wound is very dirty, rinse under cold running water.

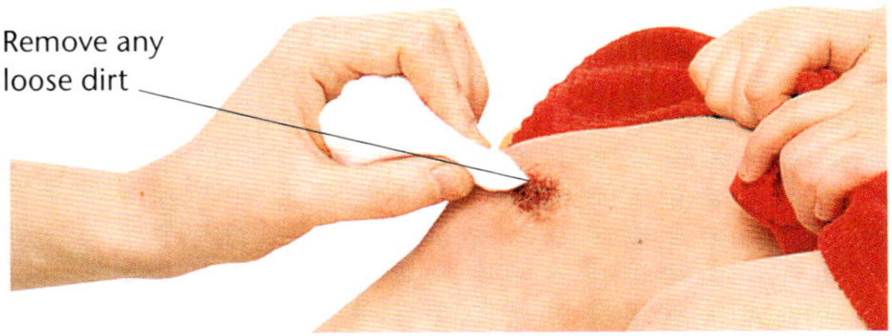

2 Try to remove any loose particles of dirt or gravel with the corner of a piece of gauze or cold running water. This may cause slight bleeding.

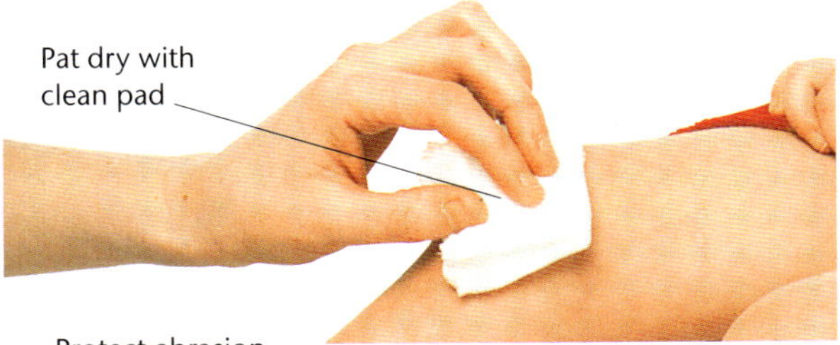

3 Apply direct pressure with a clean pad to stop any bleeding. Pat the wound dry with clean pieces of gauze.

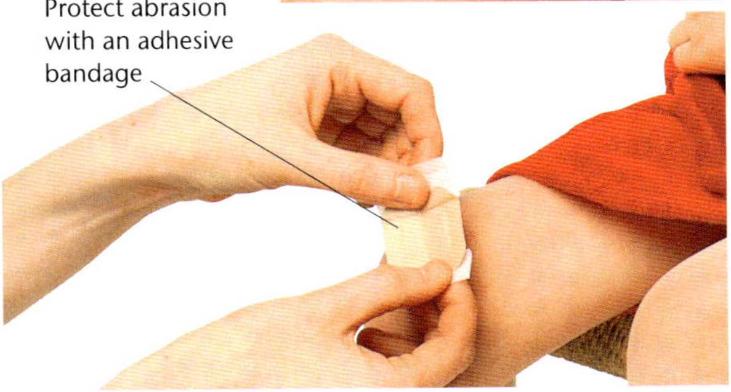

4 Apply an antibiotic cream and cover with an adhesive bandage that has a pad large enough to cover the wound and the area around it.

! IMPORTANT

- **Do not** clean or cover cuts with cotton wool or any fluffy material; it may stick to the wound and delay healing.
- **Loosen** particles of dirt by rinsing the wound under cool running water.
- **If** particles are deeply embedded, *see opposite* and TAKE YOUR CHILD TO THE DOCTOR OR HOSPITAL.
- **Check** that your child's tetanus immunization is up to date.

Tetanus

This is a dangerous infection that is present in the soil. If it is transferred into a wound, tetanus germs release toxins (poisons) into the nervous system. Tetanus is best prevented through scheduled childhood vaccination. Babies receive this as part of their immunization program. Every child should be given a tetanus booster before starting school.

see also

- Infected wound, *p.42*

IMPORTANT

- **Do not** try to remove objects that are embedded in a wound because you may cause further damage and bleeding.

Tetanus

This is a dangerous infection caused by a bacterium present in the soil. If these bacteria are transferred into a wound, they may multiply and release toxins (poisons) into the nervous system. Tetanus is best prevented through vaccination. Babies receive this as part of their immunization program. Every child should be given a tetanus booster before starting school.

Infected wound

A wound is infected if there is increasing pain and soreness; swelling, redness, and a feeling of heat around the injury; or there is pus or oozing. If there is an absess or pus draining from the wound, cover it with clean gauze and take your child to the doctor. If there are signs of advanced infection, such as fever, swollen glands, and faint red lines extending from those glands, take your child to the hospital.

1. If red and crusty, apply antibiotic ointment and cover the wound with an adhesive dressing.

2. Cover with clean gauze a wound that has pus or oozing.

   TAKE YOUR CHILD TO THE DOCTOR

3. If there are other symptoms of advanced infection,

   TAKE YOUR CHILD TO THE HOSPITAL

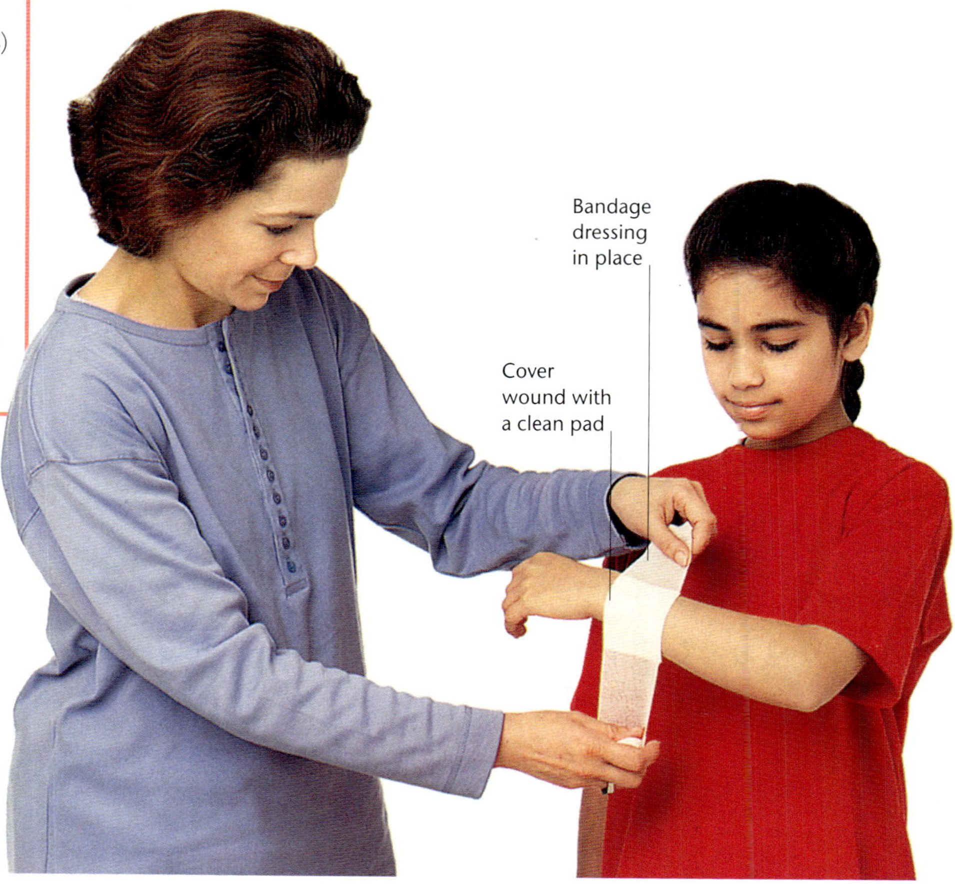

Blisters

If a blister is caused by friction (for example, a badly fitting shoe), treat as here. You can buy special padded blister bandages.

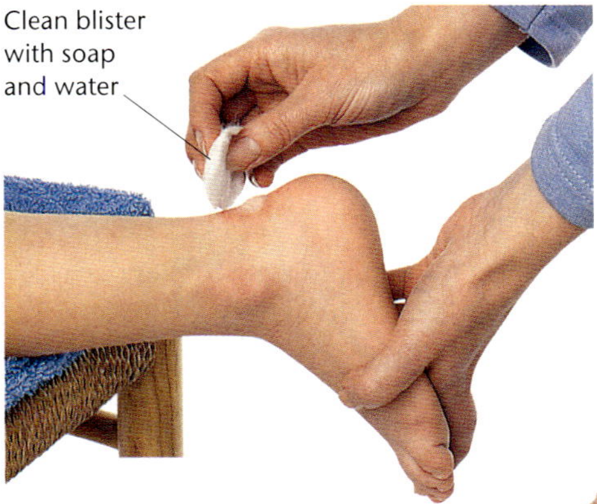

1. Clean the blister thoroughly with soap and water. Rinse it with clean water.

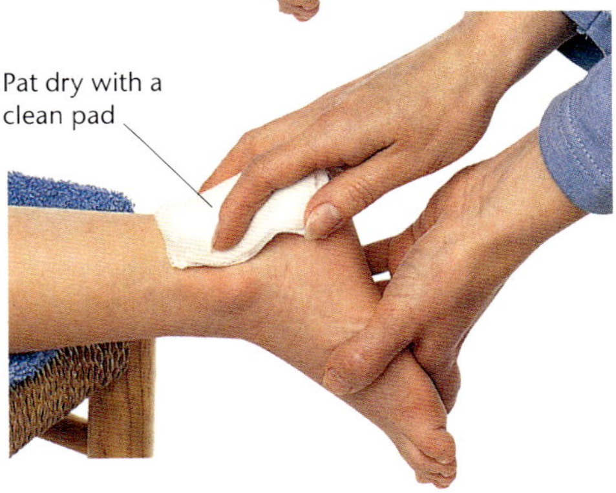

2. Thoroughly dry the blister and the surrounding skin. Pat it gently with a clean gauze pad or paper tissues.

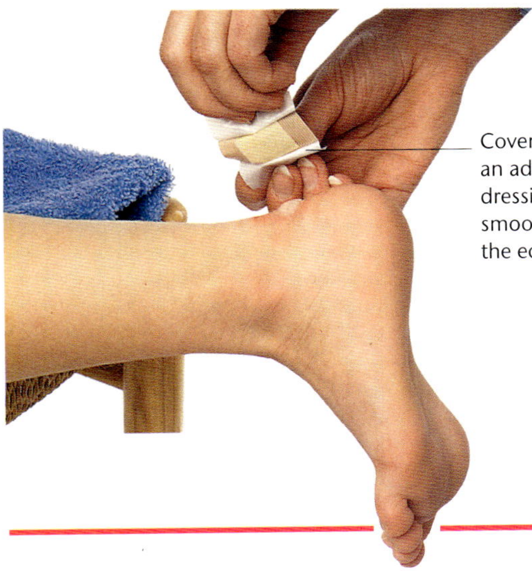

3. Ideally cover it with a blister bandage if you have one; if not, a normal one will do. The adhesive bandage needs to have a pad large enough to cover the entire blister. Make sure the edges are smooth, to prevent another blister from developing.

IMPORTANT

- **If** the blister is very large, cover it with a clean, nonfluffy dressing, held in place with adhesive tape or a bandage.
- **Do not** deliberately break a blister because this can cause it to become infected.
- **Do not** use this method for a blister caused by a burn; treat these as described on pages 52–53.

see also

- Burns and scalds, *p.52*

IMPORTANT

- **Do not** try to remove objects in the eye, except an eyelash or speck of dirt. Small objects like dirt can be flushed out of the eye using running water for 10 minutes.
- **If** he cannot keep his eyes still, cover both of them.
- **Put** the dressing over the eyebrow and closed eyelid, not the eyeball.

Eyebrow or eyelid wounds

A wound to the eyebrow or eyelid may be associated with a more serious eye injury or infection, which can damage the child's sight. If you do not suspect any other injury, follow the steps below, but if there is any chance of eye trauma or objects embedded in the eye, take the child to the hospital immediately.

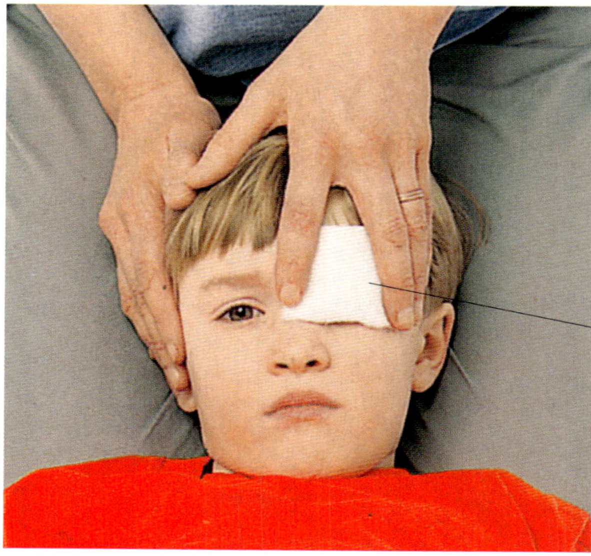

Lay a sterile dressing over injured eye

1 Help your child lie down and cradle his head in your lap to keep it still—make sure he can hear you. He may be in pain; tell him not to rub or move either of his eyes.

2 Reassure your child and lay a sterile dressing over the injured eye.

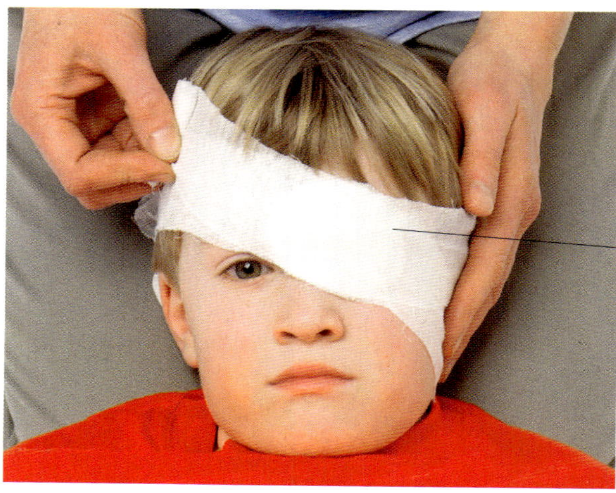

Secure dressing with gauze bandage

3 Secure the dressing with a gauze bandage wrapped around his head. Fasten in place with tape away from the injured eye.

4 Keep him lying on his back if bleeding.

TAKE YOUR CHILD TO THE HOSPITAL

see also

- Chemical burn to eye, *p.56*
- Object in eye, *p.76*

Nosebleed

Children get nosebleeds from a blow to the nose, dry air, or from picking it. Bleeding usually stops quickly, but it can alarm young children.

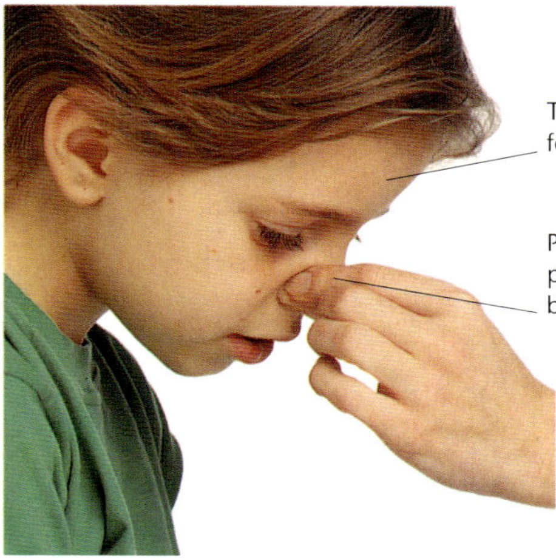

1 Help your child sit down with her head well forward. Ask her to breathe through her mouth, then pinch the fleshy part of her nose for 10 minutes. Then release the pressure.

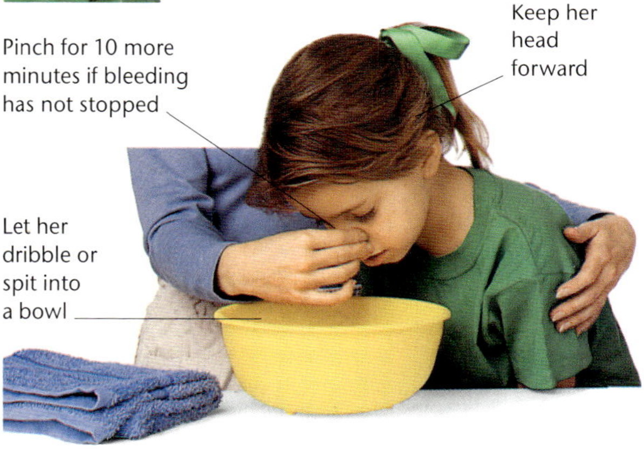
Keep her head forward
Pinch for 10 more minutes if bleeding has not stopped
Let her dribble or spit into a bowl

2 Tell your child to spit out any excess fluid in her mouth. If the bleeding has not stopped, pinch it again for another 10 minutes, then release pressure. If the nose is still bleeding, pinch it again for up to 10 minutes.

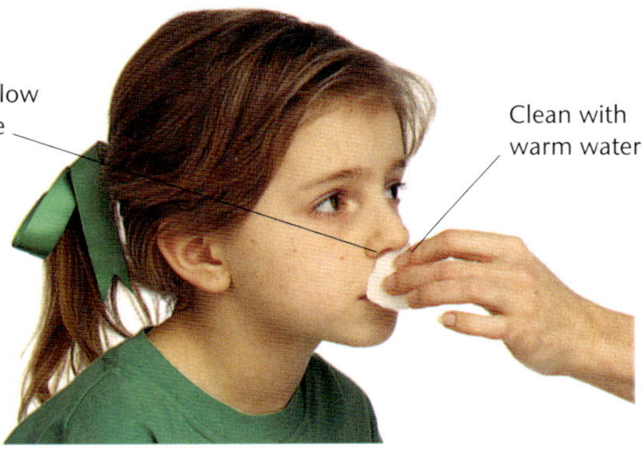

3 Once the bleeding has stopped, use some cotton dipped in lukewarm water to clean your child's face. Advise her to rest and not to blow her nose. If your child picks at (or blows) her nose within the next few hours, the bleeding may start again.

! IMPORTANT

- **If** there is blood or blood-stained watery fluid coming from the nose following a head injury, CALL 911 OR YOUR LOCAL EMS.
- **If** the nosebleed is severe or goes on for more than half an hour, TAKE YOUR CHILD TO THE HOSPITAL.

see also

- Head injury, *p.60*

IMPORTANT

- If the bleeding follows a head injury and there is blood or watery blood-stained fluid draining from the ear, CALL 911 OR YOUR LOCAL EMS.
- If the injury is caused by an earring being ripped out, your child may need stitches. TAKE YOUR CHILD TO THE HOSPITAL.

Bleeding from inside the ear

Help your child into a semiupright position, with his head tilted toward the injured side to allow blood to drain away. Put an absorbent pad over the ear and bandage it lightly in place. Do not plug the ear. SEEK MEDICAL ADVICE.

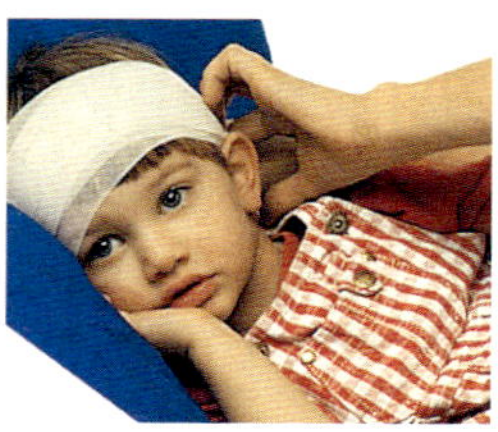

see also

- Head injury, *p.60*
- Object in ear, *p.77*

Ear wound

Outer ear wounds can bleed profusely, which can be alarming. If blood is coming from inside the ear, check that your child has not inserted something into it. If bleeding follows a head injury, CALL 911 OR YOUR LOCAL EMS.

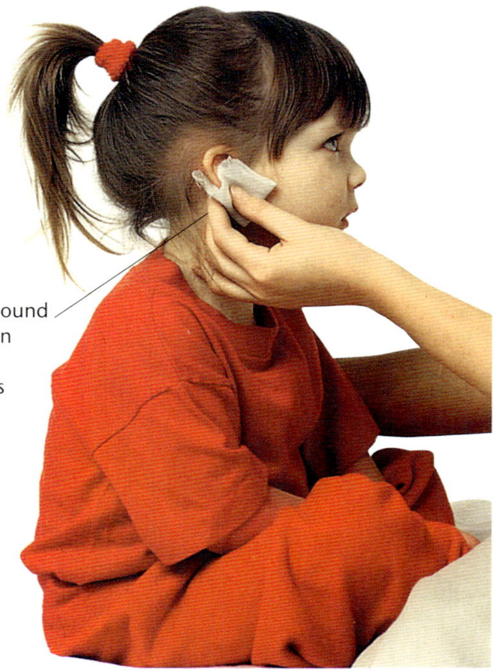

Press on wound over a clean pad for 10 minutes

1 Help your child sit down and gently pinch the wound with your thumb and forefinger over a clean piece of gauze. Keep pressing for 10 minutes.

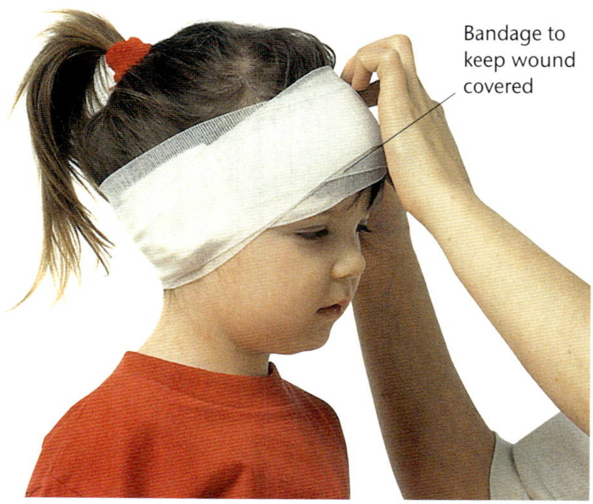

Bandage to keep wound covered

2 Cover the injured ear with a sterile dressing and lightly bandage it in place.

SEEK MEDICAL ADVICE

Mouth wound

These wounds can be the result of a child biting the inside of his mouth in a fall, for example, or from the loss of a tooth. Make sure your child does not inhale blood because this can result in breathing problems.

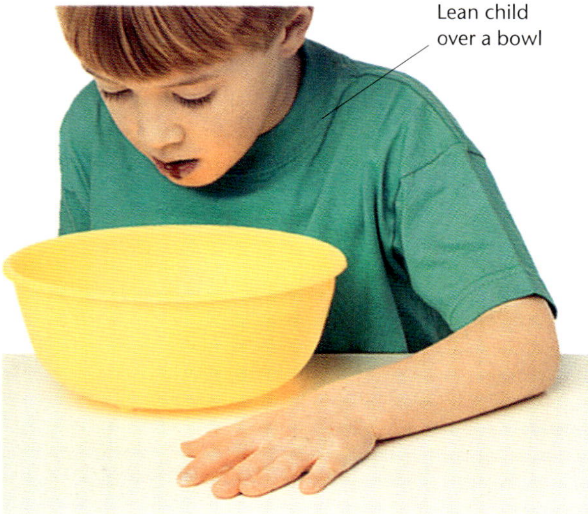

Lean child over a bowl

1 Help your child sit down with his head over a bowl. Encourage him to spit out any blood.

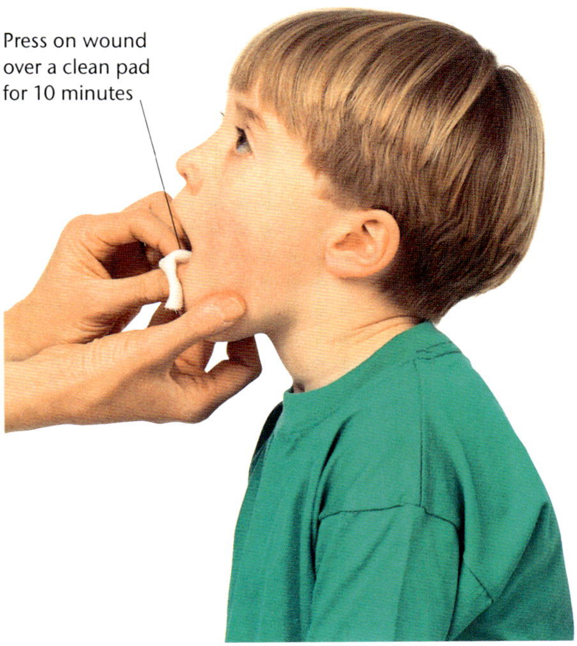

Press on wound over a clean pad for 10 minutes

2 Place a pad over the wound and pinch it between your thumb and forefinger, maintaining the pressure for 10 minutes. Your child may be able to do this for himself.

SEEK MEDICAL ADVICE

! IMPORTANT

- **Do not** wash out his mouth—it may disturb a blood clot.
- **If** he loses an "adult" tooth, it may be possible for a dentist to replant it. Do not clean the tooth. Handle the tooth by the crown (white part), not the root. Put the tooth back in the socket if you can. If you can't, keep it moist by putting it in milk or saliva. Take your child to the dentist or the ER.
- **Ensure** a baby tooth has not been inhaled or swallowed. A dentist should check the gum.

Bleeding from tooth socket

Ask your child to sit down and support her jaw. Place a pad over the tooth socket, making sure that it is higher than the adjacent teeth. Tell her to bite hard on the pad. A younger child may need you to hold the pad in place.

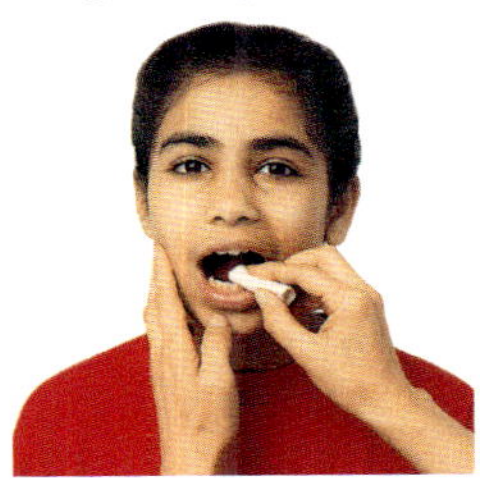

! IMPORTANT

- **Get** to a hospital quickly. It may be possible to reattach an amputated part using microsurgery when both the child and the severed part reach the hospital in time.
- **Never** wash the severed part or allow it to come into direct contact with ice.
- **Do not** apply gauze to open wounds.

Amputation

Whether a injury causes partial or total amputation, the part can often be reattached. Your child will need an anaesthetic so don't give him anything to eat or drink because it may delay surgery.

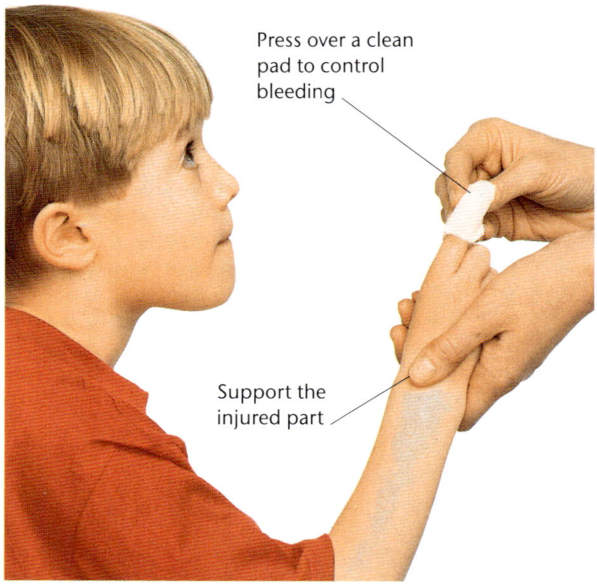

1 Control the blood loss by pressing firmly on the injury using a sterile dressing or clean pad. If necessary, treat for shock; help your child lie down and raise his legs above his heart.

2 Bandage or tape the dressing firmly in place. You can cover a finger with a gauze finger bandage to protect it.

CALL 911 OR YOUR LOCAL EMS

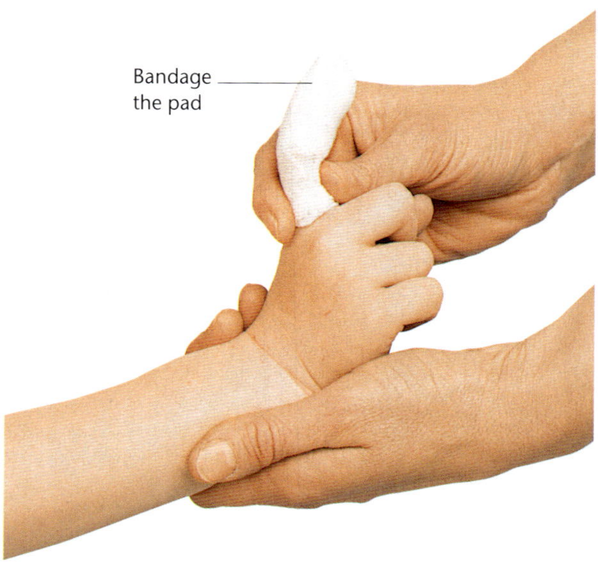

3 Tell the 911 operator or EMS dispatcher it is an amputation. Monitor your child for signs of shock while waiting. If possible, put the severed part in a plastic bag and keep it cool, *see left*.

Care of the amputated part

Preserve the severed part until you get to the hospital. Wrap it in plastic wrap or a plastic bag, then in a soft fabric, such as a cotton handkerchief or piece of gauze. Place the wrapped part in a plastic bag filled with ice cubes; the part must not touch the ice. Put the whole package in another bag or container. Mark with the time of injury and the child's name then give it to the emergency personnel.

see also

- Severe bleeding, *p.38*
- Shock, *p.36*

Internal bleeding

Suspect this when signs of shock develop without obvious blood loss. There may also be "pattern bruising" around the injury with marks from clothes or crushing objects because bleeding may be occurring in the lungs or abdomen.

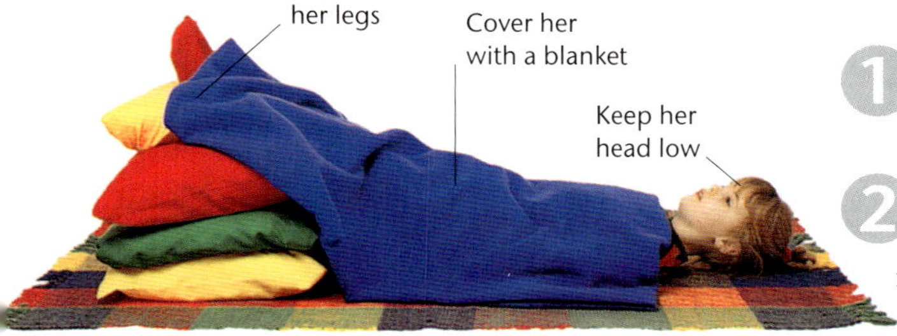
Raise and support her legs
Cover her with a blanket
Keep her head low

CALL 911 OR YOUR LOCAL EMS

1. Help her lie down; raise her legs.
2. Monitor breathing, pulse, and level of response while waiting for help, *p. 14*.

IMPORTANT

- **If the child is unresponsive, open her airway and check breathing. If breathing, place in the recovery position; if she is not breathing, begin CPR immediately with 30 chest compressions.**

see also

- Shock, *p.36*
- Unresponsive baby, *pp.19–21*
- Unresponsive child, *pp.22–27*

Crush injury

A crush injury can be serious because it may cause internal bleeding and broken bones as well as open wounds. If you suspect broken bones, support the injury but do not move your child unless he is in immediate danger.

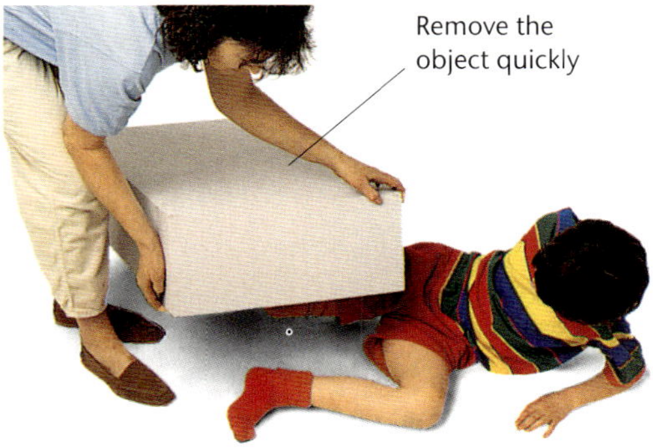
Remove the object quickly

CALL 911 OR YOUR LOCAL EMS

1. If the incident has only just happened, remove the heavy object from the child quickly.

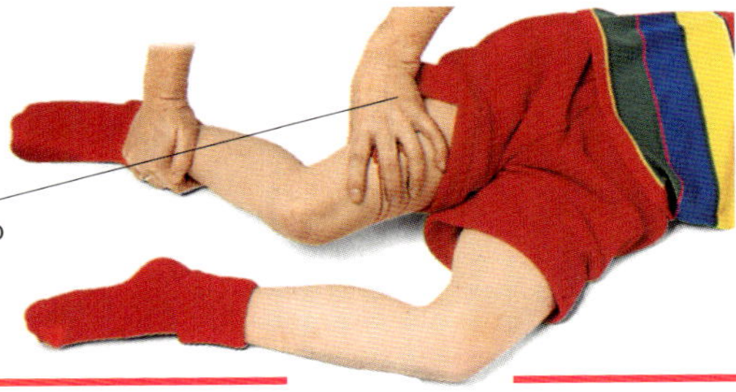
Press on wound to control bleeding

2. Control any bleeding by pressing firmly on the wound, with your hand or a clean pad. Support the injured part, but do not move it. Watch for signs of shock.

IMPORTANT

- An object that is crushing any part of the airway/chest/abdomen and impairing breathing should **always** be removed immediately.
- If the object is **NOT** impairing breathing and your child has been crushed for a prolonged period, call 911/EMS first before attempting to remove the object, as it may cause toxic fluids from the damaged muscles to be released into the body.

see also

- Severe bleeding, *p.38*
- Shock, *p.36*
- Leg injury, *p.64*

Chest wound

A wound to the chest can cause serious internal injuries. The lungs are particularly vulnerable, and breathing problems, shock, and collapsed lungs may follow an injury. If the wound is not obviously bleeding, leave it exposed—don't cover it with a dresssing.

IMPORTANT

- **Monitor** your child for signs of shock.
- **If** your child becomes unresponsive and is not breathing normally, begin CPR with 30 compressions immediately. CALL 911 OR YOUR LOCAL EMS.
- **If** you need to place him in the recovery position, place him so that he is lying on his injured side to support his chest and help the good lung function.

CALL 911 OR YOUR LOCAL EMS

1. Help your child to sit down in a semi-upright position.

2. If the wound is obviously bleeding, apply direct pressure with your hand—over a dressing if there's one available. Support the child in the same position until help arrives.

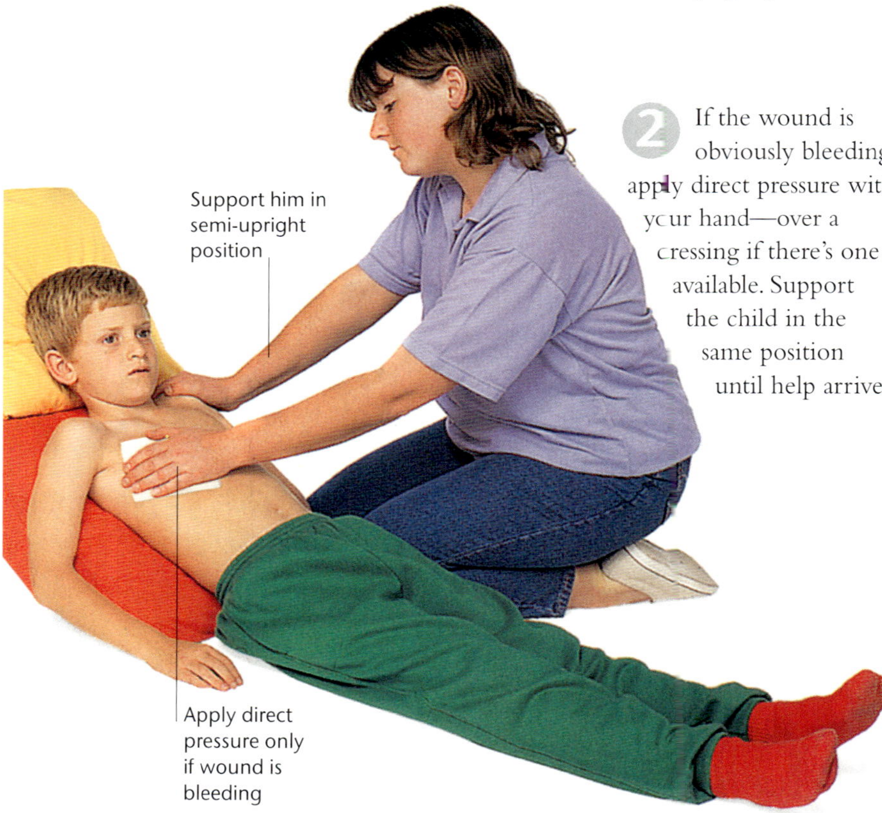

3. Tape the dressing in place on three sides only, leaving one side open to allow for air to escape when he breathes out.

4. Monitor his breathing, pulse, and level of response while you wait for help to arrive. If he becomes short of breath, release pressure and remove dressing.

see also

- Checking vital signs, *p.14*
- Severe bleeding, *p.38*
- Shock, *p.36*
- Unresponsive child, *pp.22–27*

Abdominal wound

A child with an abdominal wound is likely to develop the signs of shock. There is high risk of internal as well as external bleeding because internal organs may be damaged, so this is an emergency.

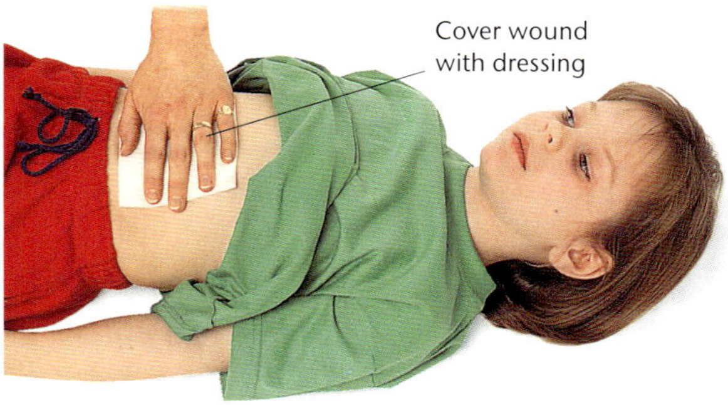

1 Help your child lie down and loosen any tight clothing around her waist. Cover the injury with a large sterile dressing and, if needed to stop bleeding, apply pressure over the pad.

CALL 911 OR YOUR LOCAL EMS

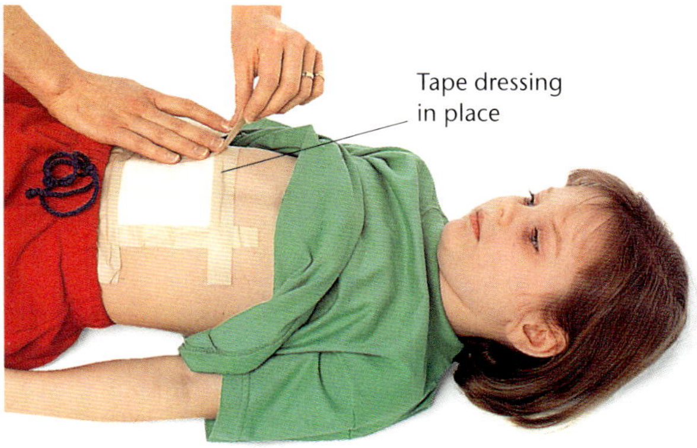

2 If your child has a major abdominal wound, just cover the wound with a sterile dressing. Raise and support her knees by placing a pillow under them—this eases the strain on the abdomen.

3 Secure the dressing lightly in place with tape; use hypoallergenic tape if possible.

4 Monitor her breathing, pulse, and level of response while you wait for help to arrive. Treat for shock if necessary. Continue to reassure her and watch for any change in her condition while waiting for help.

! IMPORTANT

- **Monitor** your child for signs of shock.
- **If** your child becomes unresponsive and is not breathing normally, begin CPR with 30 compressions immediately. CALL 911 OR YOUR LOCAL EMS.
- **If** intestines are protruding from wound, do not apply pressure. Follow steps 2–4.

see also

- Checking vital signs, *p.14*
- Severe bleeding, *p.38*
- Shock, *p.36*
- Unresponsive child, *pp.22–27*

Burns and scalds

It is very important to cool the burn as quickly as possible to stop the burning, minimize damage, and reduce pain. You must always seek medical advice or take a child to the hospital following any burn—however small—because there is risk of infection.

IMPORTANT

- **If** cooling with a shower, make sure it is cool or cold and that the pressure is set to low.
- **Do not** immerse young children in cold water because this can overcool the child and result in hypothermia.
- **If** no cold water is available, use another cool liquid such as milk.
- **Never** put lotions, lard, butter, or oil on a burn or scald.

Thermal burns to the mouth and throat

Burns in this area are very serious as they cause swelling and inflammation of the air passages, giving a serious risk of suffocation. Act quickly. If necessary, loosen clothing from around her neck.

- **If** your child becomes unresponsive and is not breathing normally, begin CPR with 30 compressions immediately. CALL 911 OR YOUR LOCAL EMS.

1 Start cooling the burn as quickly as possible to stop burning and minimize swelling. Flood the affected area with cool or cold water. Help the child to sit or lie down on a rug to make sure the burned area does not come into contact with the ground.

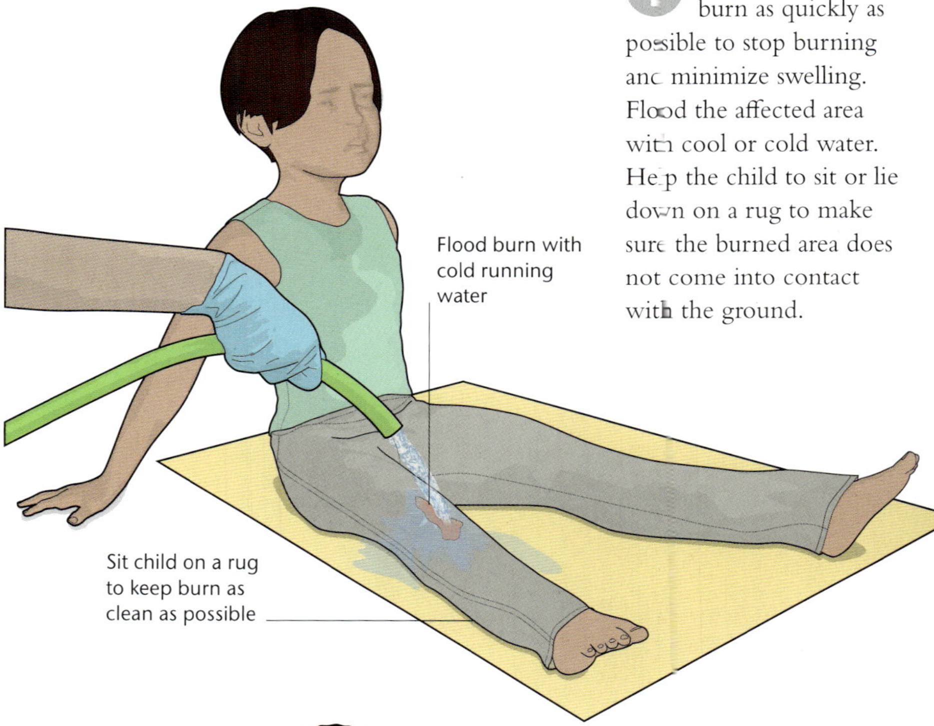

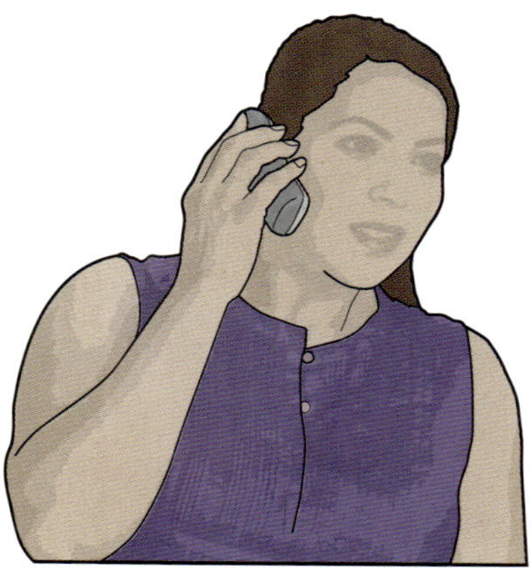

2 Continue cooling the burn for at least 10 minutes or until the pain stops.

TAKE YOUR CHILD TO THE HOSPITAL

OR

CALL 911 OR YOUR LOCAL EMS

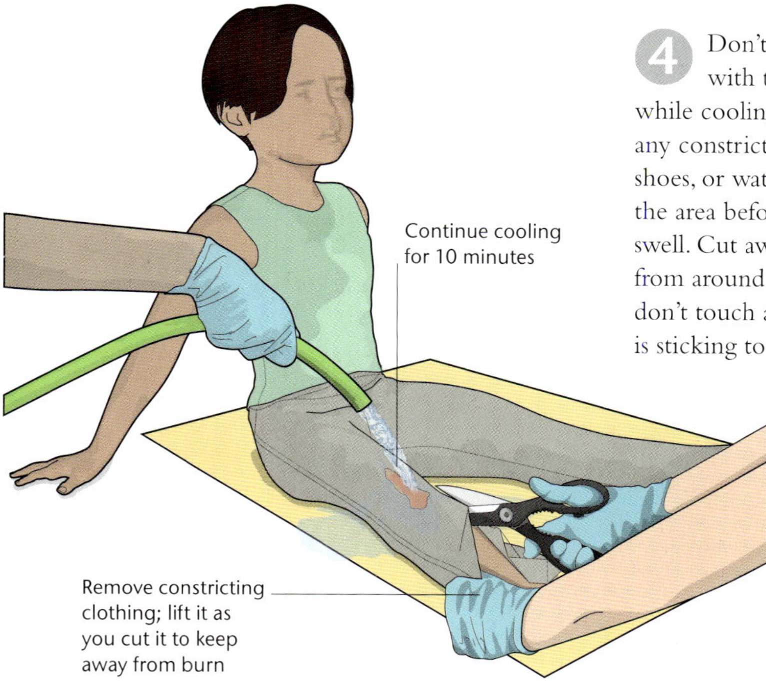

4 Don't interfere with the burn but while cooling it, remove any constricting clothing, shoes, or watches from the area before it starts to swell. Cut away clothing from around the burn, but don't touch anything that is sticking to it.

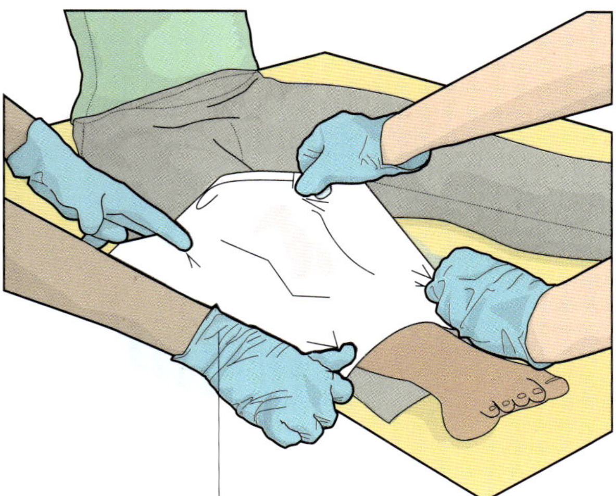

5 Once the burn is cooled, cover it with a nonadhesive dressing such as gauze, or plastic wrap. Lay it lengthwise along the limb; don't wrap it around a limb, which will swell. Monitor breathing, pulse, and level of response while you are waiting for help to arrive.

see also

- Checking vital signs, *p.14*
- Fire, *p.11*
- Shock, *p.36*
- Unresponsive baby, *pp.19–21*
- Unresponsive child, *pp.22–27*

! IMPORTANT

- **Do not** remove any clothing or material that is sticking to the burned area because this may cause further injury.
- **If** you have no plastic wrap, use a sterile dressing or any clean, nonfluffy material.
- **Do not** give your child anything to eat or drink because an anesthetic may be needed.
- **If** your child becomes unresponsive and is not breathing normally, begin CPR with 30 compressions immediately. CALL 911 OR YOUR LOCAL EMS.

Using a plastic bag

You can use a clean plastic bag to protect an injured hand or foot. Secure it loosely with a piece of tape that is applied to the bag; don't put tape on the child's skin.

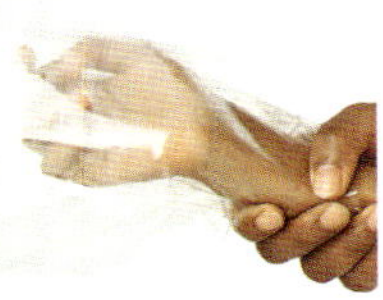

! IMPORTANT

- **Do not** touch your child until you are sure the electrical current has been turned off.
- **Seek** medical advice for all burns to children.
- **Do not** immerse young children in cold water because this can overcool the child and result in hypothermia.
- **If** child becomes unresponsive and is not breathing normally, begin CPR immediately with 30 chest compressions; if breathing, place in the recovery position. CALL 911 OR YOUR LOCAL EMS.

Electrical burn

An electric shock from a low-voltage source can result in burns. These may occur at both the point of entry and the point of exit of the current.

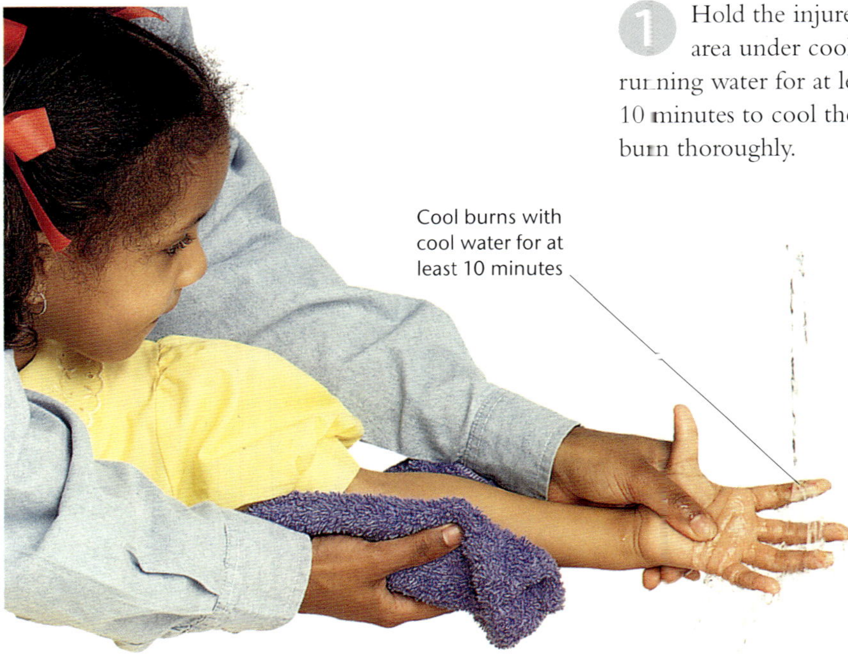

Cool burns with cool water for at least 10 minutes

1 Hold the injured area under cool running water for at least 10 minutes to cool the burn thoroughly.

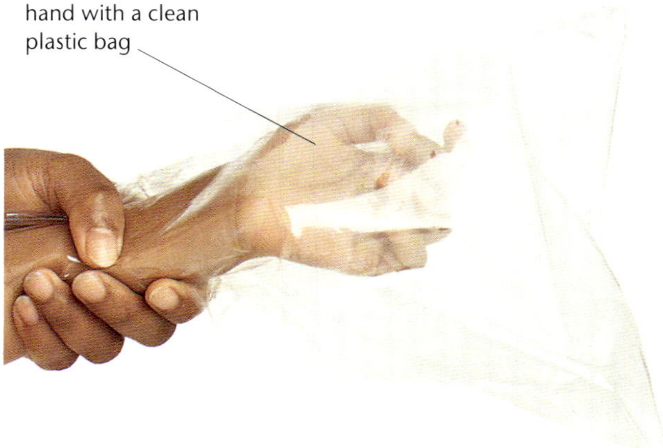

Cover burns on a hand with a clean plastic bag

2 If the burn is on a hand or foot, a clean plastic bag can be used, bandaged below the burn or clean material such as a pillowcase.

TAKE YOUR CHILD TO THE HOSPITAL

OR

CALL 911 OR YOUR LOCAL EMS

see also

- Electrical injury, *p.12*
- Unresponsive baby, *pp.19–21*
- Unresponsive child, *p.22–27*

Chemical burn to skin

Chemical burns can be caused by household agents such as oven cleaner or paint stripper. These burns can be serious and there will be fierce, stinging pain, redness or staining, followed by blistering and peeling of skin.

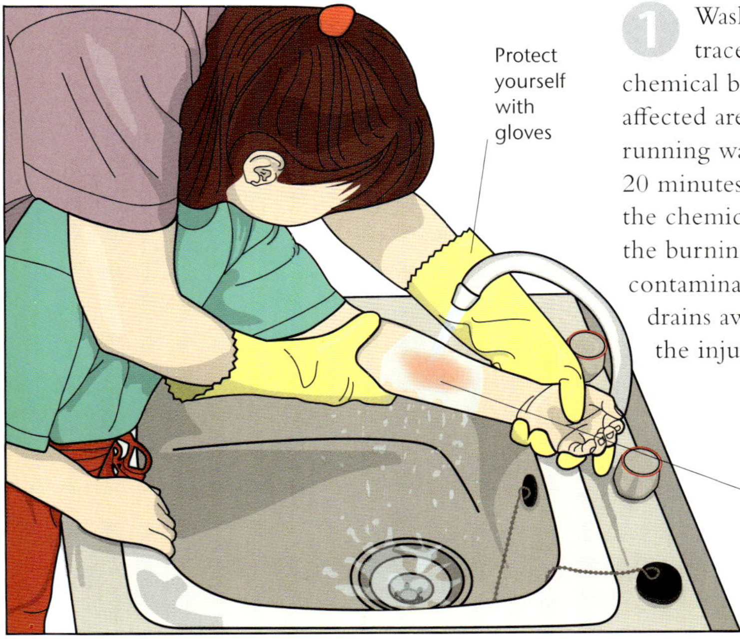

1 Wash away all traces of the chemical by holding the affected area under cool running water for at least 20 minutes to remove the chemicals and stop the burning. Make sure contaminated water drains away from the injury.

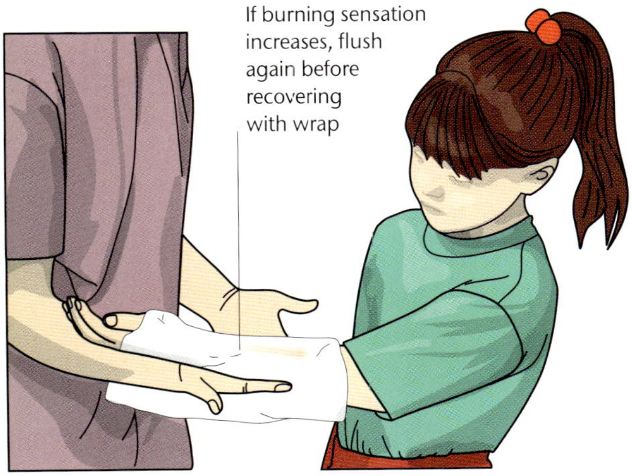

2 Once the burn is cooled, it can be covered very lightly with a nonadhesive dressing or plastic wrap, which will protect from infection and prevent it from drying out.

TAKE YOUR CHILD TO THE HOSPITAL

OR

CALL 911 OR YOUR LOCAL EMS

IMPORTANT

- **Call** your provincial Poison Control Centre for guidance.
- **Note** the name of the substance that caused the burn and give the information to the hospital staff.
- **Always** wear protective gloves when treating your child, and beware of chemical fumes.
- **If** plastic wrap is not available, a clean, nonfluffy material can be laid over the burn to protect from infection.

see also

- Chemical burn to eye, *p.56*
- Fume inhalation, *p.33*
- Swallowed chemicals, *p.57*

Chemical burn to eye

Splashes of chemicals in the eye can cause scarring or even blindness. Your child may have a chemical burn if he complains of fierce pain in the eye; he has difficulty opening the affected eye; the surface of the eye is watery; or there is redness and swelling in and around the eye.

IMPORTANT

- **Do not** let your child touch his eye. The eye will be shut in spasm and pain, so gently pull the eyelids open.

Using pitcher of water

If you can't hold your child under a faucet, you may find it easier to use a pitcher to pour water over the affected eye. Get a helper to support your child with her head tilted down and to one side. Do not splash the unaffected eye with the contaminated water.

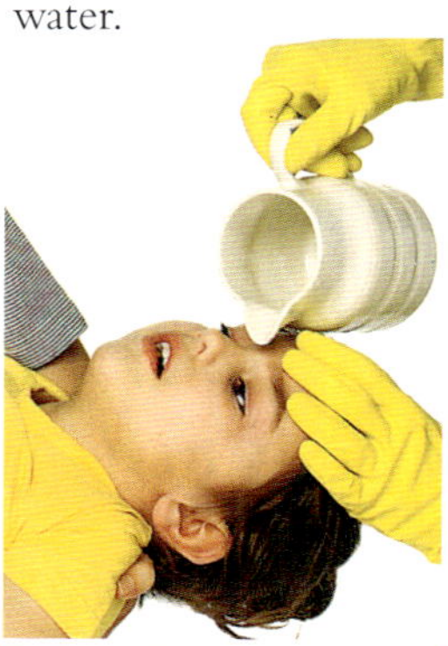

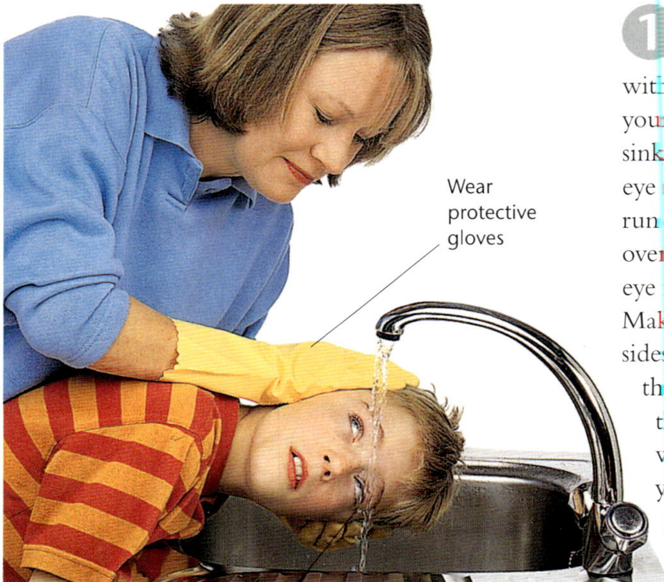

Wear protective gloves

Rinse eye with cold water for 10 minutes

1 Protect yourself from the chemical with rubber gloves. Hold your child's head over a sink, with the unaffected eye uppermost. Gently run cool or tepid water over the contaminated eye for at least 10 minutes. Make sure that both sides of the eyelid are thoroughly washed and that the contaminated water drains away from your child's face.

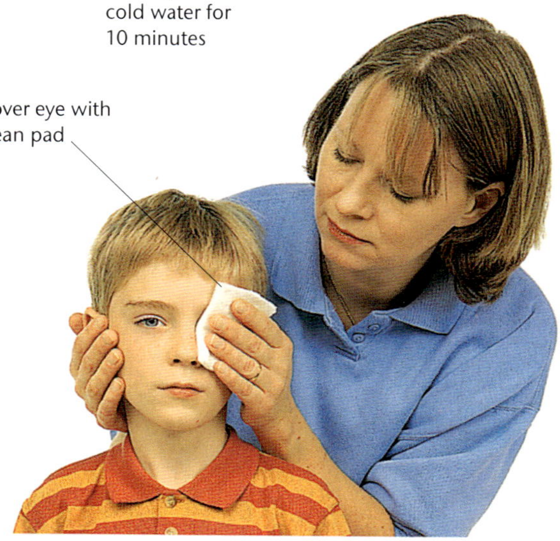

Cover eye with clean pad

2 Once the injured eye is thoroughly washed, cover it with a large sterile dressing. Hold the dressing in place until you get medical aid.

TAKE YOUR CHILD TO THE HOSPITAL

OR

CALL 911 OR YOUR LOCAL EMS

Swallowed chemicals

If you think your child has swallowed a poison, try to find out what, when, and how much she has taken. Be aware too that some chemicals also give off dangerous fumes.

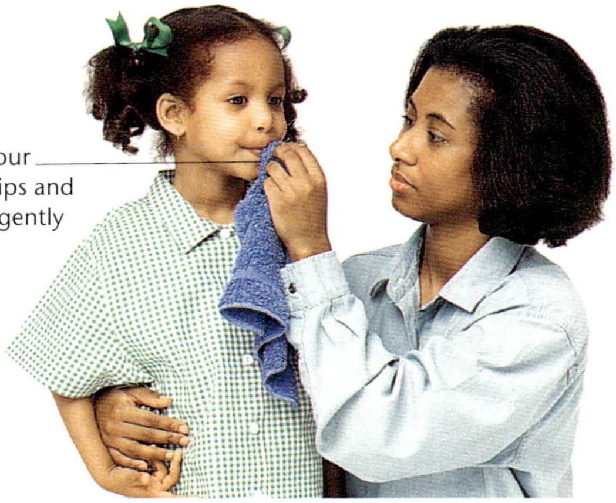
Wash your child's lips and mouth gently

1. Wipe away any residual chemical from around your child's mouth and face.

CALL THE POISON CONTROL CENTRE

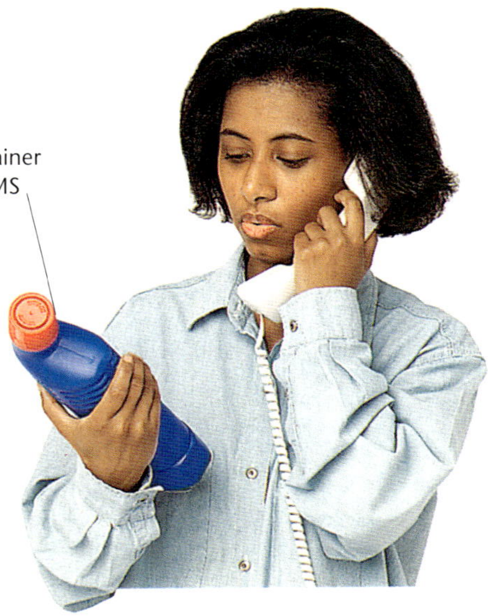
Keep container to show EMS

2. Find out what chemical your child swallowed, when, and if possible how much, then call your provincial Poison Control Centre for guidance on appropriate treatment.

IMPORTANT

- **Do not** try to make your child vomit because this can cause further harm.
- **Do not** give your child anything to drink, unless recommended to do so by your provincial Poison Control Centre.
- **If** your child becomes unresponsive, open her airway and check for breathing. If breathing, put her in the recovery position. If not breathing, begin CPR immediately. CALL 911.
- **If** you need to give rescue breaths and there are chemicals on the child's mouth, protect yourself by using a face shield or pocket mask.

see also

- Chemical burn to eye, *opposite*
- Fume inhalation, *p.33*
- Unresponsive baby, *pp.19–21*
- Unresponsive child, *pp.22–27*

> **IMPORTANT**
> - **Do not** make your child throw up because it can cause more harm.
> - **Even** a small amount of alcohol may harm a young child.
> - **If** your child becomes unresponsive and is not breathing normally, begin CPR immediately with 30 chest compressions.
>
> CALL 911 OR YOUR LOCAL EMS.

see also
- Unresponsive baby, *pp.19–21*
- Unresponsive child, *pp.22–27*

Drug or alcohol poisoning

If your child has taken medication, the container may be nearby. If he drank alcohol, there may be a smell of alcohol and he may be staggering and throw up. He may also have a flushed and moist face; slurred speech; deep, noisy breathing; and a pounding pulse.

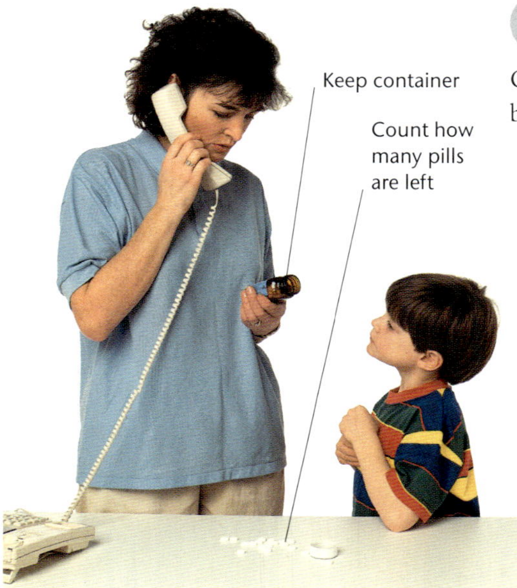

1. Try to find out what he has taken, when, and how much. Check the label on the medicine bottle.

CALL THE POISON CONTROL CENTRE

IF UNRESPONSIVE, CALL 911

2. If he drank alcohol, let your child rest where you can watch him while waiting for help to arrive. Give him a bowl in case he throws up. If he falls asleep, try to wake him to make sure he can be easily roused.

> **IMPORTANT**
> - **Do not** make your child vomit. This can cause further harm.

Plant poisoning

Many plants are poisonous in large quantities. Small pieces or one or two berries are unlikely to be fatal but can cause stomach upset.

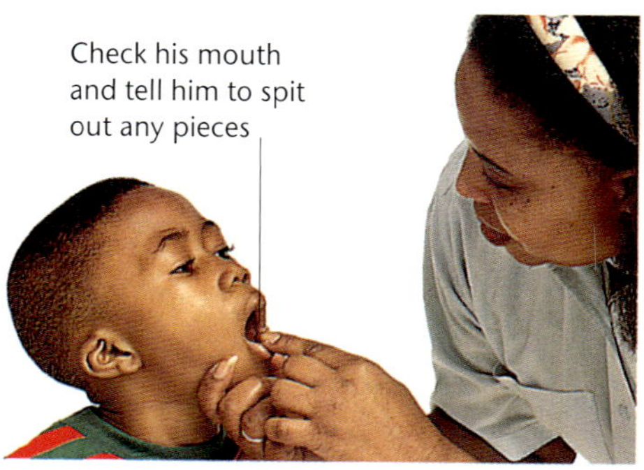

1. Try to find out what your child ate, when, and how much—keep a sample of the plant.

CALL THE POISON CONTROL CENTRE

2. Look inside your child's mouth. Pick out any remaining pieces of plant or berries.

Scalp wound

This type of wound can bleed profusely. If the wound was caused by a blow to the child's head, watch for any change in her condition, especially her level of response, while waiting for emergency help.

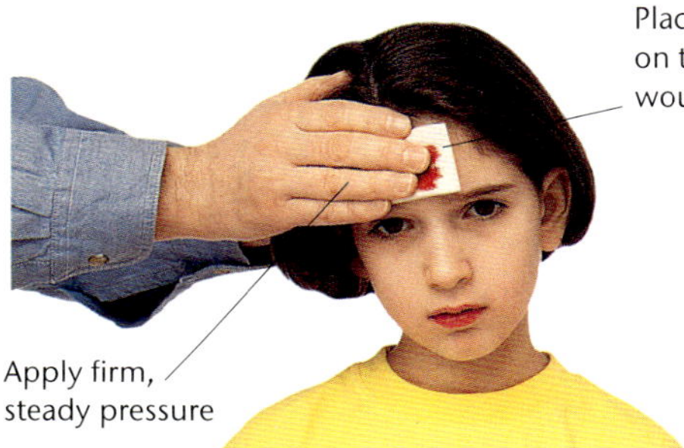

1. Cover the injury with a clean pad or sterile dressing that is larger than the wound. Press firmly on the pad and the wound to control the bleeding. Place another pad on top, if necessary, and keep pressing on the wound.

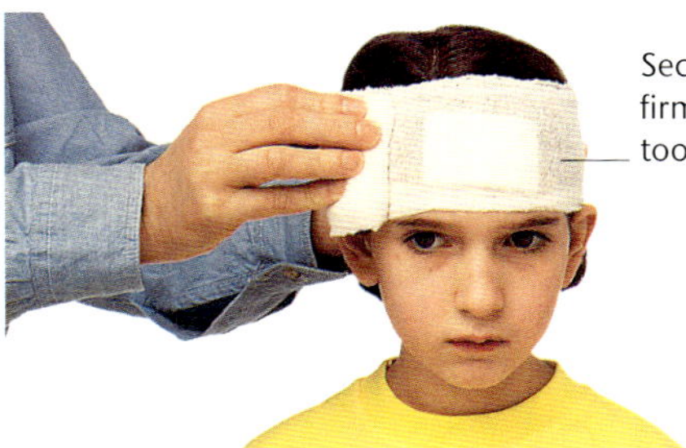

2. Bandage the dressing firmly in place. If the bleeding continues, apply pressure again with your hand.

3. Help your child lie down with her head and shoulders slightly raised.

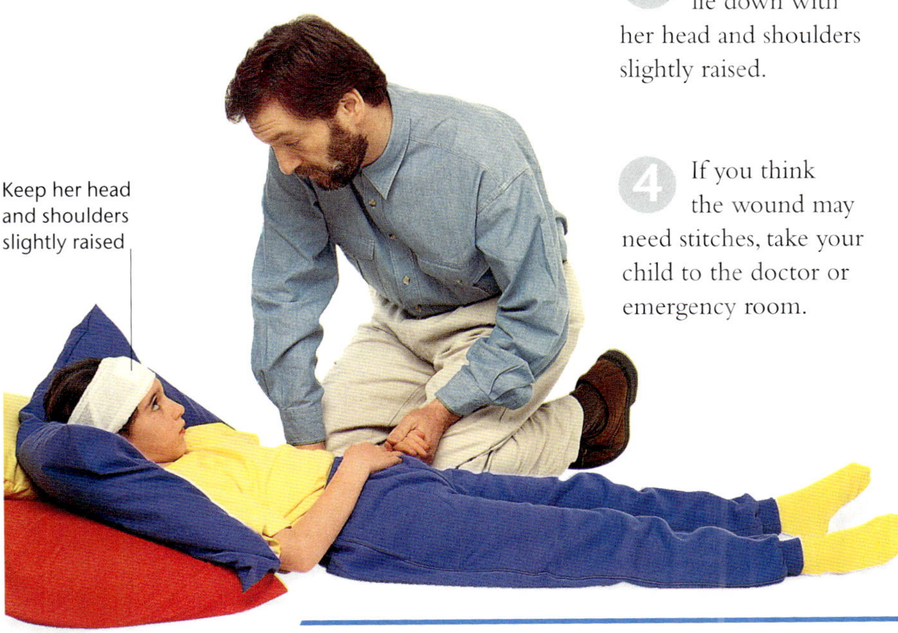

4. If you think the wound may need stitches, take your child to the doctor or emergency room.

IMPORTANT

- **If** blood continues to seep through the first and second dressings, add another and apply more pressure to stop the bleeding.
- **If** the bleeding is massive, uncontrollable, or there is a chance of brain injury, **call 911 or your local EMS.**
- **If** your child becomes unresponsive and is not breathing normally, begin CPR immediately with 30 chest compressions.
CALL 911 OR YOUR LOCAL EMS.

see also

- Head injury, *p.60*
- Severe bleeding, *p.38*
- Shock, *p.36*
- Unresponsive baby, *pp.19–21*
- Unresponsive child, *pp.22–27*

IMPORTANT

- **Never** shake a baby or child to assess her reactions.
- **If** a head injury occurs during an athletic activity, do not allow your child to continue to play until she has been assessed by a healthcare professional.

Signs of worsening head injury

Seek urgent medical advice if after a head injury you notice any of the following:

- She becomes disoriented and/or increasingly drowsy;
- She complains of vision problems;
- She is vomiting;
- She complains of a persistent or worsening headache;
- She is confused, with loss of memory, dizziness;
- She has difficulty speaking and/or walking and problems with balance;
- She suffers a seizure;
- She is unable to stop crying or be consoled.

Head injury

If your child has a minor bump to the head, she may simply have a bruise with no other sign of injury. If, however, the child has suffered a more serious blow, the brain can be shaken inside the skull and she may be dazed or temporarily unresponsive—this is concussion. Your child may have a headache, feel dizzy, complain of nausea, and may not remember what happened.

If there has been a severe blow to the head, there may be bleeding or swelling within the skull that can press on the brain, which is a serious condition. A child may seem unaffected at first, but as time goes by (minutes, hours, or even days) her condition can worsen, and so it is very important to watch her and monitor her condition looking for signs of a worsening head injury (*see box, left*).

1 If the child is dazed, help her lie down on the floor (protect her from the cold). Don't sit her on a chair because she may fall off and hurt herself.

2 If your child was "knocked out," even briefly,

SEEK MEDICAL ADVICE

3 Make her rest and watch her closely. Check her for signs of a worsening head injury (*left*), reassure her, and stay with her. If she does not recover completely or shows any sign of deterioration,

CALL 911 OR YOUR LOCAL EMS

4 You can apply a cold pack (*see p.108*) to the injury for up to 20 minutes at a time.

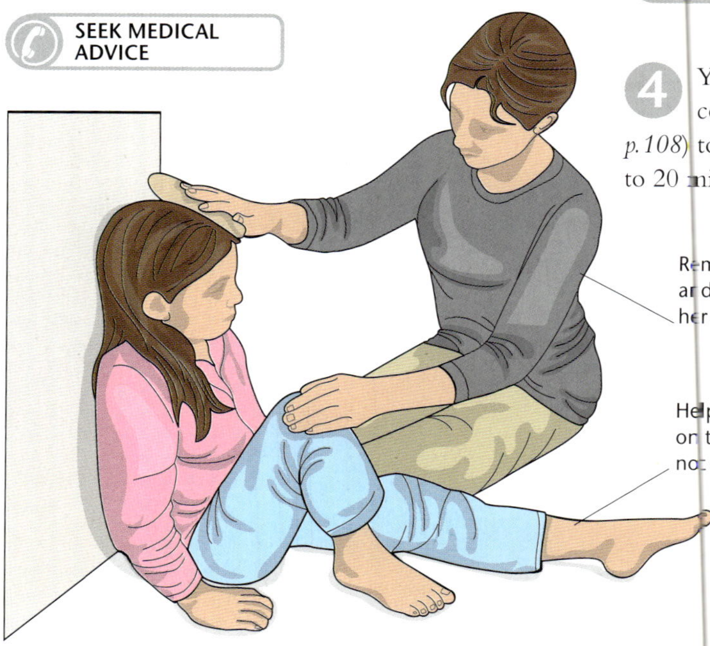

Checking a child's level of response

Your child could be awake following an injury, completely unresponsive, or somewhere between the two. She may deteriorate over minutes, hours, or even days. It is important to assess her condition and monitor any changes so that you can tell the emergency personnel or hospital staff.

- Is she alert? Are her eyes open and does she respond normally when you talk to her?
- Does she only respond to voice by answering simple questions or obeying instructions? Does she open her eyes?
- Does she respond only to pain, for example, by opening her eyes if you flick her foot or tap her shoulder?
- Is she completely unresponsive?

Note any response or change of response, and the time.

IMPORTANT

- **Suspect** skull fracture if the level of response is impaired, there is blood or watery fluid coming from the nose or ear; there is a soft area on the scalp; and/or distortion of the face or head.
- **Remember**, there's a possibility of a spinal injury with any head injury.
- **If** you suspect a neck injury, support the head and neck (*see p.63*).

If your child becomes unresponsive

Do not move your child because there could be an associated back or neck injury, and moving her could result in damage to the brain or spinal cord.

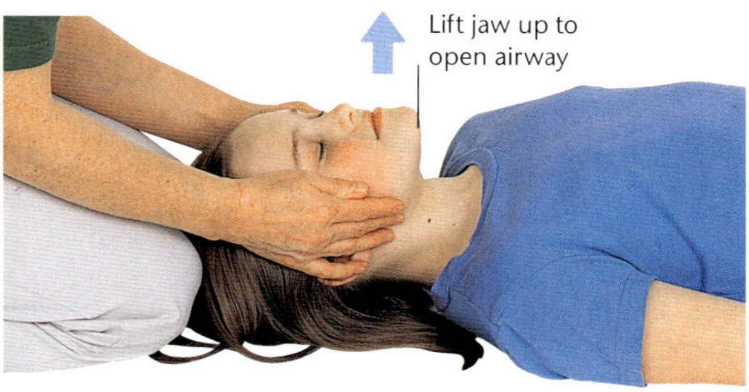

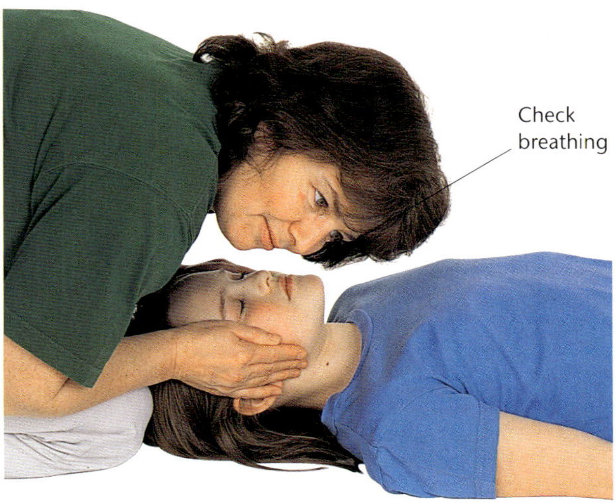

1. Kneel behind her head and rest your elbows on the ground or your knees. Open her airway using the **jaw thrust method**: place one hand on either side of her face, with your fingertips on the angles of her jaw. Gently lift the jaw up to open the airway (don't tilt her head back).

2. Check her breathing. If she is breathing, continue to support her jaw to keep the airway open. If she is not breathing, begin CPR immediately. Ask someone else to call 911.

CALL 911 OR YOUR LOCAL EMS

see also

- Checking vital signs, *p.14*
- Cold packs, *p.108*
- Scalp wound, *p.59*
- Spine injury, *p.63*
- Unresponsive baby, *pp.19–21*
- Unresponsive child, *pp.22–27*

IMPORTANT

- **If** pinching her nose hurts too much, simply ask her to sit forward over the bowl and give her a soft pad or towel to soak up the blood.

Nose or cheekbone injury

The main risk with fractures to the nose or cheekbones is that the swelling can affect the air passages, causing breathing problems. There may also be bleeding from the child's nose or mouth.

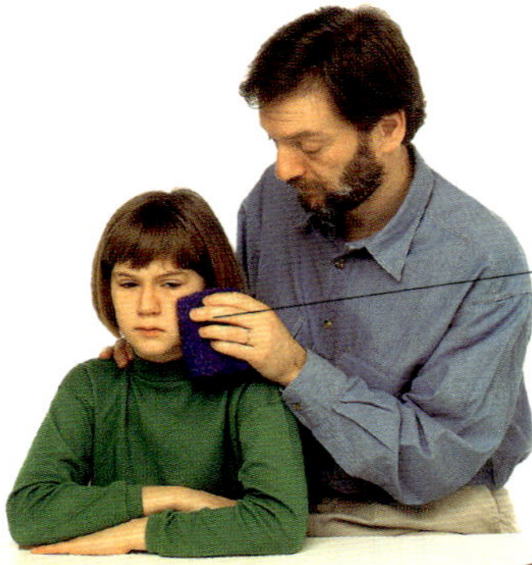

Apply cold compress to injury

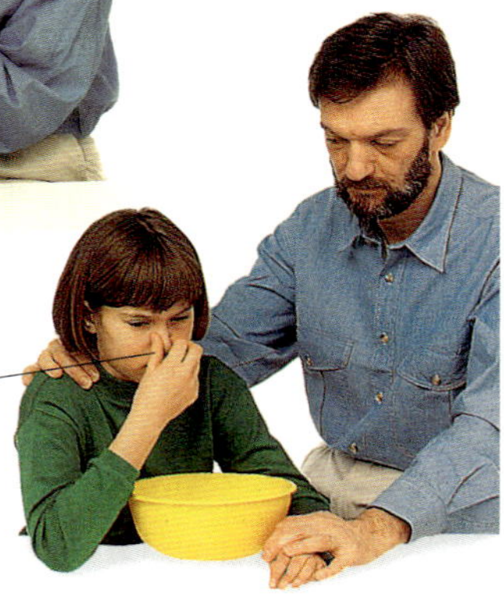

Pinch nostrils together to stop bleeding

1 Help your child sit down and apply a cold pack (see *p.108*) to the injured area to help minimize the swelling. Hold the cold pack in place for about 20 minutes.

2 If your child's nose is bleeding, ask her to sit with her head well forward and to pinch the fleshy part of her nose to help control bleeding. If any bones are broken,

TAKE YOUR CHILD TO THE HOSPITAL

see also

- Nosebleed, *p.45*
- Unresponsive baby, *pp.19–21*
- Unresponsive child, *pp.22–27*

IMPORTANT

- **If** your child becomes unresponsive and is not breathing normally, begin CPR immediately with 30 chest compressions. CALL 911 OR YOUR LOCAL EMS.

Jaw injury

A broken jaw will be tender and swollen, with loss of normal mobility. Her teeth may be out of line.

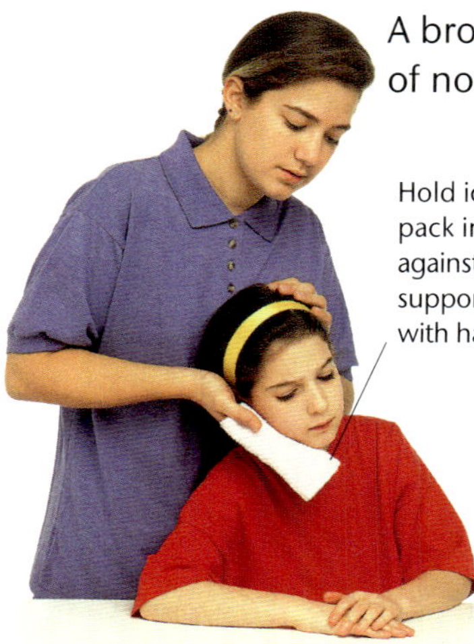

Hold ice pack in cloth against jaw; support jaw with hand

1 Help your child to sit with head well forward. Tell her to spit out any loose teeth and not to swallow any blood or saliva.

2 Hold an icepack gently under her injured jaw, and support it in this position until you get to the hospital. Do not bandage the pad in place in case she vomits.

TAKE YOUR CHILD TO THE HOSPITAL

see also

- Unresponsive baby, *pp.19–21*
- Unresponsive child, *p.22–27*

Spine injury

If a child lands on his neck or back in a fall or falls awkwardly and complains of back pain or tingling in any part of his body, suspect spine injury. Support him in the position found to prevent further damage.

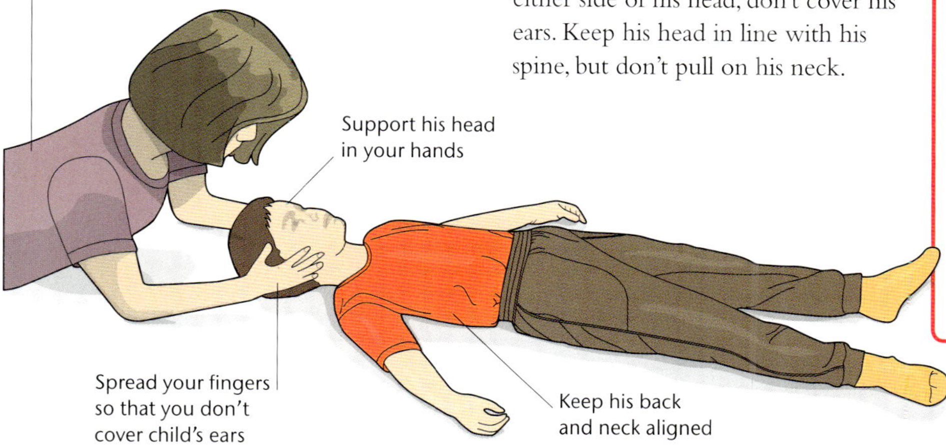

1 Reassure your child and tell him not to move. Lie behind his head, rest your elbows on the ground, and place your hands on either side of his head; don't cover his ears. Keep his head in line with his spine, but don't pull on his neck.

CALL 911 OR YOUR LOCAL EMS

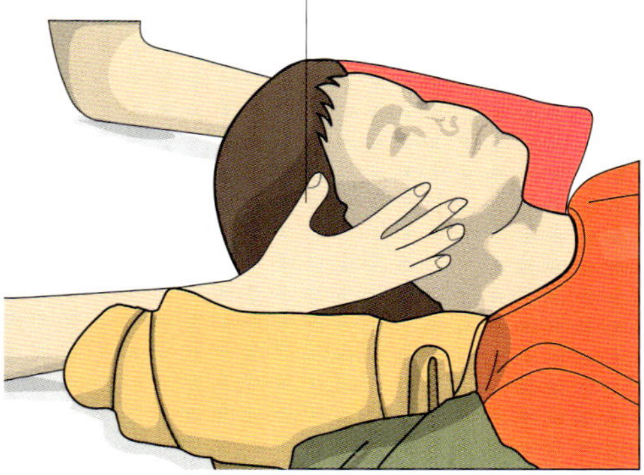

2 Keep his head and neck supported in the same position until help arrives. Ask someone to put rolled blankets or towels around his neck and shoulders for extra support.

3 Continue to keep his head steady. Monitor breathing, pulse, and level of response while waiting for help to arrive, and perform CPR if needed.

IMPORTANT

- **Do not** move the injured child from the position in which you find him unless his life is in danger.
- **If** you do have to move him, take care not to twist or bend the neck or spine.
- **If** your child becomes unresponsive, open airway using the jaw thrust technique *(p.61)* and check breathing. If breathing, maintain jaw thrust and keep the head, neck, and spine aligned; if not, begin CPR immediately, with 30 compressions. CALL 911 OR YOUR LOCAL EMS.

see also

- Checking vital signs, *p.14*
- Head injury, *p.60*
- Unresponsive baby, *pp.19–21*
- Unresponsive child, *pp.22–27*

Pelvic injury

IMPORTANT

- **Do not** move the child.
- **Do not** bandage if it causes pain.
- **If** you see signs of shock or bleeding but no visible wound, treat for shock but do not raise her legs.
- **Do not** give the child anything to eat or drink because an anesthetic may be needed.

see also

- Shock, *p.36*

If your child has a broken pelvis, she will be unable to stand, have pain around the hip and groin, and possible bleeding from the urinary orifice.

CALL 911 OR YOUR LOCAL EMS

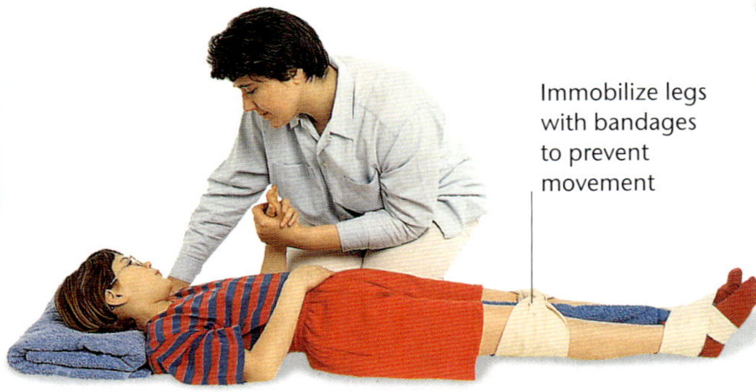

Pad between child's legs and immobilize them with a figure-eight bandage around feet and ankles and a broad-fold bandage around both knees (*see opposite*). Monitor her while you wait, *see p.14*.

Leg injury

IMPORTANT

- **If** there is a wound, treat bleeding and cover with a sterile dressing.
- **Do not** attempt to straighten the injured leg.
- **Do not** give the child anything to eat or drink because an anesthetic may be needed.

see also

- Severe bleeding, *p.38*
- Shock, *p.36*
- Check circulation, *p.105*

Suspect a break if your child is in severe pain. He needs an X-ray or scan to confirm whether or not a bone is broken. Treat the leg in the position found to prevent broken bone ends causing further internal injury.

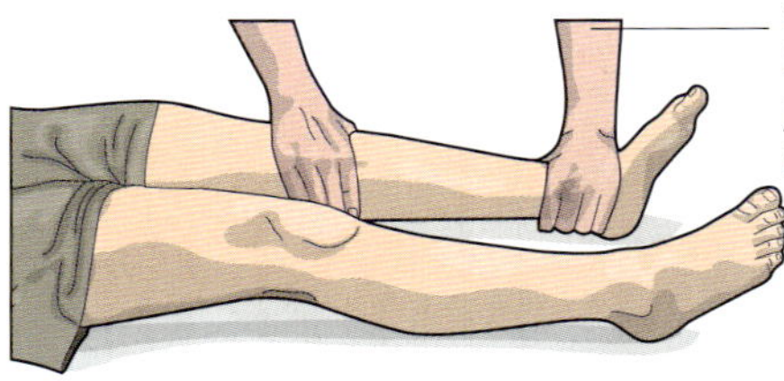

1 Make your child comfortable and keep him still. Keep his leg in the position you found it by supporting the ankle and knee joints.

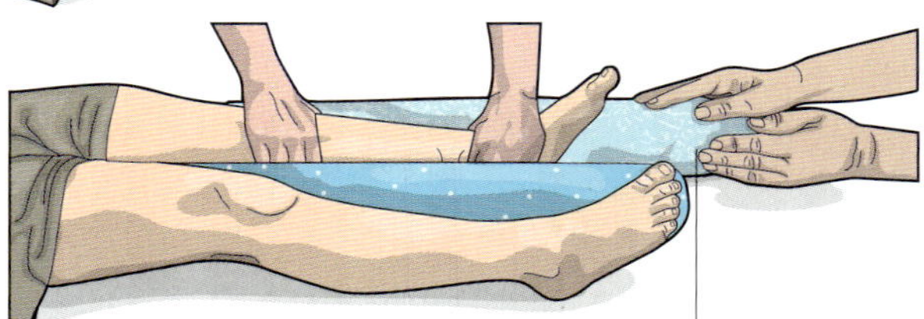

2 Support the joints until help arrives. Ask a helper to place padding along the outer side of the limb and between the legs. Cover your child with another blanket to keep him warm. If you suspect shock, raise only the *uninjured* leg.

CALL 911 OR YOUR LOCAL EMS

How to splint an injured leg

If you are going to have to wait for help, you can splint the injured leg for extra support.

1. Maintain support at the joints. Ask a helper to place padding such as a rolled-up towel or small blanket between the thighs, knees, and ankles. Bring the *uninjured* leg to the broken one.

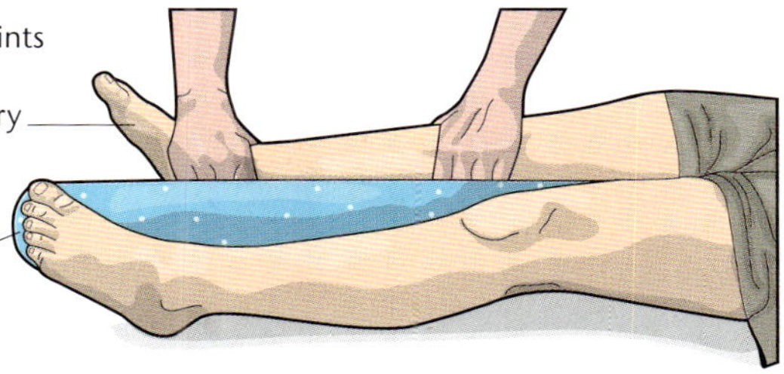

2. Slide bandages through the hollows under the legs. Place a narrow-fold bandage at the ankle and broad-fold bandages under the knees and below the fracture. Secure the bandage at the ankles first.

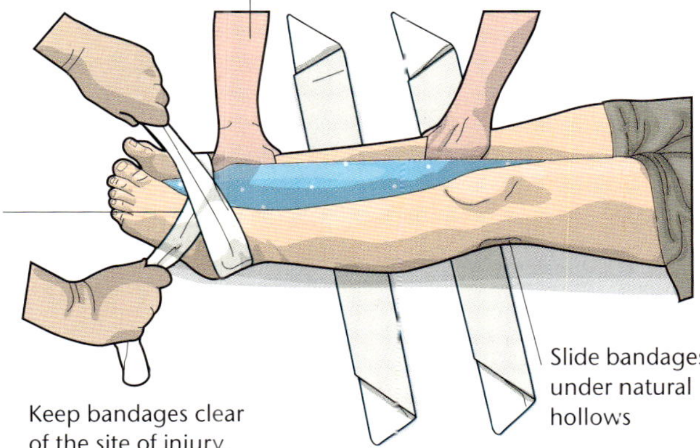

3. Secure the broad-fold bandages at the knee then below the injury site, and above if there is room. Tie all knots against the *uninjured* leg. Check circulation to ensure bandages are not too tight (*see p. 105*).

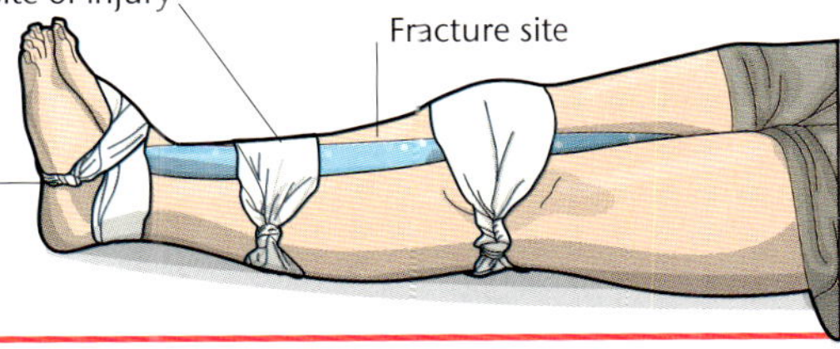

Making broad-fold and narrow-fold bandages

1.

Take a triangular bandage

2.

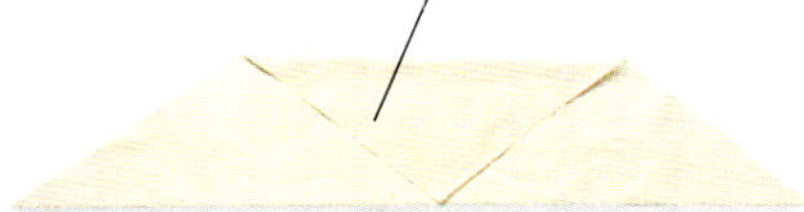
Fold top point over to touch the base

3.

Fold bandage in half to make a broad-fold bandage

Broad-fold bandage

4.

Fold bandage in half again to make a narrow-fold bandage

Narrow-fold bandage

IMPORTANT

- Follow the RICE procedure:

R Rest injured part.

I Place **ice** on the injury (**do not** place ice directly on skin).

C Provide **compression** by bandaging the area lightly.

E Elevate injured part.

- If you suspect a major injury, take your child to the hospital in the treatment position. CALL 911.

see also
- Cold packs, *p.108*
- Leg injury, *p.64*

Knee injury

This type of injury can be very painful, and your child may not be able to move it. The area around the knee joint can swell very quickly.

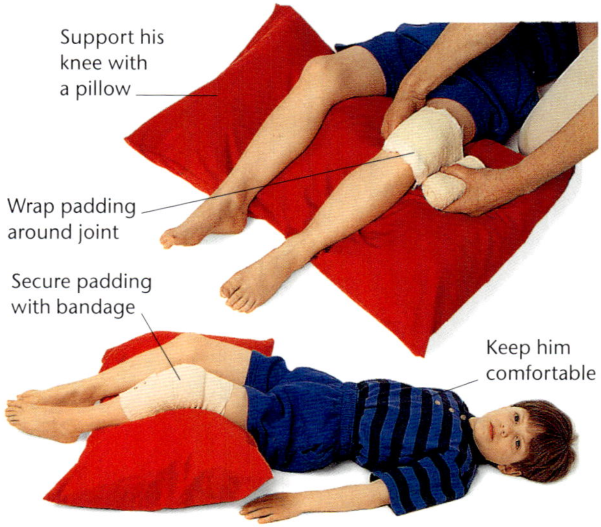

1. Reassure your child and help him lie down. Place a pillow under his legs to support them in the most comfortable position. Place a cold pack on the knee. Then wrap a layer of soft padding around it.

2. Secure the padding with a bandage.

SEEK MEDICAL ADVICE

IMPORTANT

- Follow the RICE procedure:

R Rest injured part.

I Place **ice** on the injury (**do not** place ice directly on skin).

C Provide **compression** by bandaging the area lightly.

E Elevate injured part.

see also
- Cold packs, *p.108*
- Leg injury, *p.64*

Foot injury

Your child's foot may be bruised, swollen, and stiff and she may not be able to stand. If caused by crushing, one or more bones may be broken.

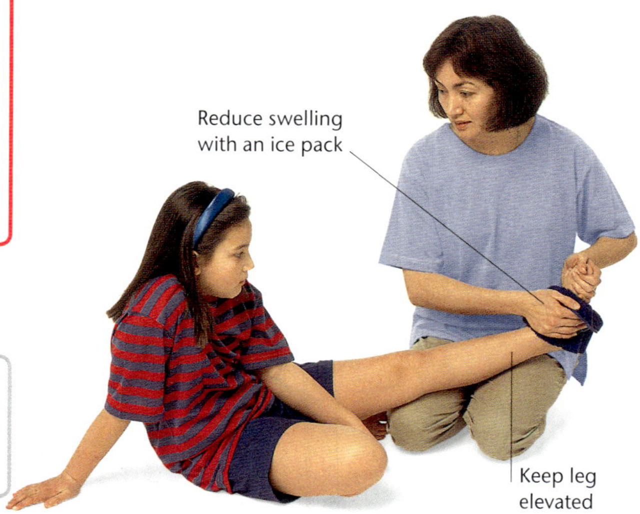

1. Sit the child down to rest the injury.

2. Place a cold pack on the injury, then provide compression by bandaging it lightly.

3. Elevate the injury to reduce bruising, pain, and swelling.

SEEK MEDICAL ADVICE

Ankle injury

The most common injury is a sprain. Suspect a sprain if your child can't take her full weight on her foot after a fall, or she has twisted, or wrenched, her ankle. She may need an X-ray or scan.

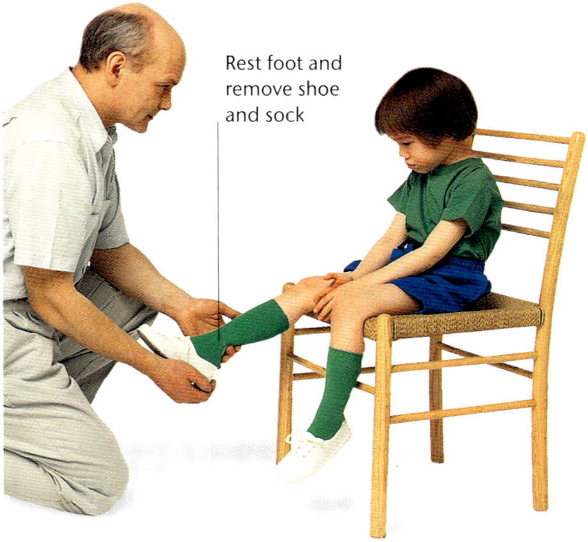

1 Help your child sit down to rest her foot. Gently remove her shoe and sock before the injured area swells.

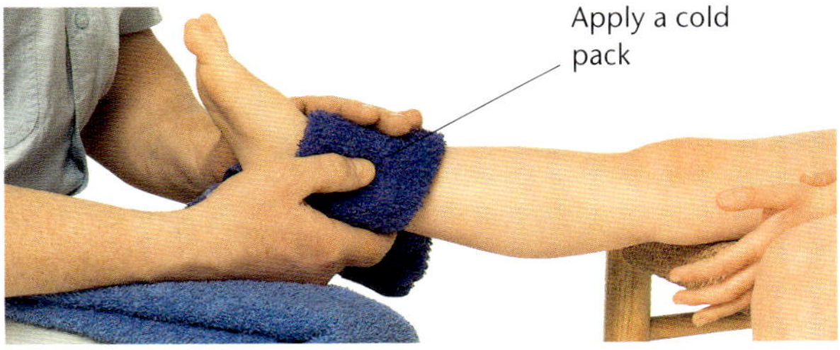

2 Place a cold pack on the injury to minimize swelling.

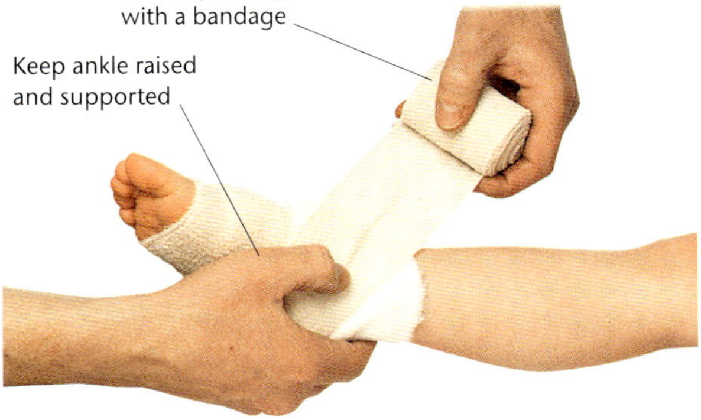

3 Provide compression: wrap a thick layer of soft padding such as cotton around the ankle and secure it with a bandage. Make sure that the bandage is not too tight.

SEEK MEDICAL ADVICE

4 Elevate the injury to help reduce bruising, pain, and swelling.

IMPORTANT

- **If** the pain is very severe or you think a bone could be broken, wrap the ankle as shown below and TAKE YOUR CHILD TO THE HOSPITAL or CALL 911.
- Follow the RICE procedure:

R Rest injured part.

I Place **ice** on the injury (**do not** place ice directly on skin).

C Apply **compression** by loosely bandaging the injured part.

E Elevate injured part.

see also

- Check circulation, *p.105*
- Cold packs, *p.108*
- Leg injury, *p.64*

IMPORTANT

- **If** putting a sling on the child causes further pain, stop and support the affected arm by hand instead.

Collarbone injury

A collarbone may be broken by indirect force, for example, if a child falls onto her outstretched hand, or by a blow to her shoulder. There will be tenderness in your child's shoulder and arm—increased by attempts to move it—and her head may be turned and inclined to the injured side.

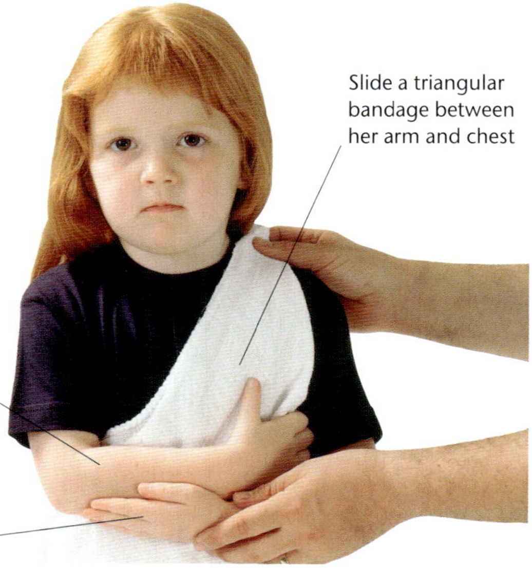

1 Help your child sit down and gently bring the arm on the injured side across her chest. Ask her to support her arm with her hand. Slide a triangular bandage between the child's arm and her chest, with the point of the bandage extending past her elbow.

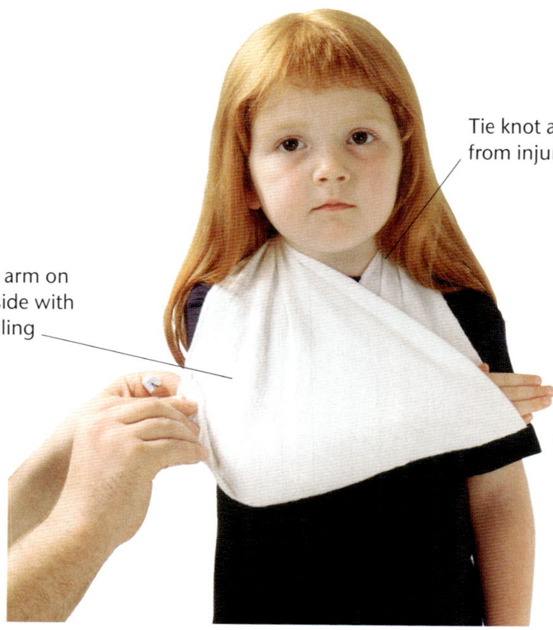

2 Support your child's arm in an arm sling to minimize swelling and discomfort. Make sure the knot is not over the site of injury.

3 For additional immobilization and comfort you can place soft padding between the arm and the sling, then tie a broad-fold bandage around the arm and body.

TAKE YOUR CHILD TO THE HOSPITAL

see also

- Triangular bandages, *p.106*

Rib injury

A child may have a broken rib following a blow to her chest, a heavy fall, or having been crushed. Symptoms include sharp pain at the fracture site, bruising, swelling, or possible wound on the injured side, and pain when breathing.

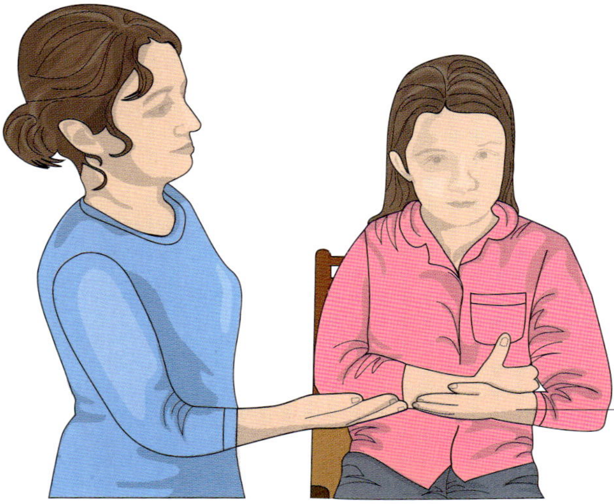

1 Help your child sit down and gently bring the arm on the injured side across her chest. Ask her to support her arm with her hand; you may need to help her.

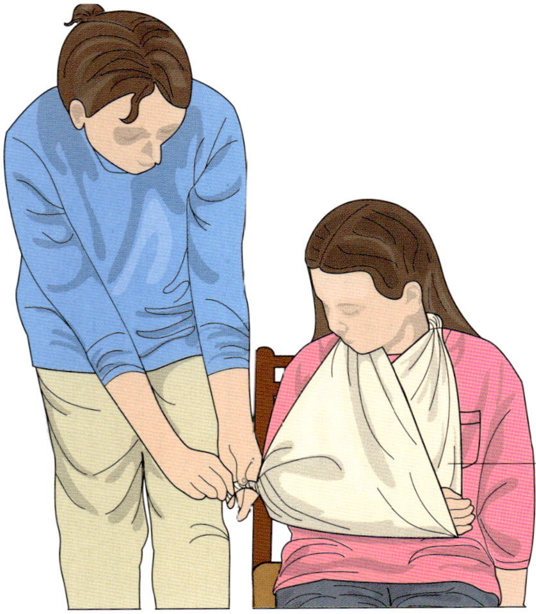

2 Support the arm on the injured side in an arm sling to minimize discomfort.

TAKE YOUR CHILD TO THE HOSPITAL

IMPORTANT

- **Do not** give the child anything to eat or drink because an anesthetic may be needed.
- **If** your child develops breathing difficulties, signs of internal bleeding, or shock, CALL 911 OR YOUR LOCAL EMS.
- **If** your child becomes unresponsive and has abnormal breathing, begin CPR immediately with 30 compressions. CALL 911 OR YOUR LOCAL EMS.

see also

- Chest wound, *p.50*
- Internal bleeding, *p.49*
- Shock, *p.36*
- Triangular bandages, *p.106*
- Unresponsive child, *pp.22–27*

Arm injury

The treatment here is for injuries to the upper arm, forearm, and wrist. Move the arm as little as possible to minimize pain.

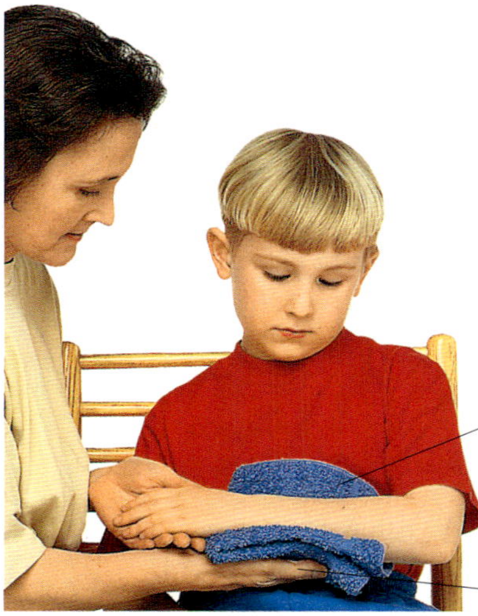

1 Help your child sit down. Support the arm and encourage him to help. Place a soft pad around the injury and between his arm and his chest.

2 For extra support place the arm in a sling and knot it on the uninjured side.

SEEK MEDICAL ADVICE

IMPORTANT

- **Do not** give the child anything to eat or drink because he may need an anesthetic.
- **If** the child cannot bend his arm treat as for elbow injury below.
- **Ice** or a cold compress may be applied to reduce swelling.

see also

- Collarbone injury, p.68

Elbow injury

Suspect an elbow injury if your child is unable to bend her arm, pain is increased by any attempts at movement, or there is swelling around the elbow. Keep the injury still because bone ends can damage blood vessels.

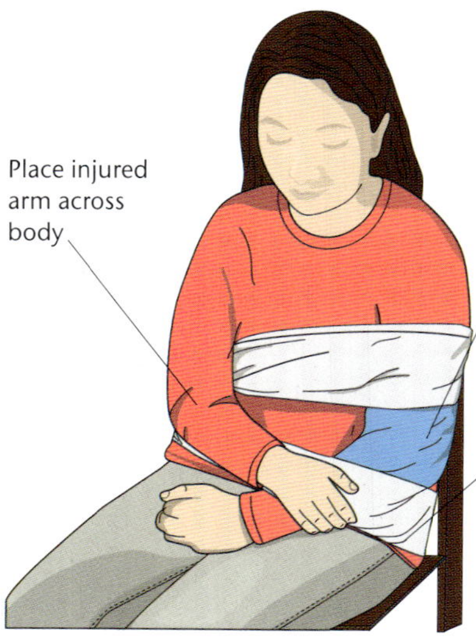

1 Help the child sit down, holding her arm across her body. Pad around the injury.

2 Apply broad-fold bandages around the body and arm above and below the elbow. Check circulation at the wrist regularly.

SEEK MEDICAL ADVICE

IMPORTANT

- **Do not** give the child anything to eat or drink because she may need an anesthetic.
- **Do not** straighten or bend the child's elbow.
- **If** bandaging causes pain, help the child lie down with her arm in a comfortable position across her body. CALL 911 OR YOUR LOCAL EMS.
- **Ice** or a cold compress may be applied to reduce swelling.

see also

- Check circulation, *p.105*
- Triangular bandages, *p.106*

Hand injury

This type of injury can be very painful. There may be several broken bones, and often a joint is dislocated. If your child's hand was crushed, there may also be an open wound.

> **! IMPORTANT**
>
> - **If** there is a wound, control the bleeding by pressing a clean dressing or pad over the site of the wound.

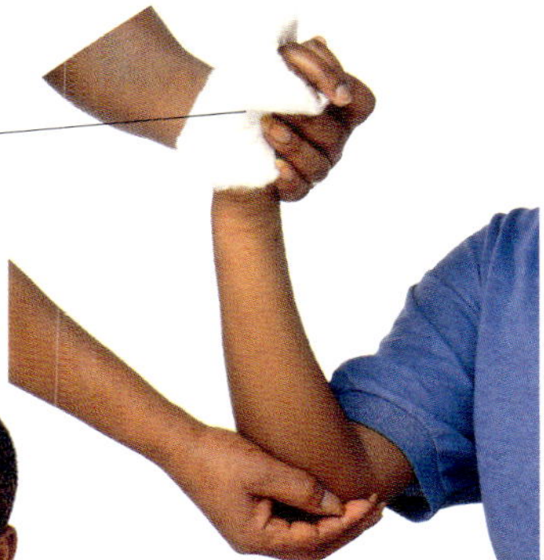

Wrap hand in soft padding

1 If there is no wound, wrap the injured hand in soft padding. Raise your child's hand into a comfortable position.

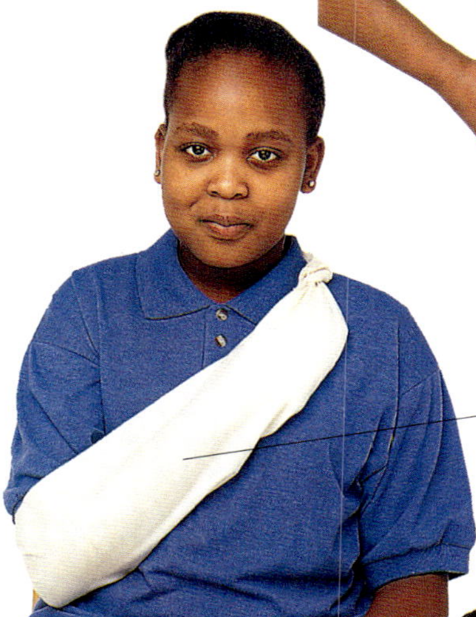

Support hand and arm in elevation sling

2 Place your child's arm in an elevation sling (*see p.107*) to reduce swelling and provide extra comfort on the trip to the hospital.

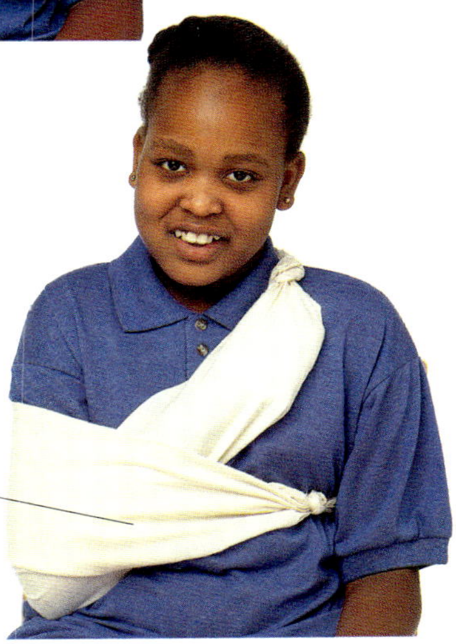

Tie broad-fold bandage around arm and body

3 For extra support, tie a broad-fold bandage (*see p.65*) around the arm and body; secure it with a knot on the uninjured side.

SEEK MEDICAL ADVICE

Jammed fingers

Hold the fingers under cold running water for a few minutes to relieve the pain and minimize swelling. If the fingers still hurt, apply a cold pack for 10 minutes (*see p.108*).

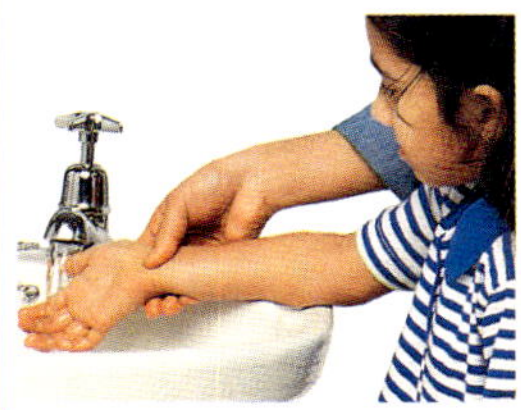

see also

- Crush injury, *p.49*
- Finger injury, *p.72*
- Severe bleeding, *p.38*
- Triangular bandages, *p.106*
- Elevation sling, *p.107*

IMPORTANT

- **If** pain or bleeding is severe, there is missing tissue, or a fingernail is damaged, TAKE YOUR CHILD TO THE HOSPITAL.

Finger injury

Injury to a finger is common in children and can vary from simple cuts or abrasions to broken bones or tendon damage if, for example, the finger is shut in a door. It is important to get the injury checked because there are several blood vessels, tendons, and nerves in the finger that can be damaged, leading to deformity, bruising, and loss of sensation.

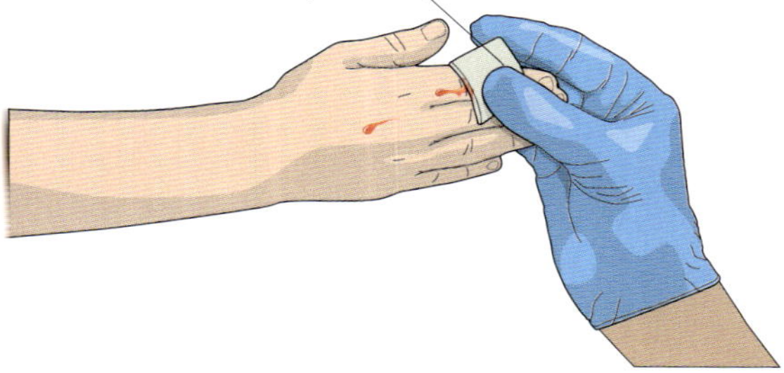

1 Apply direct pressure over a sterile or clean pad to control any bleeding. Stop if this causes pain because there may be an underlying fracture.

2 Raise and support the finger, or ask your child to hold it up, to help relieve the pain and control the bleeding.

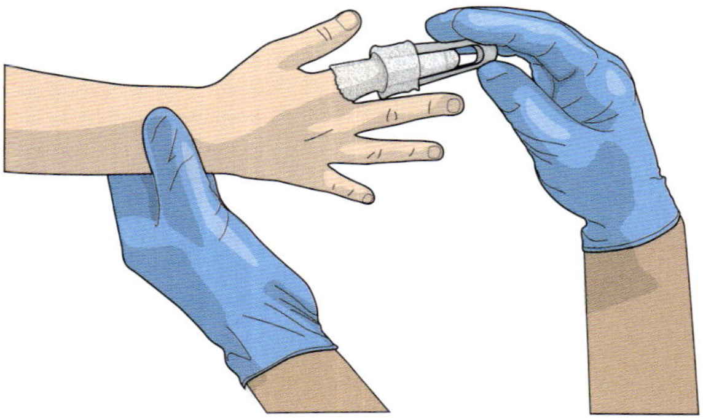

3 Secure the dressing with a bandage—a tube gauze bandage is ideal. For extra comfort, splint the finger to the next uninjured one.

SEEK MEDICAL ADVICE

OR

TAKE YOUR CHILD TO THE HOSPITAL

4 Support the arm in a raised position in an elevation sling (*see p.107*) if it makes your child more comfortable.

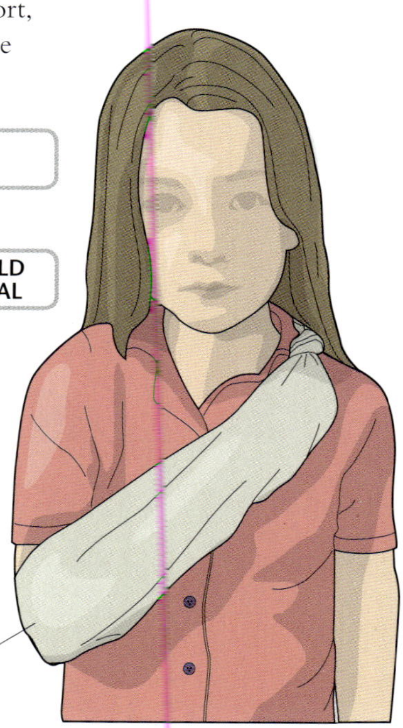

see also

- Amputation, *p.48*
- Crush injury, *p.49*
- Severe bleeding, *p.38*
- Triangular bandages, *p.106*
- Elevation sling, *p.107*

Cramp

This is a painful muscle spasm that often affects the muscles in the foot, calf, or thigh. A cramp can occur after strenuous exercise or as a result of dehydration through excessive sweating. You can relieve the pain by stretching the affected muscles, then massage them to "relax" the spasm. Give your child water to drink to ease dehyration.

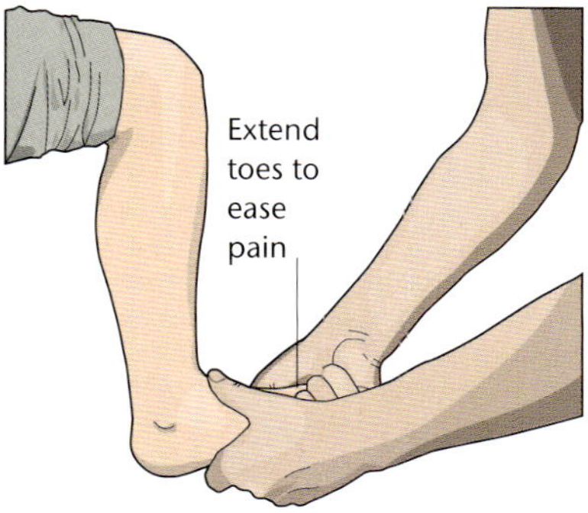

For a cramp in the foot, encourage your child to sit in a chair while you support the affected foot. Extend the toes upward to stretch the muscles. Once the spasm has passed, massage the underside of the foot with your fingers.

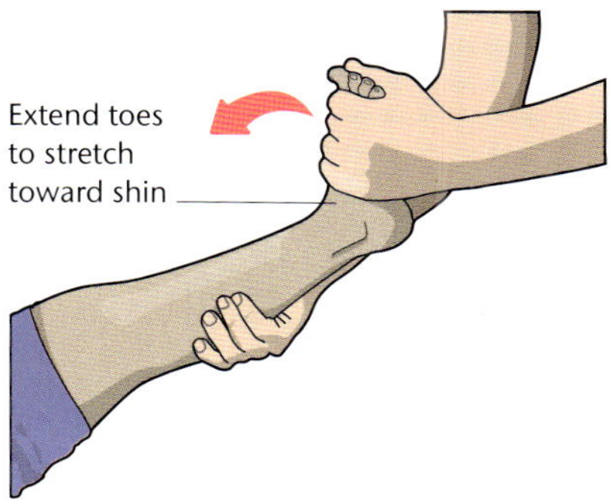

For a cramp in the calf muscles, sit or lay the child down and help her straighten her leg while you support her foot. Extend her foot toward her knee to stretch the calf muscles. Once the spasm has passed, massage the back of her leg to relax the muscles.

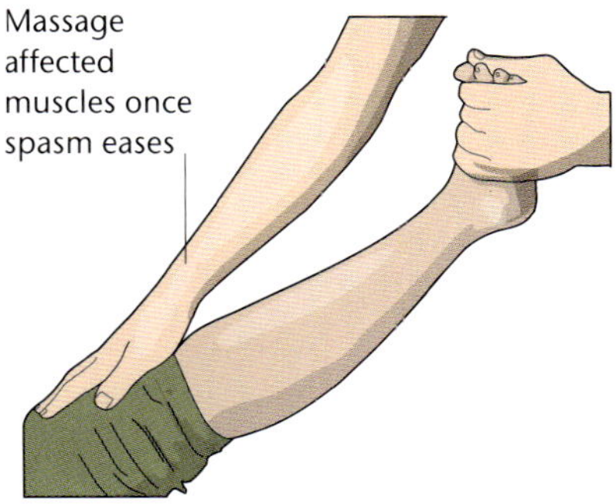

For a cramp in the front of the thigh, help your child lie down, then raise and support her leg. Bend her knee to stretch the muscles. Then, once the spasm has passed, massage the affected muscles.

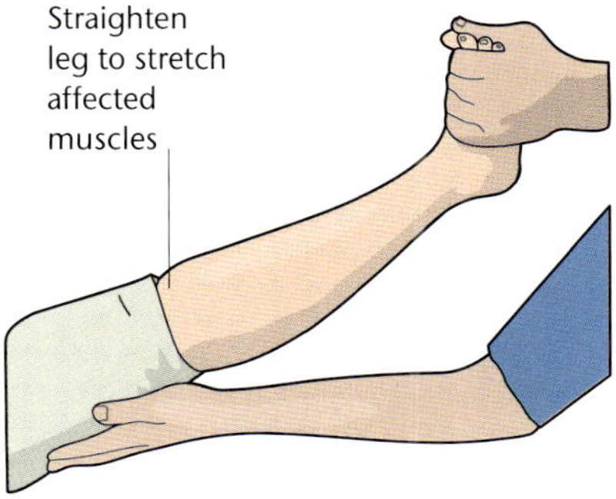

For a cramp in the back of the thigh, raise and support her leg, and straighten her leg to stretch the muscles. Once the spasm has passed, massage the affected muscles.

IMPORTANT

- **If** symptoms don't ease, SEEK MEDICAL ADVICE.

see also

- Heat exhaustion, *p.88*

IMPORTANT

- **If** you think your child has a fractured arm, support it in a sling and take her to a doctor.
- **If** bruising is severe or extensive, SEEK MEDICAL ADVICE.

Cold packs

Applying a cold pack to an injury helps minimize swelling and discomfort by reducing blood flow to the area. Make one by filling a plastic bag two-thirds full of ice and a small amount of water, or use a bag of frozen fruit or vegetables; wrap the bag in a cloth so that the ice does not make direct contact with the skin. You can also use cloth wrung out in cold water (*see p. 108*).

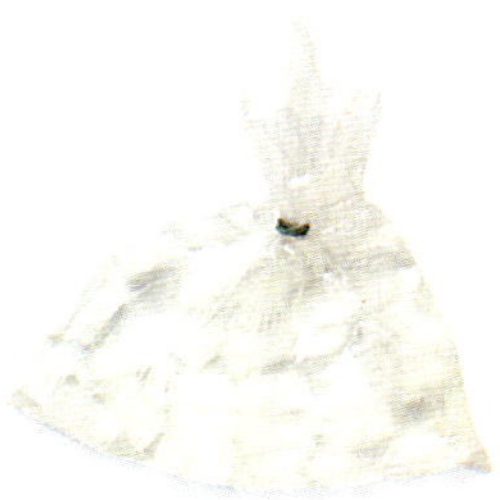

Leave a cold pack in place on an injury for 20 minutes, ideally uncovered.

Bruises and swelling

After a fall or bump, bruising and swelling may develop rapidly. Resting, cooling, and raising the injury will minimize discomfort.

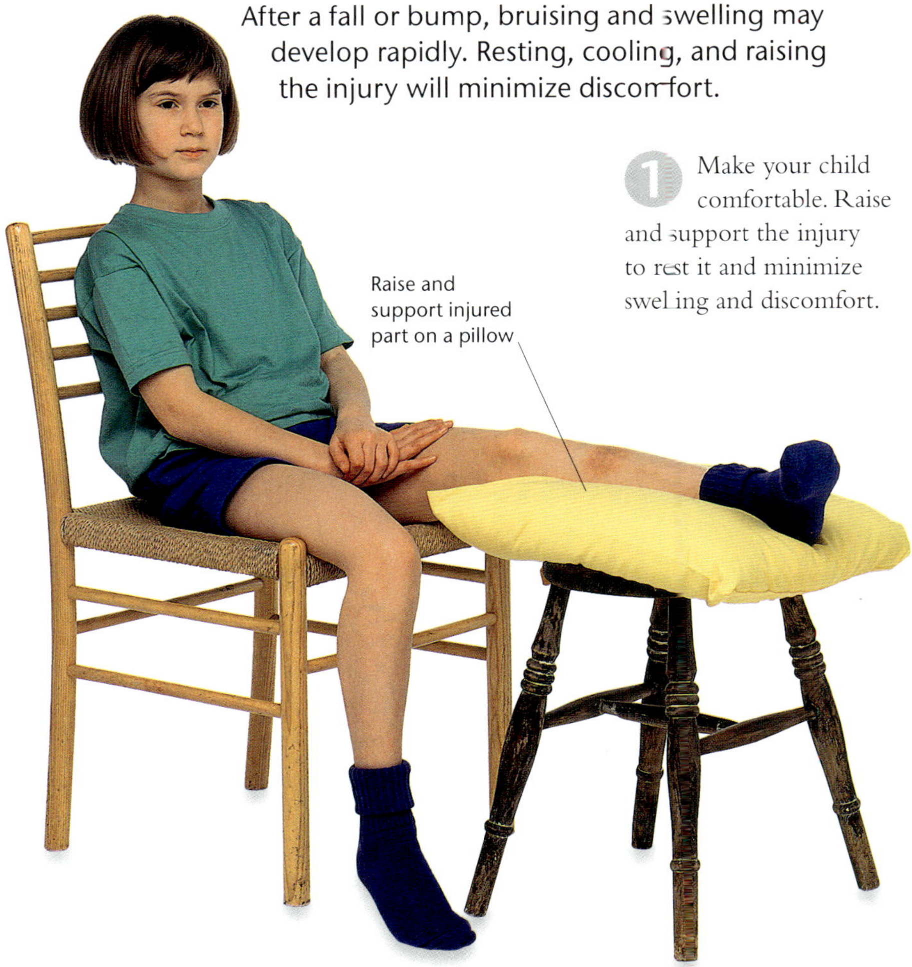

1 Make your child comfortable. Raise and support the injury to rest it and minimize swelling and discomfort.

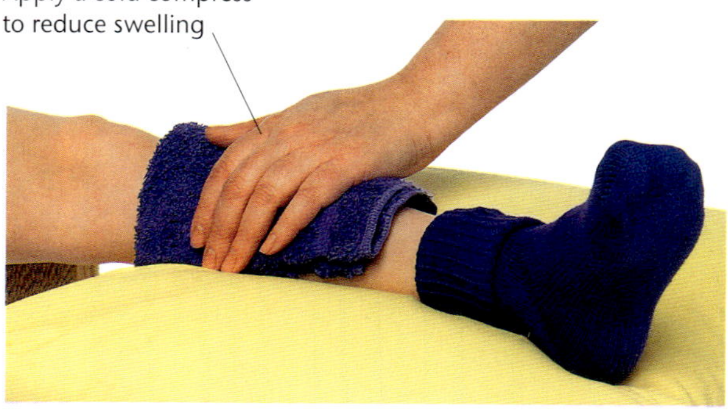

2 To reduce swelling, hold a cold pack against the injury for no more than 20 minutes (*see left*).

Splinter

There is always a risk of infection with splinters. They are often dirty and the bacteria can be carried deep into the skin. Children are most likely to get splinters in their hands and knees because they crawl on the floor.

IMPORTANT

- **If** your child is not immunized against tetanus infection, SEEK MEDICAL ADVICE.
- **Do not** poke at the area with a needle to remove the splinter.
- **If** you cannot remove the splinter, or if it breaks off, SEEK MEDICAL ADVICE.

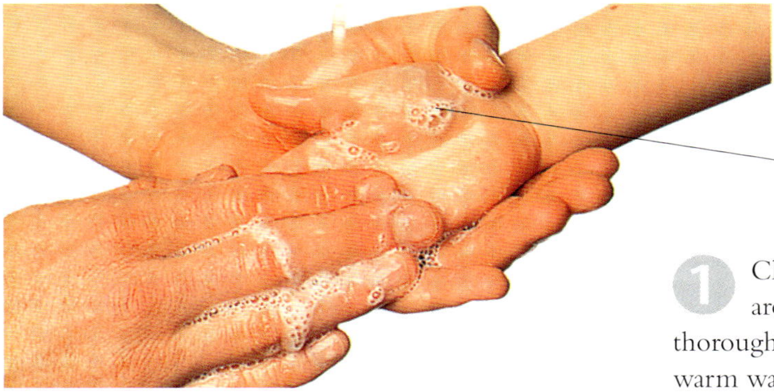

1 Clean the area around the splinter thoroughly with soap and warm water.

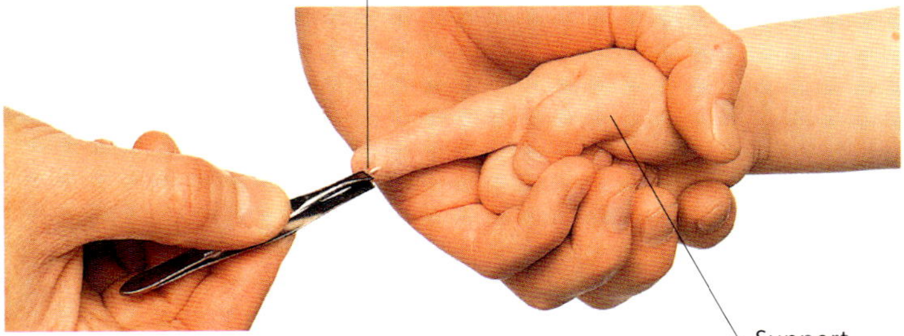

2 Grasp the splinter as close to the skin as possible, and carefully draw it back out at the same angle it went in.

3 Clean the area again, washing well with soap and water.

see also

- Infected wound, *p.42*
- Tetanus, *p.42*

Object in eye

Tiny hairs or specks of dust on the surface of the eye can be very uncomfortable for a child. Anything on the surface can generally be washed off easily; try to keep your child from rubbing her eye.

! IMPORTANT

- **Do not** touch, or attempt to remove, any foreign object that is sticking to, or embedded in, the eye.
- Tell your child to keep his eyes still, and cover the affected eye with a sterile dressing, being careful not to put pressure on the eye. TAKE YOUR CHILD TO AN OPHTHALMOLOGIST OR THE HOSPITAL.

Examine the eye

Separate eyelids gently

Ask her to look right, left, up and down

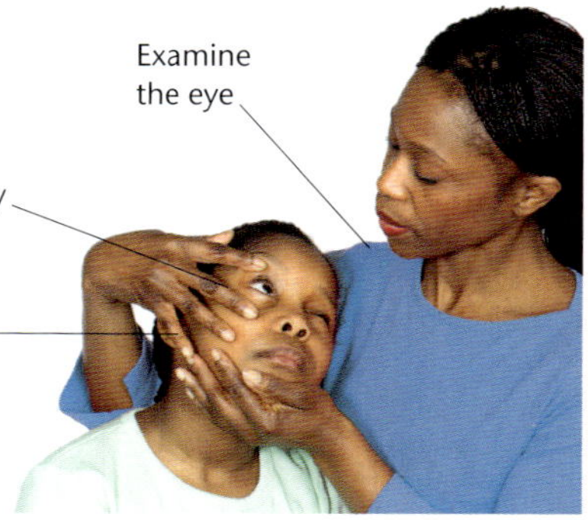

1 Encourage your child to blink several times to produce tears, which may wash the object out.

2 Help your child sit down, facing the light. Separate the eyelids of the affected eye. Ask her to look right, left, up, and down. Examine her eye thoroughly.

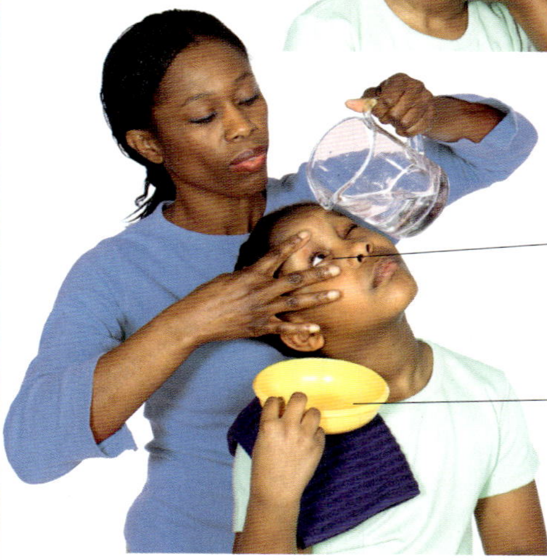

Try to wash out foreign object

Use a bowl to catch water

3 If you can see the foreign object on the surface of the eye, try to rinse it off using a pitcher of clean water. Tilt her head and aim for the inner corner so that water will wash over her eye. Or, try lifting it off with a damp swab or the corner of a handkerchief.

Lift upper eyelid over lower lid

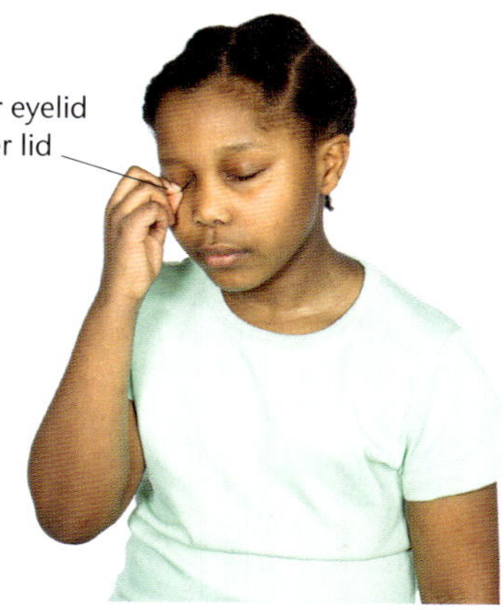

4 If an object is under the eyelid, you can ask an older child to clear it by lifting the upper eyelid over the lower one. You will need to do this for a toddler or young child; if necessary, wrap her in a towel first to stop her from grabbing your arms.

If an object has been removed

- **If** a hankerchief is used, be very careful not to scratch the surface of the eye.
- **If** eye is still red or sore TAKE HIM TO THE OPHTHALMOLOGIST OR HOSPITAL.

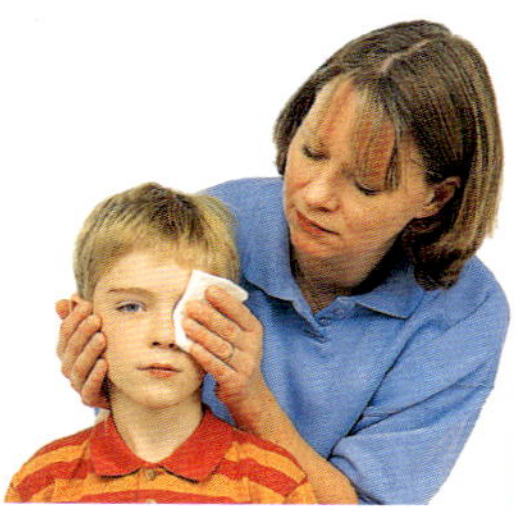

see also

- Eyebrow or eyelid wounds, *p.44*

Object in ear

Children often push things into their ears. A hard object may become stuck, which can cause pain and mechanical hearing loss, which will be resolved when it is removed.

> **IMPORTANT**
> - **Do not** attempt to remove the object.

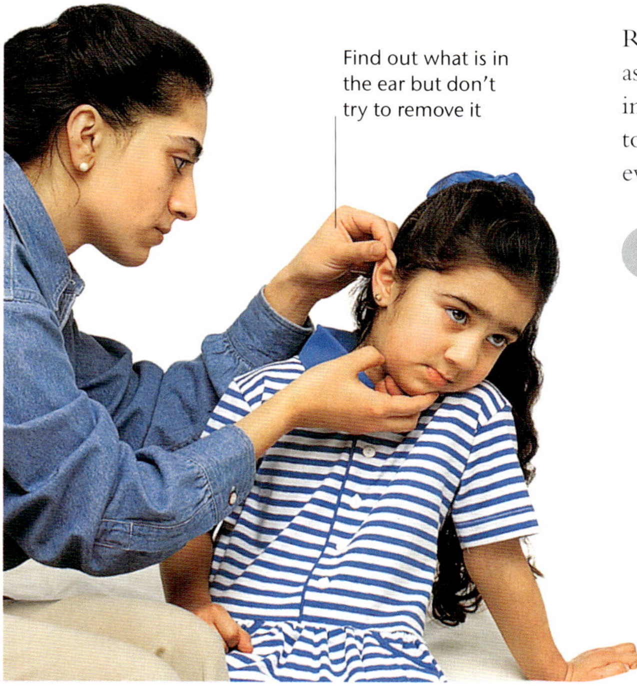
Find out what is in the ear but don't try to remove it

Reassure your child and ask her what she put into her ear. Don't try to remove the object, even if you can see it.

TAKE YOUR CHILD TO A DOCTOR, AN EAR DOCTOR, OR THE HOSPITAL

If there is an insect in the ear

If an insect flies or crawls into your child's ear she may be very alarmed.

1. Help her sit down. Support her head with the affected ear uppermost.

2. Gently flood the ear with tepid water so that the insect floats out.

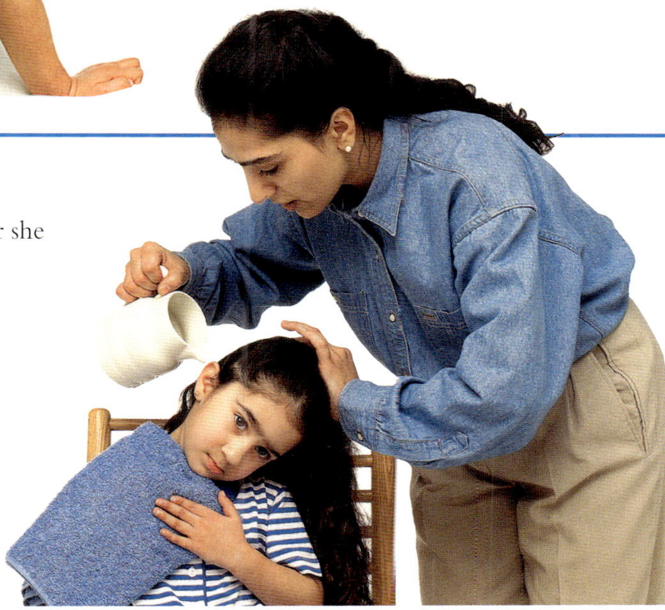

Object in nose

IMPORTANT

- **Do** not attempt to remove the object, even if you can see it.

If your child has something stuck in his nose, his breathing may be difficult or noisy and his nose may be swollen. Smelly or blood-stained discharge from the nose indicates an object has been present for a while.

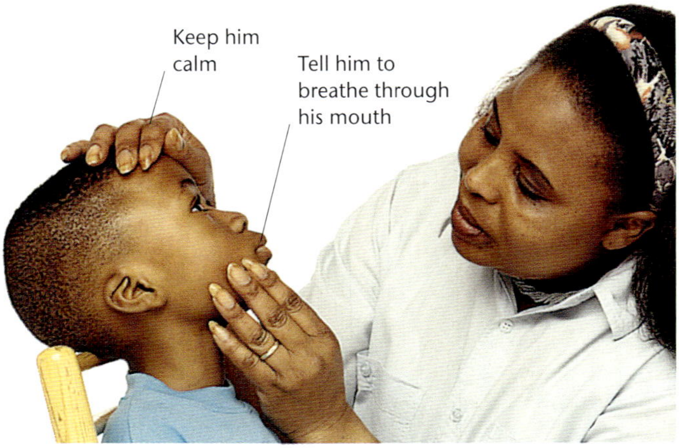

1. Reassure your child and try to find out what he put in his nose. Tell him not to touch it.

2. Tell your child to breathe through his mouth until the object is removed.

TAKE YOUR CHILD TO THE DOCTOR

Swallowed object

IMPORTANT

- **If** the object is sharp or large, don't give your child anything to eat or drink. TAKE YOUR CHILD TO THE HOSPITAL.
- **If** he has swallowed a battery or a magnet, CALL THE POISON CONTROL CENTRE AND TAKE YOUR CHILD TO THE HOSPITAL.
- **If** your child shows any symptoms such as
  - vomiting,
  - abdominal pain,
  - trouble breathing,
  - persistent cough,
  - vomiting or coughing up blood,

  TAKE HIM TO THE HOSPITAL OR CALL 911.

Young children often put small objects in their mouths and may swallow them. Most objects will pass straight through the digestive system. Small button batteries are dangerous because they contain corrosive chemicals. If you have any doubt about what your child swallowed and how to treat it, call your provincial Poison Control Centre.

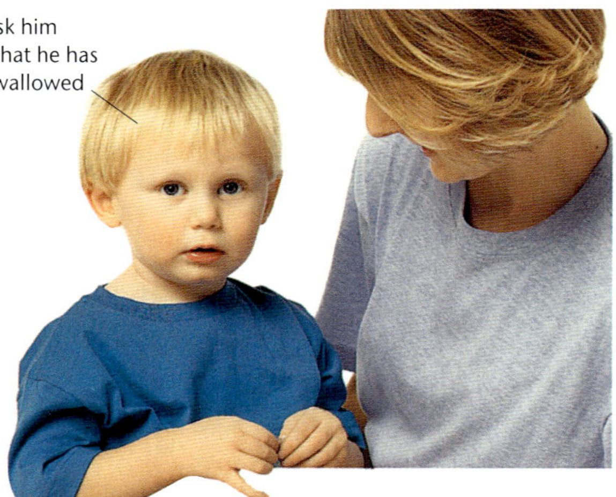

1. Reassure your child. Try to find out what the child has swallowed.

2. If the object is small and smooth like a pebble, there is little danger.

SEEK MEDICAL ADVICE

Animal and human bites

The main risk with any bite is infection; sharp pointed teeth can carry germs through the skin and into the tissues. Severe wounds with torn edges may need advanced medical care. Rabies is rare but possible; teach your child to watch out for wild animals and pets behaving strangely.

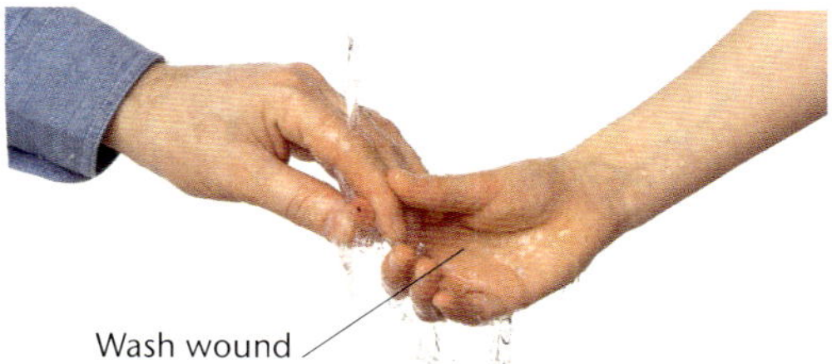

Wash wound with soap and warm, running water

1. Wash the wound thoroughly, using soap and warm water. Rinse the wound under running water for at least five minutes to wash away any dirt.

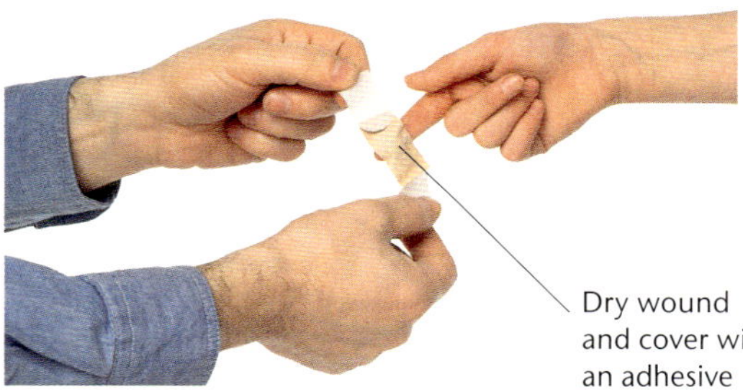

Dry wound and cover with an adhesive bandage

2. Gently but thoroughly, pat the wound dry with a clean pad or tissue. Cover it with an adhesive bandage or a small sterile dressing.

SEEK MEDICAL ADVICE

IMPORTANT

- **If** the bleeding is severe, treat it; then, if there are signs of shock, CALL 911 OR YOUR LOCAL EMS.
- **If** you think your child may have been bitten by a rabid animal, take him to the hospital immediately.
- **Make** sure child's tetanus immunization is up to date.

see also

- Severe bleeding, *p.38*
- Infected wound, *p.42*
- Shock, *p.36*

For a serious animal bite

1. If bleeding is severe, apply direct pressure over the wound, preferably over a sterile dressing or clean, nonfluffy pad.

CALL 911 OR YOUR LOCAL EMS

2. Cover the wound with a sterile dressing or pad and bandage firmly in place to help maintain direct pressure; make sure the bandage is not too tight (*see p.105*). Treat child for shock if necessary. Monitor the child's breathing, pulse, and level of reponse while waiting for help to arrive.

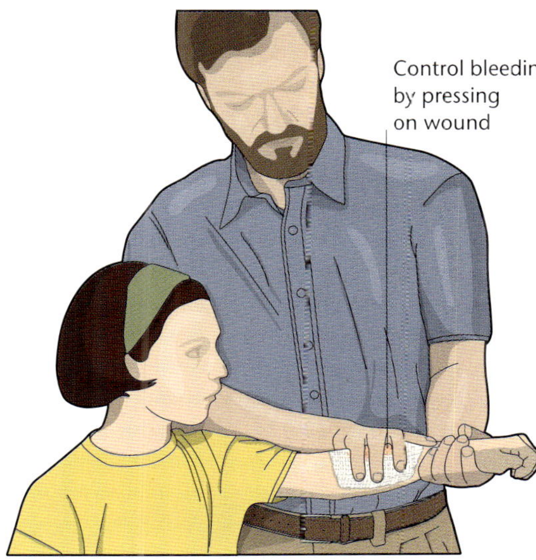

Control bleeding by pressing on wound

IMPORTANT

- **If** severe rash, face and neck swelling, vomiting, and/or breathing difficulties develop, treat for anaphylactic shock. CALL 911 OR YOUR LOCAL EMS.

If sting is in mouth

Give your child an ice cube to suck or cold water to sip and SEEK MEDICAL ADVICE. If swelling develops, CALL 911 OR YOUR LOCAL EMS.

see also

- Anaphylactic shock, *p.91*

Insect sting

Bee, wasp, or hornet stings can be very alarming for a child, but they are rarely dangerous. Your child will experience a sharp pain followed by soreness, red skin, and slight swelling around the site of the sting.

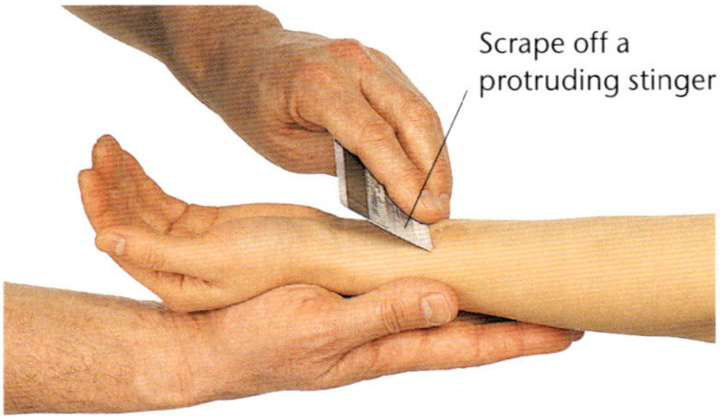

1. If the stinger is still in the skin, brush or scrape it off sideways with your fingernail or a plastic card. If that doesn't work, carefully remove it with tweezers by grabbing the base of the stinger and being careful not to squeeze the venom sac.

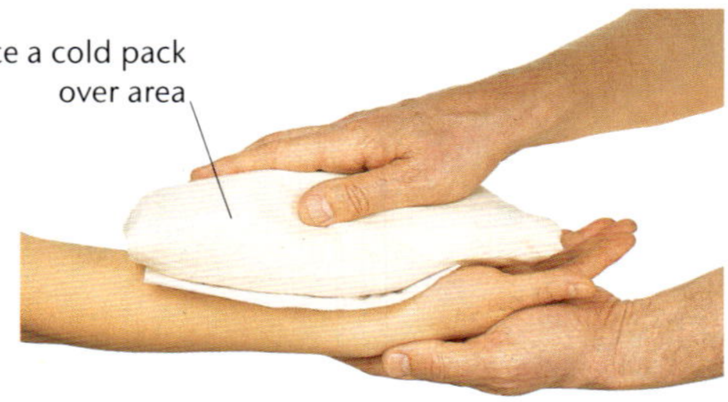

2. Wash with soap and water, then place a cold pack (*p.108*) on the site for about 20 minutes to reduce pain and swelling. Rest the injured part. If pain and swelling persist,

SEEK MEDICAL ADVICE

IMPORTANT

- **If** the rash is extensive, SEEK MEDICAL ADVICE.

Poison ivy rash

If your child brushes against poison ivy, he may develop a blotchy, red, itchy rash that may frighten him. Reassure him and soothe the rash.

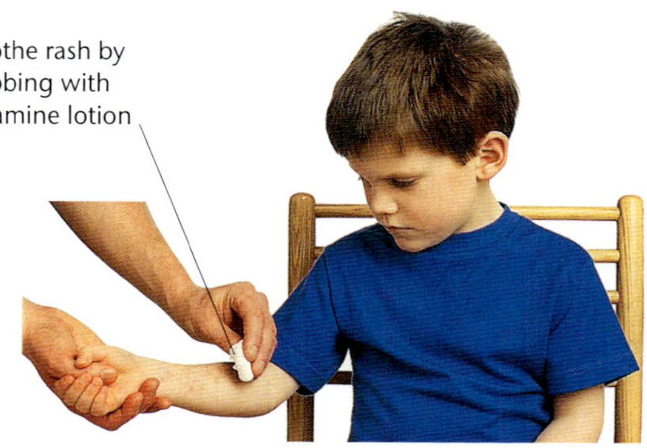

1. To relieve the itching, dab the rash with cotton soaked in calamine lotion.

2. Alternatively, place a cold pack over the rash until the pain is relieved, about 20 minutes.

see also

- Allergy, *p.90*
- Cold pack, *p.108*

Tick bite

Found in woodlands and long grass, ticks are minute, spiderlike creatures that carry viruses and bacteria, including Borrelia, which causes Lyme disease. They attach themselves to people and animals to suck blood and can swell up to the size of a watermelon seed. Always check yourself and your child after walking in areas where ticks are likely to be found.

1 Using fine-toothed tweezers, grasp the tick as close to the child's skin as possible. Pull the tick's "head" upward using steady pressure. Don't twist or crush the tick because this can leave mouth parts (and saliva) embedded in the child. If mouth parts are left behind, you can try to remove these with tweezers; seek medical advice if you cannot.

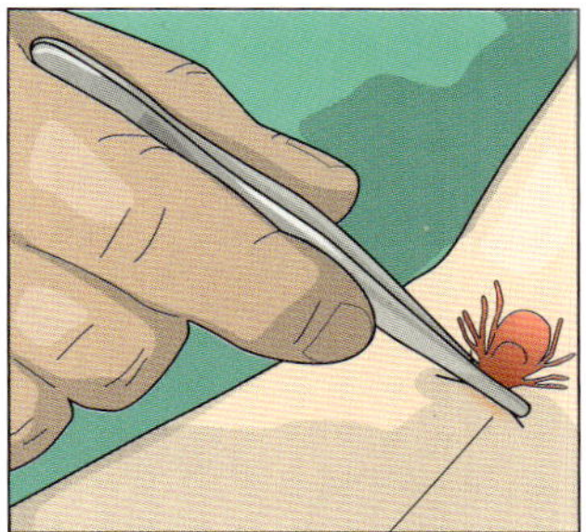

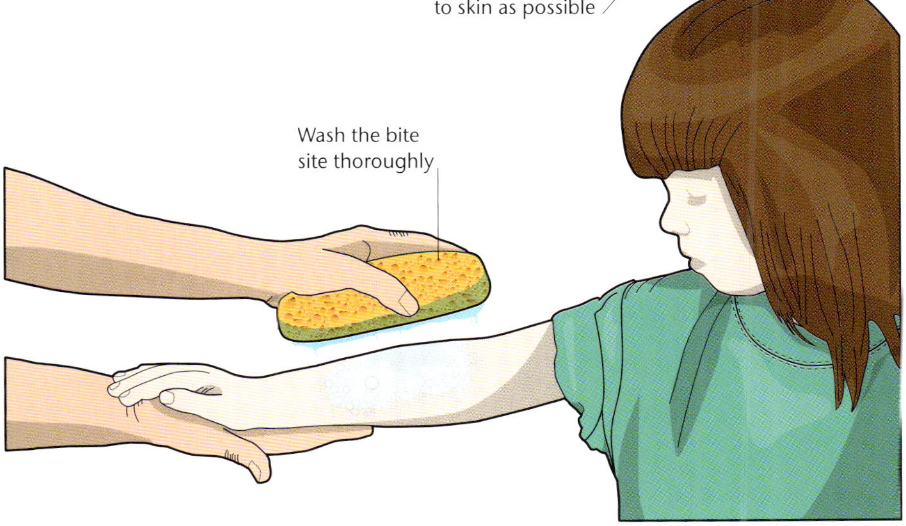

2 Wash the area around the bite with soap and water.

SEEK MEDICAL ADVICE

3 Put the tick into a sealed plastic bag and take it to your doctor, who may want to check that it is complete.

4 If your child develops a rash around the bite site or they start to display any flulike symptoms, *see box right*, seek urgent medical advice.

IMPORTANT

- **Do not** attempt to burn the tick or cover it with petroleum jelly in your attempt to remove it. You could injure the child and it may cause the tick to regurgitate infective fluid into her.
- **If** you can't remove the tick or you think mouth parts remain, SEEK URGENT MEDICAL ADVICE.

Lyme disease

The first sign of this may be a circular rash at the site of the bite that can develop up to 30 days later. The rash is described as looking like a bull's-eye. In some cases, however, this rash never appears, so if there are any other symptoms, such as fever, joint aches, headache, or weakness, SEEK URGENT MEDICAL ADVICE.

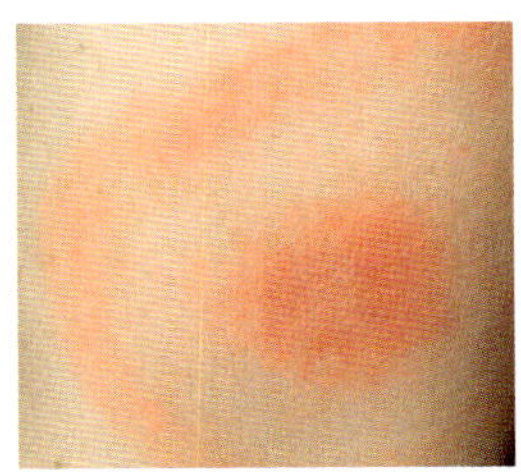

see also

- Fever *p.94*

> **! IMPORTANT**
> - **If** the sting is caused by Portuguese Man-of-War, immerse the area in hot water (40°C/104°F) for 10 minutes and SEEK MEDICAL ADVICE.
> - **If** the skin is very red and painful, TAKE HER TO THE HOSPITAL.
> - **If** the injury is extensive or your child develops anaphylactic shock, CALL 911 OR YOUR LOCAL EMS.

> *see also*
>
> - Anaphylactic shock, *p.91*
> - Checking vital signs, *p.14*
>

Jellyfish sting

Jellyfish and sea anemone venom is contained in stinging cells that stick to a child's skin. Stings from marine creatures in temperate waters may not be dangerous, but those in tropical waters can cause severe poisoning. Vinegar or seawater should be used to flush the stung area.

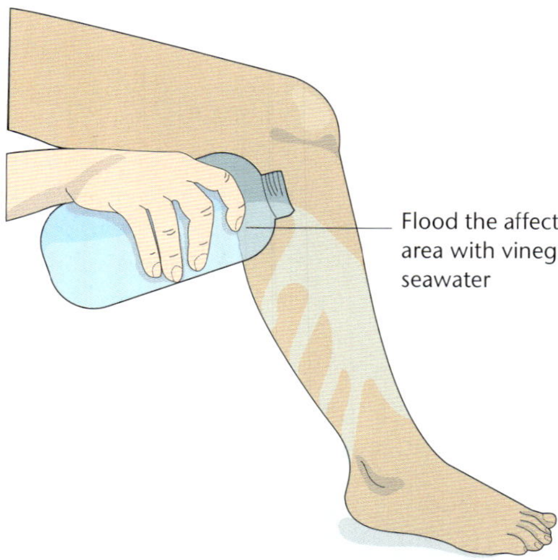

1. Pour vinegar if available or seawater over the affected area for at least 30 seconds to incapacitate the stinging cells.

2. When the stinging stops, place the affected area in very warm water, being careful not to scald your child.

CALL 911 OR YOUR LOCAL EMS

3. Monitor breathing, pulse, and level of response while you wait.

> **! IMPORTANT**
> - **Make** sure the water is not too hot.
> - **If** any spines remain embedded in the skin, or the foot starts to swell, elevate the limb and TAKE YOUR CHILD TO THE HOSPITAL

Marine puncture wound

When stepped on, the spines from a marine creatures such as catfish, lionfish, stonefish, and stingrays can puncture the skin, causing painful swelling and soreness. The spines can also break off and become embedded in a child's foot.

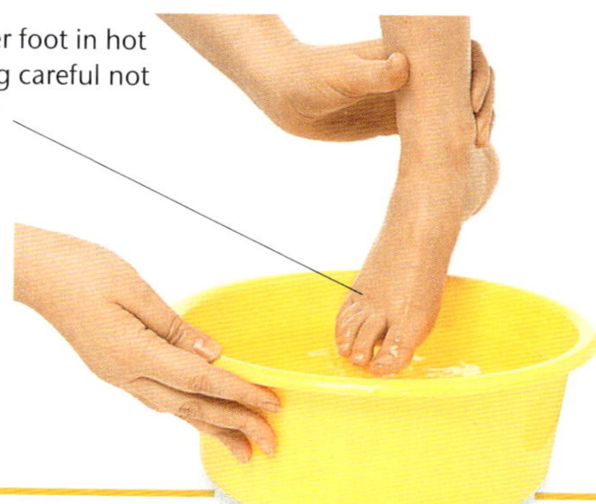

Immerse the injury in water as hot as your child can bear for about 30 minutes. Add more hot water as it cools, but be careful not to scald her.

TAKE YOUR CHILD TO THE HOSPITAL

Snakebite

The toxin in a snake's venom can be either hemotoxic or neurotoxic. Hemotoxic venoms cause bruising, swelling, and bleeding, while neurotoxins can cause tingling, numbness, oral swelling, vomiting, and also difficulty breathing.

CALL 911 OR YOUR LOCAL EMS

1. Remain calm. Help the child lie down and stay still. Keep the affected part lower than the level of the heart.

2. Gently wash the wound with warm water.

3. Place a pad over the site and put a pressure bandage on top. Immobilize the bitten part with broad-fold bandages.

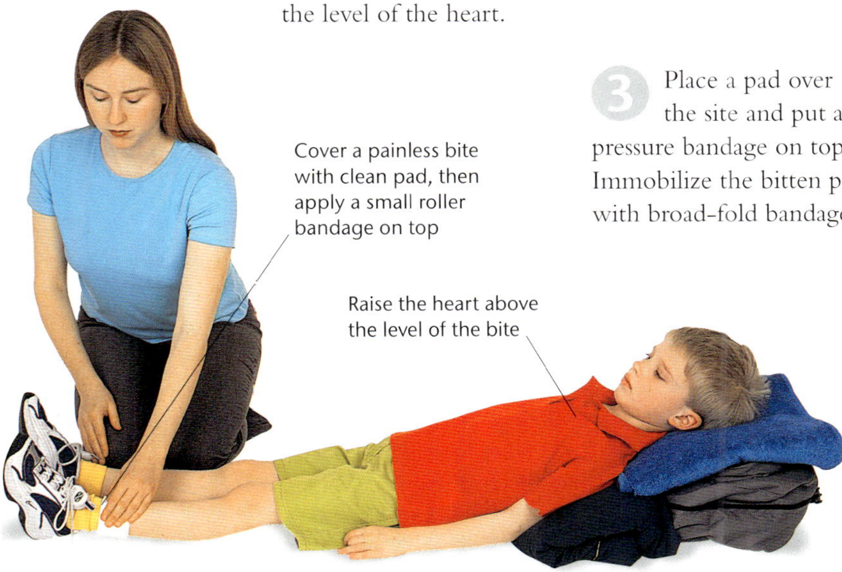

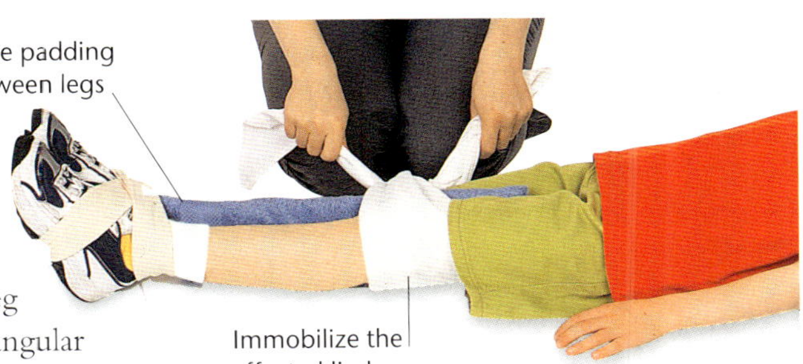

4. Immobilize a leg with folded triangular bandages and padding; use a sling if the arm is affected.

IMPORTANT

- **Do not** let your child walk around; keeping him still prevents the venom from spreading.
- **Do not** apply a tourniquet, cut out the wound, or try to suck out the venom.
- **If** possible, give an accurate description of the snake to the emergency services personnel, but never try to capture it.
- **If** your child develops a severe allergic reaction, treat as for anaphylactic shock.
- **If** your child becomes unresponsive and is not breathing normally, begin CPR immediately, with 30 compressions. CALL 911 OR YOUR LOCAL EMS.

see also

- Anaphylactic shock, *p.91*
- Checking vital signs, *p.14*
- Triangular bandages, *p.65* and *p.106*
- Unresponsive baby, *pp.19–21*
- Unresponsive child, *p.22–27*

IMPORTANT

- **Do not** put a source of direct heat, such as a hot water bottle, next to the child's skin because it may cause a burn.
- **If** your child becomes unresponsive and isn't breathing normally, begin CPR with 30 compressions immediately. CALL 911 OR YOUR LOCAL EMS.

Hypothermia

This develops if the body temperature falls below 35°C (95°F), and if it falls further it is very serious. An older child is most likely to develop it outside in poor weather conditions, especially if there is a high wind-chill factor, or if a child falls into cold water. For babies, *see opposite*. If your child has had cold exposure and is shivering, she may have mild hypothermia. As she gets colder and the shivering stops, her condition is more serious. She may become listless, confused, or unresponsive.

For a child outside

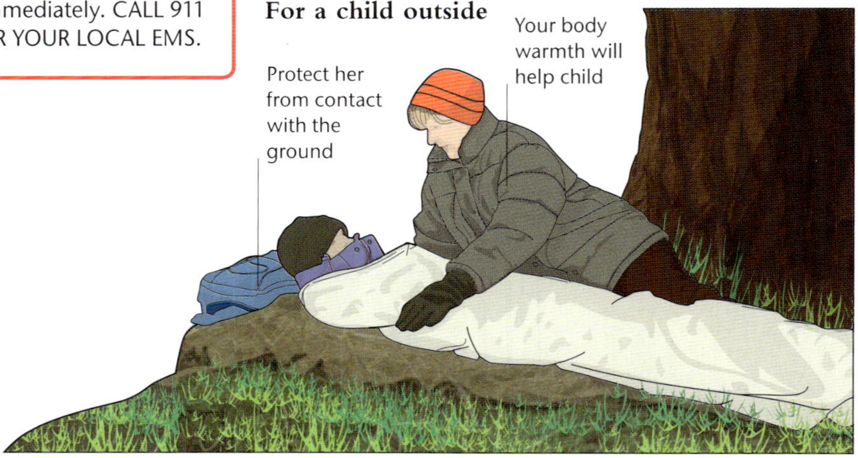
Protect her from contact with the ground
Your body warmth will help child

Take your child to a shelter. If there isn't one nearby, lay her on a layer of dry insulating material such as soft brush or moss and protect her from the wind. Wrap her in a dry sleeping bag and a foil blanket if available. Use your body to keep her warm, too.

CALL 911 OR YOUR LOCAL EMS

For a child indoors

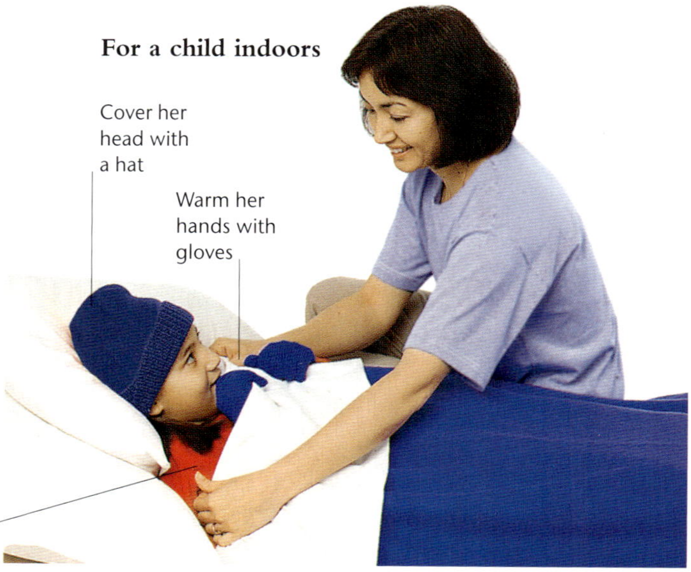
Cover her head with a hat
Warm her hands with gloves
Remove wet clothes

1 If you can get to a shelter or your child is indoors, remove any wet clothes and replace them with dry ones. Cover her with plenty of blankets—you can put her in bed. Cover her head with a hat and make sure that the room is warm. Stay with her.

SEEK MEDICAL ADVICE

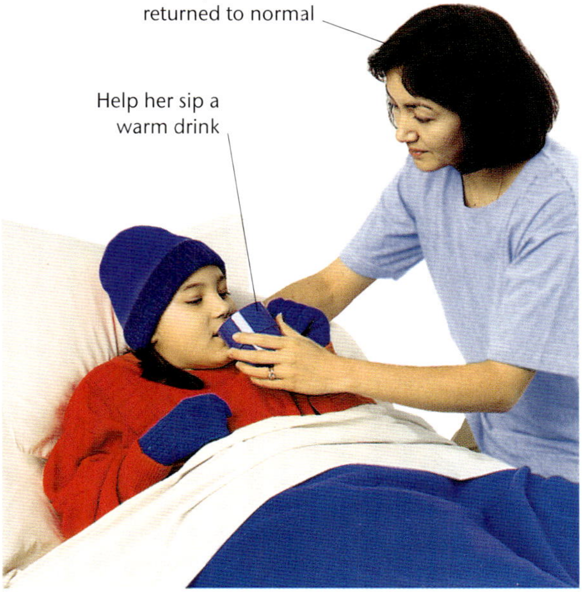

2 Warm the centre of her body first (armpits, chest, groin, and neck), using an electric blanket, body heat, hot water bottles, or layers of blankets/towels.

3 Give your child a warm drink and some high-energy foods, such as chocolate. Monitor her breathing, pulse, temperature, and level of response. Do not leave her alone until you are sure that her temperature has returned to normal.

IMPORTANT

- **Do not** put a source of direct heat, such as a hot water bottle, next to the child's skin because it may cause a burn.
- **If** your child becomes unresponsive and isn't breathing normally, begin CPR with 30 compressions immediately. CALL 911 OR YOUR LOCAL EMS.

see also

- Checking vital signs, *p.14*
- Unresponsive baby, *pp.19–21*
- Unresponsive child, *pp.22–27*

Hypothermia in babies

A baby's temperature regulation is not fully developed. He can lose body heat rapidly and develop hypothermia in a cold room. Suspect hypothermia if you are in a cool or cold environment and your baby's skin feels cold; he is limp and unusually quiet; and he refuses to feed.

CALL 911 OR YOUR LOCAL EMS

1 Rewarm a baby by warming the room or taking him to a warm room. Wrap him in blankets.

2 Put a hat on his head and cuddle him against your body so that he is warmed by your body heat.

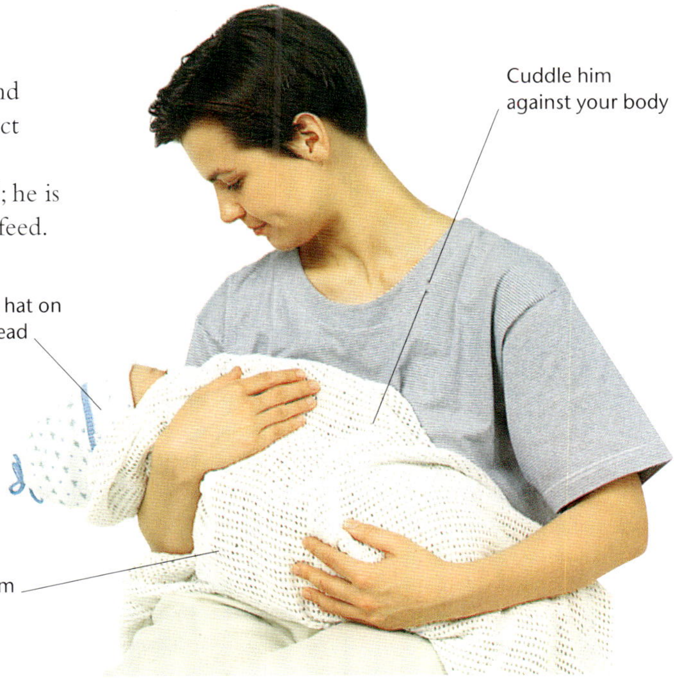

IMPORTANT

- **Do not** warm by rubbing because it can damage the skin and surrounding tissues
- **Do not** use direct heat, such as hot water bottles or an open flame, to rewarm skin.
- **Never** burst blisters.

If the skin is broken

If there are any open wounds or the frozen skin is broken, cover the area with a soft gauze dressing and bandage it lightly in place. TAKE YOUR CHILD TO THE HOSPITAL.

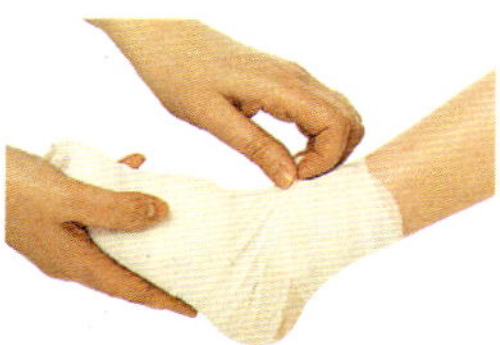

Frostbite

If children are exposed to extreme weather conditions, the tissues of the fingers, toes, and other extremeties may freeze. Your child may have frostbite if she has pins and needles, with numbness and hard, stiff skin that is turning white and waxy. Shelter your child before treating her.

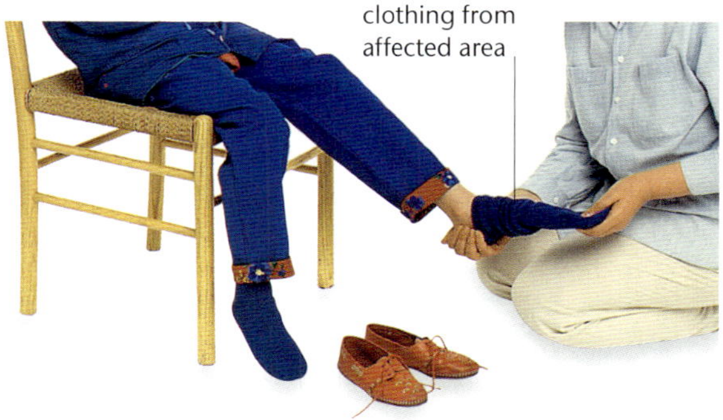

Gently remove clothing from affected area

CALL 911 OR YOUR LOCAL EMS

1. While you are still outside, advise your child to put her hands under her armpits to use her body warmth to prevent her condition from worsening.

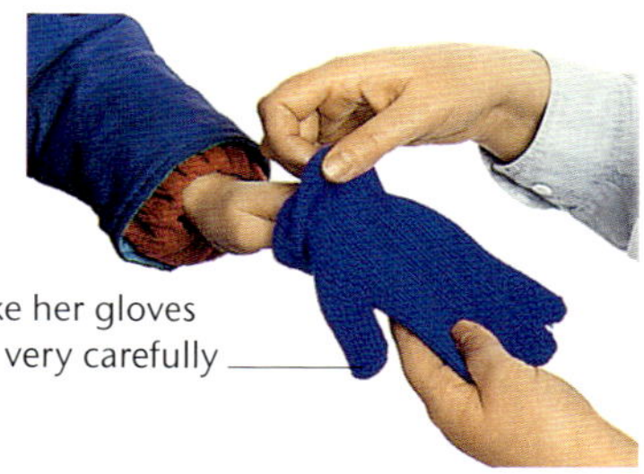

Take her gloves off very carefully

2. Once in a warm shelter, help her sit down, then start treatment. Gently remove constrictions from the affected area such as shoes, socks, and/or gloves and rings. Undo her coat. Start warming the affected area with your hands, in your lap, and/or in the child's armpits; don't rub them.

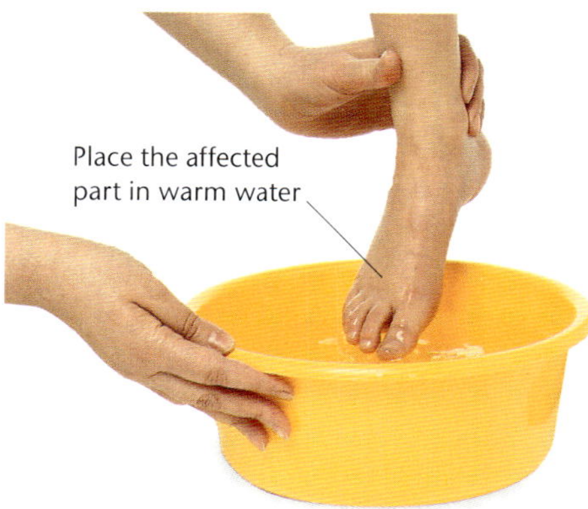

Place the affected part in warm water

3. Place the affected part(s) in warm water—it should be around 40°C (104°F). This may be painful. Pat dry and cover with a light gauze bandage.

4. After warming, raise the affected area to reduce swelling. Give your child the recommended dose of acetaminophen (not aspirin) to ease the pain while you wait for help to arrive.

Sunburn

Sunburn is red, and may be itchy or tender. Babies and young children are very vulnerable: keep them in the shade; apply sunscreen; put on a hat, and cover with protective clothing in hot weather.

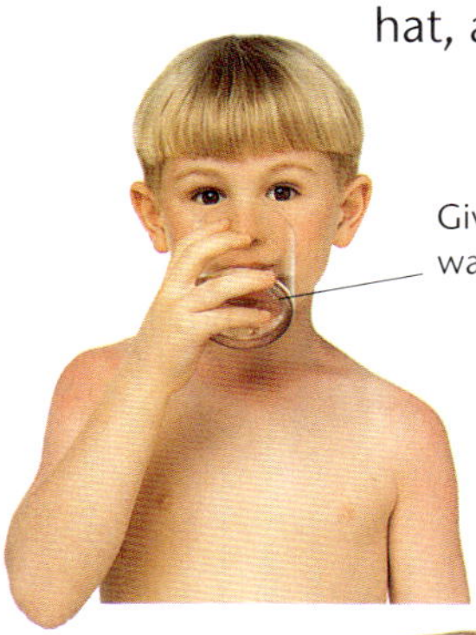

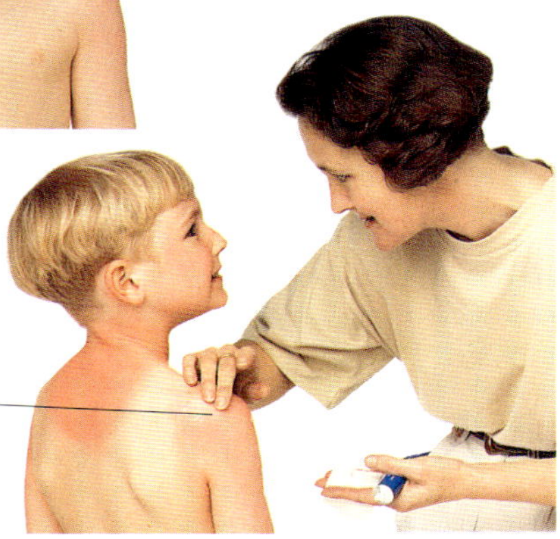

1. Move your child into the shade or into a cool room and give him a cold drink. Cool the skin with cold water compresses.

2. Apply an aloe vera cream or gel to soothe the skin. Make sure you *know* your child is not allergic to it.

IMPORTANT

- If there is blistering or other skin damage, SEEK MEDICAL ADVICE.
- If your child is restless, flushed, dizzy, or has a temperature or headache, he may have heatstroke—CALL 911 OR YOUR LOCAL EMS.

see also

- Heat exhaustion, *p.88*
- Heatstroke, *p.89*

Heat rash

This is a prickly, red rash that develops particularly around the sweat glands on the chest and back and under the arms.

1. Help your child sit down in a cool room and undress her. Sponge the affected area with cool water.

2. Pat her almost dry with a soft towel, leaving the skin slightly damp. Apply calamine lotion if the rash itches.

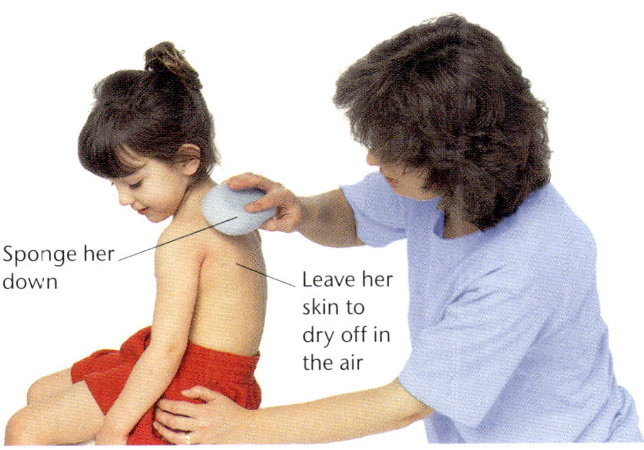

IMPORTANT

- If your baby develops heat rash, remove some of her clothes to cool her, or bathe her in tepid water. Dry her gently, leaving her skin slightly damp.
- If the rash has not faded after 12 hours, or if she develops a raised temperature, SEEK MEDICAL ADVICE.

see also

- Heat exhaustion, *p.88*

Heat exhaustion

Caused by excessive heat, whether the result of too many clothes or being left in a hot car, heat exhaustion can lead to dehydration—a loss of water and salts from the body because of excessive sweating without taking in fluids to replace what has been lost. A full, bounding pulse is a symptom.

IMPORTANT

- If a baby or very young child develops heatstroke, undress him completely in a cool room.
- If your child becomes unresponsive and is not breathing normally, begin CPR with 30 chest compressions immediately. CALL 911 OR YOUR LOCAL EMS.

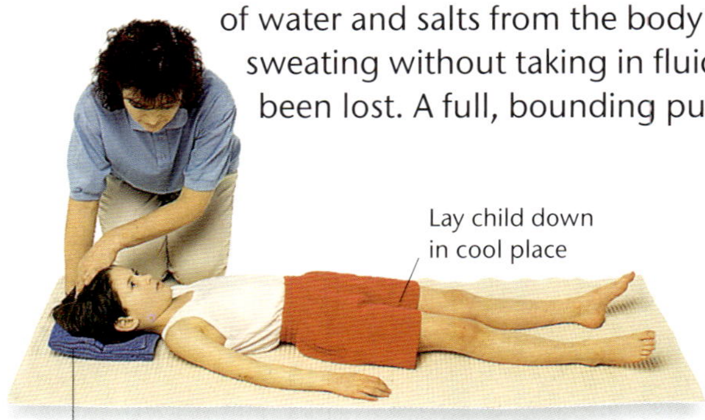

1 Take your child into the shade or into a cool room. Help him to lie down.

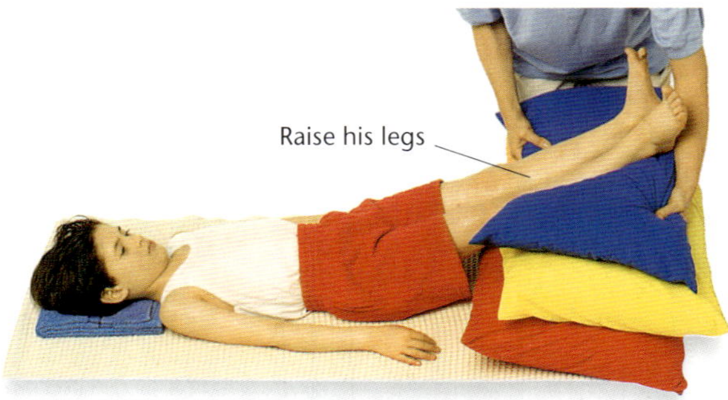

2 Raise and support your child's legs on some pillows. This improves blood supply to the brain. Encourage him to rest quietly.

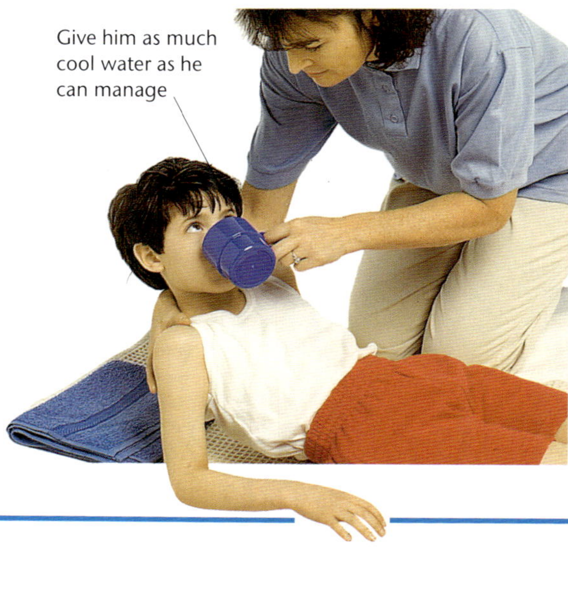

3 Help your child sip as much cool water as he can manage. Later give oral rehydration salts or an isotonic sports drink to replace salt lost from the body.

SEEK MEDICAL ADVICE

4 Monitor breathing, pulse, level of response, and temperature. If his condition worsens,

CALL 911 OR YOUR LOCAL EMS

see also

- Checking vital signs, *p.14*
- Heatstroke, *opposite*
- Unresponsive baby, *pp.19–21*
- Unresponsive child, *p.22–27*

Heatstroke

This is a life-threatening condition that develops if the body becomes overheated in hot surroundings. Treat your child for heatstroke if she develops a sudden headache; is confused; is vomiting; has hot, flushed, dry skin; is becoming unresponsive; and has a temperature of over 40°C (104°F). A rapidly weakening pulse is very serious.

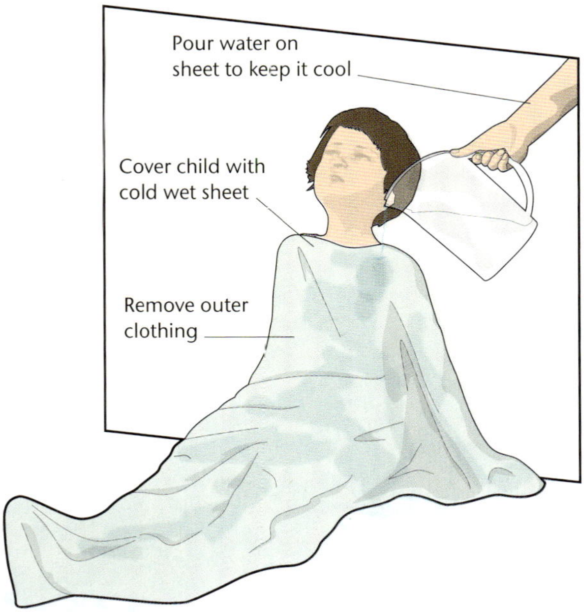

1. Quickly move child into a cool place. Remove as much outer clothing as you can.

CALL 911 OR YOUR LOCAL EMS

2. Help the child sit down on the ground. Support her with pillows and/or against a wall and wrap her in a cold, wet sheet. Gently pour more water over the sheet to keep it cool.

3. A fan, and icepacks applied to the groin and armpits, will also help cool the child.

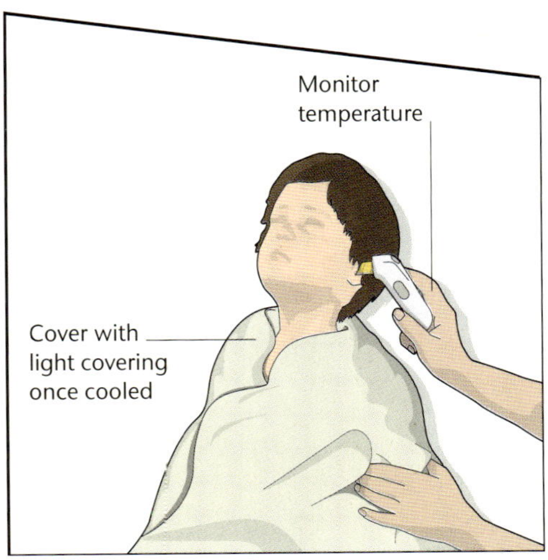

4. Once her temperature has normalized, replace wet sheet with a dry, light cover. Reassure your child and monitor breathing, pulse, level of response, and temperature while waiting for help to arrive. Repeat the cooling if her temperature starts to rise again.

IMPORTANT

- **If** a baby or very young child develops heatstroke, undress him completely in a cool room.
- **If** your child becomes unresponsive and is not breathing normally, begin CPR with 30 chest compressions immediately. CALL 911 OR YOUR LOCAL EMS.

see also

- Checking vital signs, *p.14*
- Unresponsive baby, *pp.19–21*
- Unresponsive child, *p.22–27*

IMPORTANT

- If the child's condition does not improve, the rash worsens, he develops breathing difficulties and/or swelling of the face or neck, or is vomiting or becoming distressed, treat for anaphylactic shock, *opposite*.

CALL 911 OR YOUR LOCAL EMS.

Allergy

This is an abnormal reaction in the body's defenses that occurs in response to exposure to an allergen, and symptoms vary depending on the cause. Common allergens include pollen; dust; some foods such as nuts, shellfish, and eggs; as well as insect stings or bites. Mild allergy normally develops slowly, and a child may have an itchy rash or raised blotchy areas on his skin, sneezing, and red itchy eyes. Any swelling of the feet, hands, and/or face; wheezing; and even stomach pain, vomiting, and diarrhea can be signs of a serious anaphylactic reaction.

1. Try to identify the cause and try to remove the allergen from the child or the child from the allergen. If pollen is the allergen, move him indoors. If he has a reaction to laundry detergent, remove the affected clothing.

2. Treat any symptoms. For example, soothe an itchy rash with calamine lotion. Suggest he use his asthma medication if necessary.

3. Talk to your pharmacist because some mild allergies can be controlled with over-the-counter medication formulated for children. If the symptoms persist,

SEEK MEDICAL ADVICE

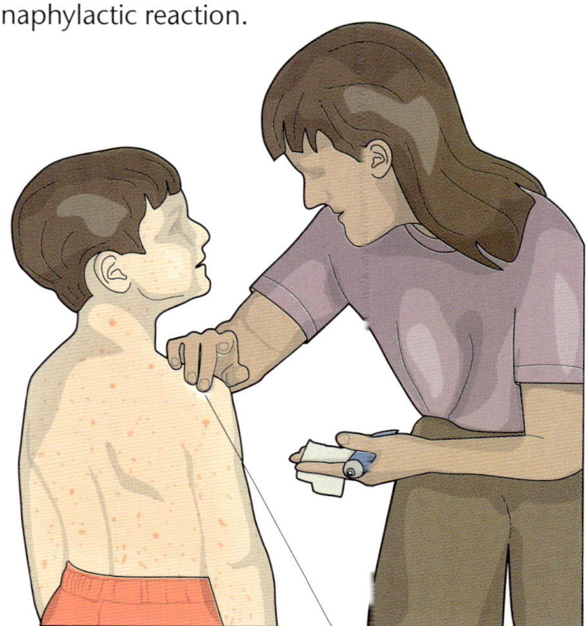

Dab calamine on itchy skin

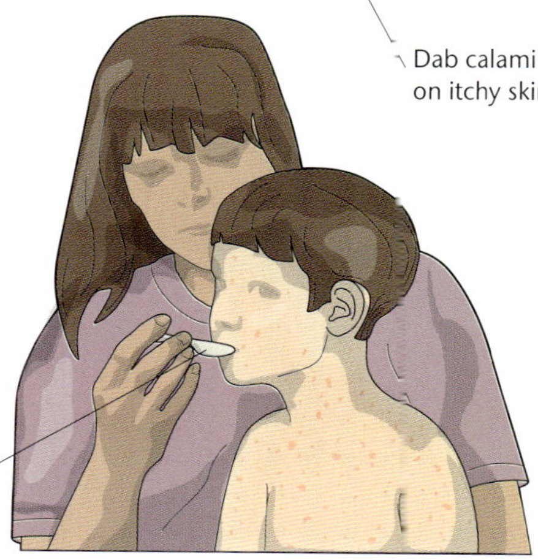

Offer recommended dose of antihistamine medication

see also

- Asthma, *p.35*
- Anaphylactic shock, *opposite*

Anaphylactic shock

This is a severe allergic reaction affecting the whole body that may develop within a few minutes of, for example, the injection of a drug, an insect sting, or ingestion of a food. It causes constriction of the air passages and swelling of the face and neck that can result in suffocation. Suspect anaphylactic shock if your child has increased difficulty breathing or swelling of the lips, face, or neck. Skin may be blotchy or flushed.

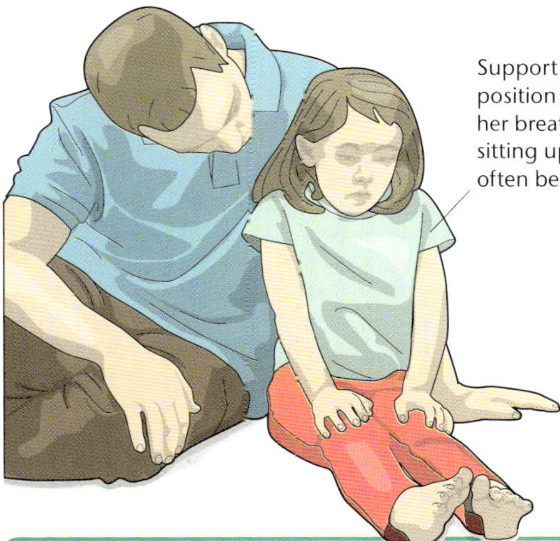

Support her in a position that helps her breathing; sitting upright is often best

CALL 911 OR YOUR LOCAL EMS.

1. Help your child into a position that helps breathing. Help with medication.

2. Monitor breathing, pulse, and level of response as you wait for emergency help. If pulse weakens and she becomes pale, treat for shock.

IMPORTANT

- **If** child has a known allergy and has her own medication, help her use it or give it to her yourself, *see below*.
- **If** your child becomes unresponsive and is not breathing normally, begin CPR with 30 chest compressions immediately. CALL 911 OR YOUR LOCAL EMS

see also

- Checking vital signs, *p.14*
- Shock, *p.36*
- Unresponsive baby, *pp.19–21*
- Unresponsive child, *pp.22–27*

Administering an auto-injector

A child with a known allergy is often prescribed medication—usually an auto-injector of epinephrine—to use in the event of a reaction.

1. Hold the injector with your fist and remove the safety cap; don't put your thumb over the end.

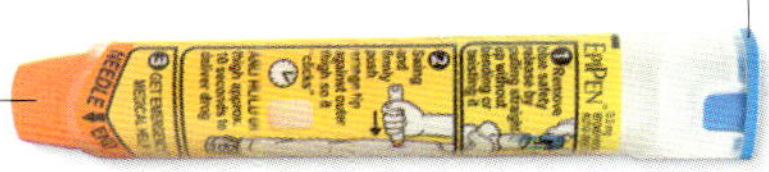

Tip

Safety cap

2. Place the tip against the child's outer thigh. Push it firmly against the thigh to release the medication; a click should be heard. Hold it in place for 10 seconds, remove it, and rub the injection site for 10 seconds. Repeat at 5-minute intervals if there's no improvement.

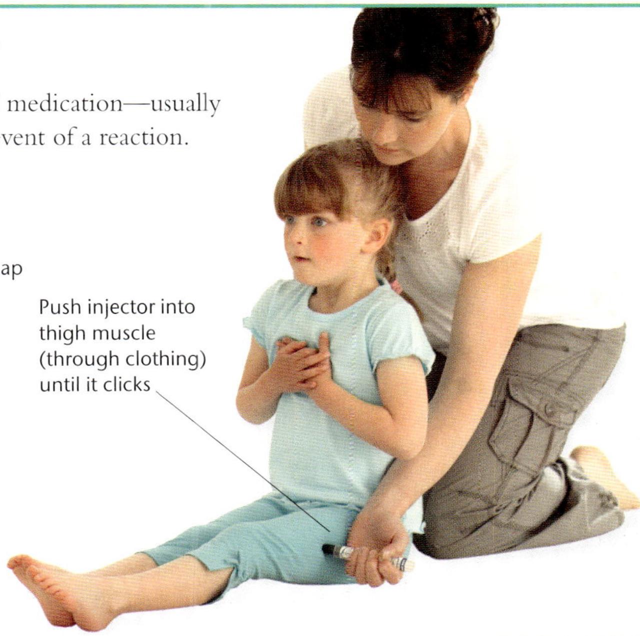

Push injector into thigh muscle (through clothing) until it clicks

Diabetic emergency

If a child with Type 1 diabetes has low blood sugar, he may be weak or hungry; confused or behaving aggressively; sweating; and very pale. He may also have a strong, pounding pulse and breathing may be shallow.

> **IMPORTANT**
>
> - **Do not** give an unresponsive child anything to eat or drink.
> - **If** your child does not improve after food or a drink, or deteriorates, CALL 911 OR YOUR LOCAL EMS.
> - **Do not** give your child a diet or low-calorie drink.
> - **Make sure** the child's doctor checks insulin dosage even if he seems to have recovered completely.

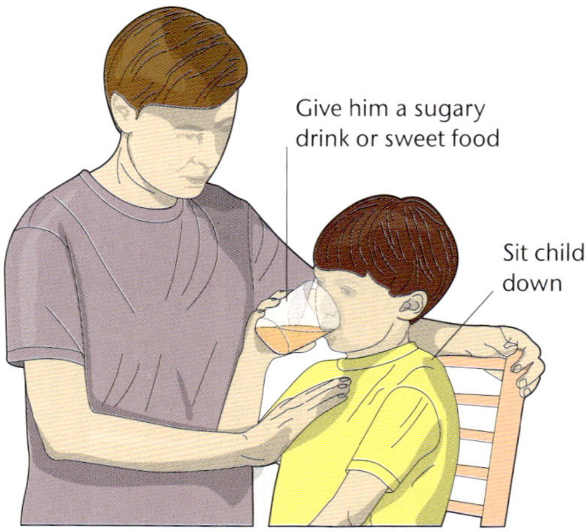

Help your child to sit down and give him 15–20ml (0.5–0.7oz) of glucose (150ml/5fl.oz orange juice, or 15ml/3tsp sugar) to raise his blood sugar levels. If he recovers, give him more. Check his glucose levels and monitor him until he is fully recovered.

SEEK MEDICAL ADVICE

If the child becomes unresponsive

If she is breathing, place her in the recovery position, *p.26*. Then,

CALL 911 OR YOUR LOCAL EMS

1. If she is not breathing normally, begin CPR immediately (*see p. 24*) with 30 chest compressions.
2. Open airway and give 2 rescue breaths.

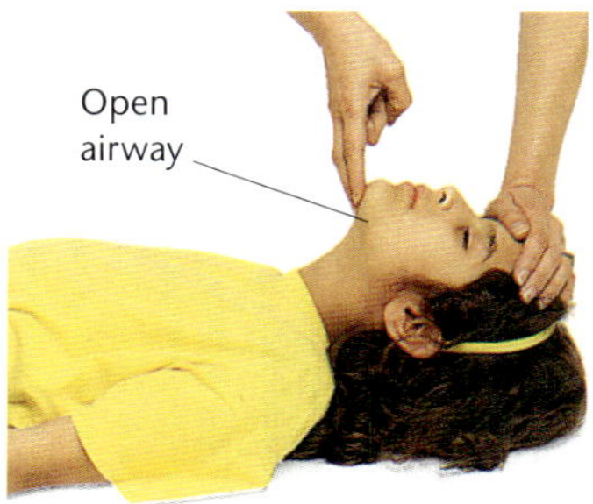

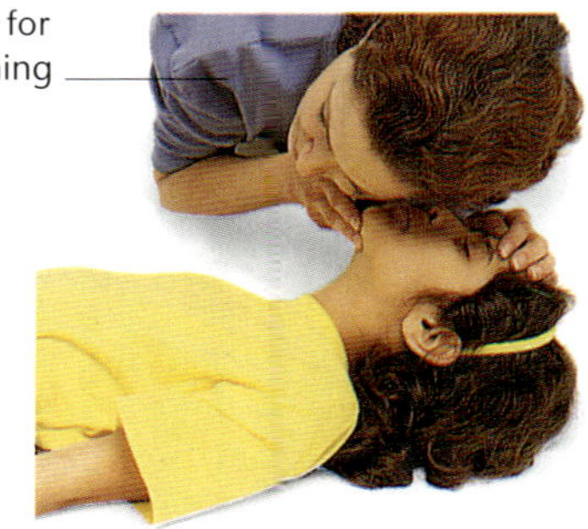

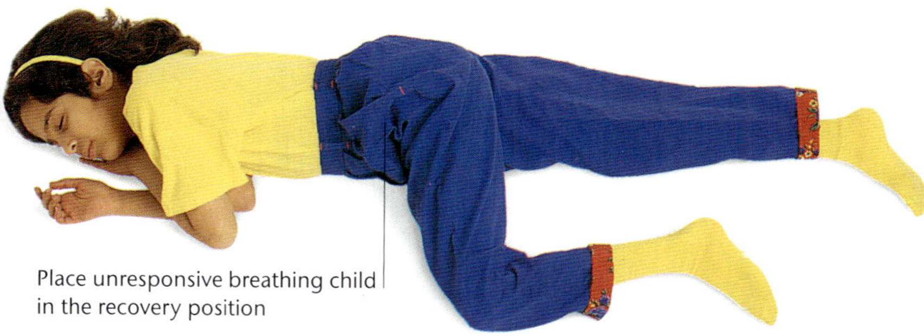

Place unresponsive breathing child in the recovery position

Fainting

Your child may be about to faint if she complains of feeling weak, sweaty, and nauseous, and is very pale. The period of unresponsiveness is brief and accompanied by a slow pulse; recovery is rapid and complete.

1 Help your child lie down and raise her legs above the level of her heart; this helps improve the blood flow to the vital organs. Support her legs on a pile of pillows or folded blankets.

2 Reassure your child and help her sit up gradually. If she starts to feel faint again, help her to lie back down until she feels better, then try again. If you are concerned about your child after the faint,

SEEK MEDICAL ADVICE

3 Offer her something to drink, such as juice.

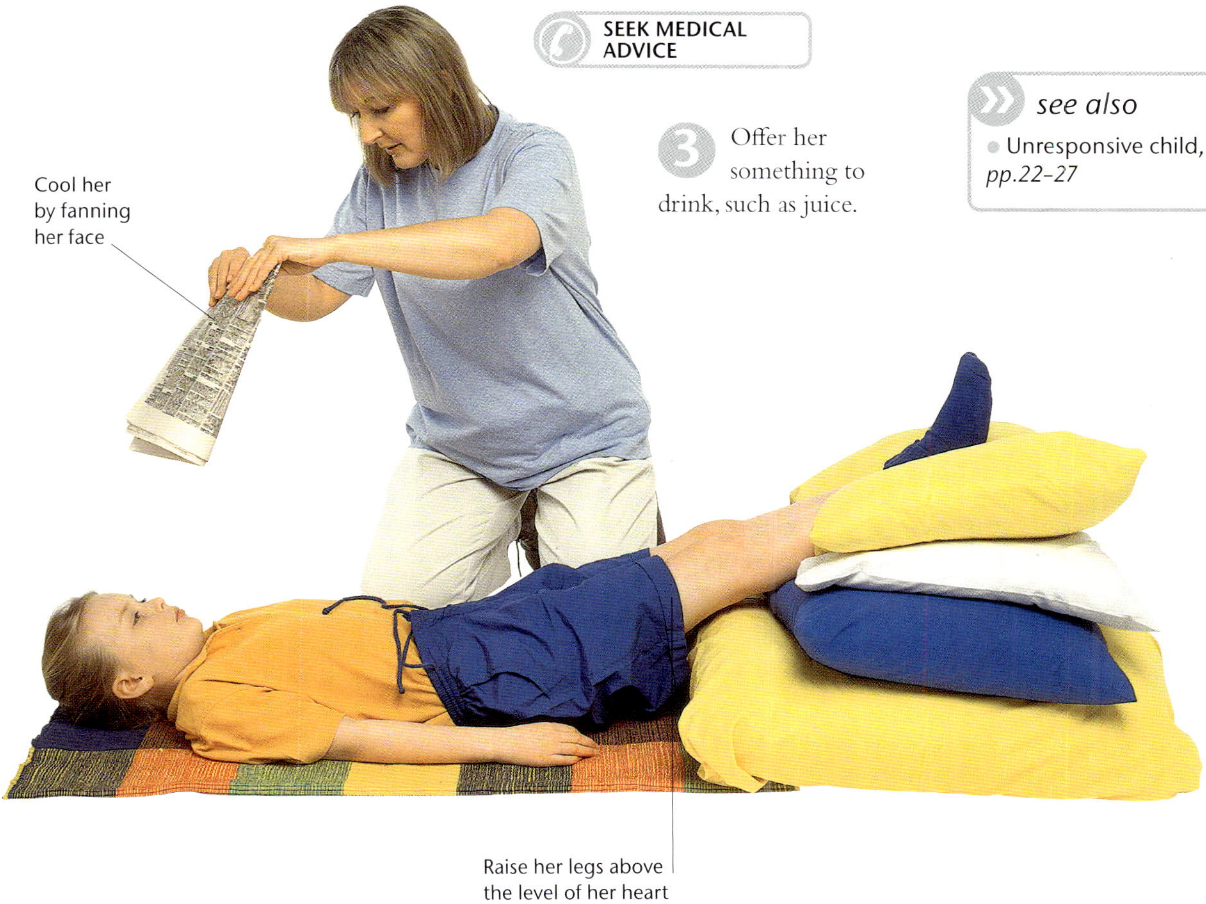

IMPORTANT

- **Do not** sit your child on a chair with her head down if she is feeling faint because she may fall off and hurt herself.
- **If** your child becomes unresponsive and is not breathing normally, begin CPR immediately with 30 compressions. CALL 911 OR YOUR LOCAL EMS.

see also

- Unresponsive child, *pp.22–27*

Fever

A body temperature that is above 38°C (100.4°F) indicates fever. An infection is the usual cause. Fevers are usually not harmful, but sometimes febrile seizures (*see p.96*) may occur. As the fever advances she will have hot, flushed skin, be sweating, and have a headache. Raised body temperature may also be caused by overheating (*see* Heatstroke, *p.89*)

IMPORTANT

- **Children under three months** old should be assessed immediately by a medical professional.
- **If** your baby is under three months old, you should not give her acetaminophen or ibuprofen syrup unless you are advised to do so by your doctor.
- **If** your child is very hot, take off as many clothes as possible; you can also sponge her with cool water.
- **If** your child complains of a severe headache, suspect meningitis. TAKE YOUR CHILD TO THE HOSPITAL or CALL 911.

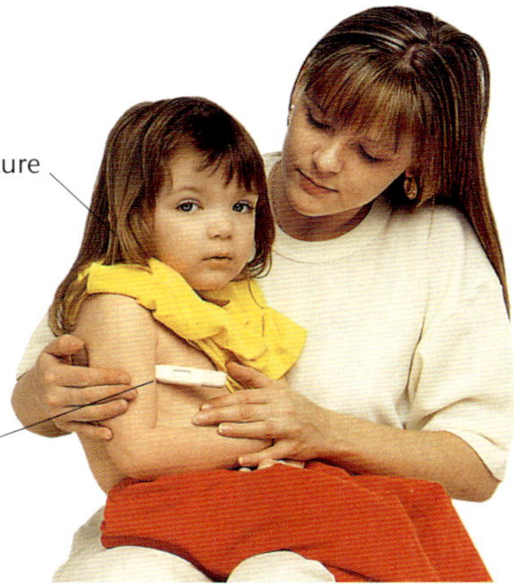

Take her temperature

Tuck the thermometer under her arm

1 Take your child's temperature. If you are using a digital thermometer, on a young child lift your child's arm and tuck the pointed end into her armpit. Fold her arm over her chest and leave the thermometer in place until it beeps; an armpit reading will be about 0.5°C (1°F) lower than under the tongue.

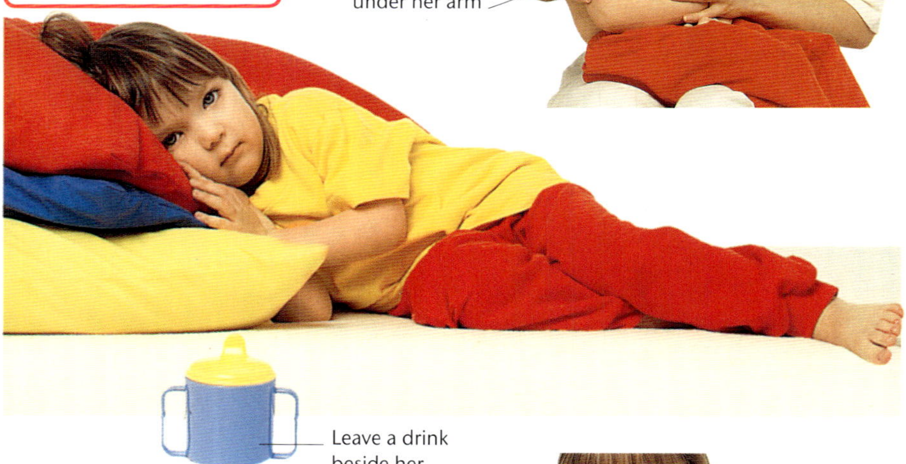

Leave a drink beside her

2 Make your child comfortable on a bed or sofa, but do not cover her. To help bring down her temperature, make sure she has plenty of water or diluted fruit juice to drink.

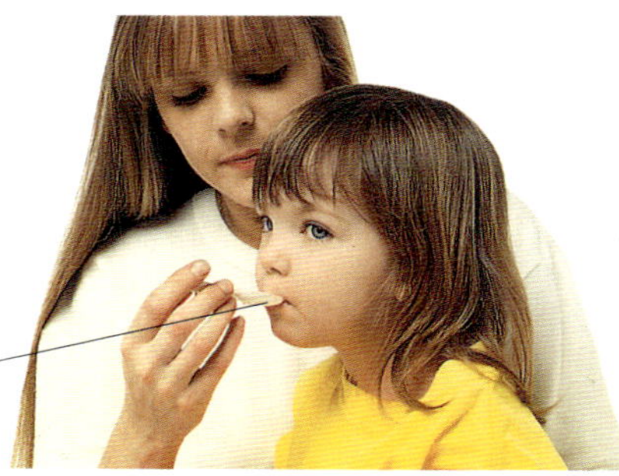

Give her the recommended dose of acetaminophen or ibuprofen syrup

3 You can give her the recommended dose of acetaminophen or ibuprofen syrup (not aspirin) to help reduce her temperature; never give aspirin to anyone under the age of 16 years.

see also

- Febrile seizures, *p.96*
- Heatstroke, *p.89*
- Meningitis, *opposite*

Meningitis

This is a life-threatening infection affecting the tissues that surround the brain. In the early stages your child may have a flulike illness with a high temperature. If his neck is stiff and his eyes are sensitive to light, he needs immediate medical evaluation. Take him to the hospital or call 911 or your local EMS. He may complain of cold hands and feet, or joint and limb pain. As infection develops he is likely to have a headache, begin vomiting, and become increasingly drowsy. Later, a red or purple rash may develop that does not disappear if pressed.

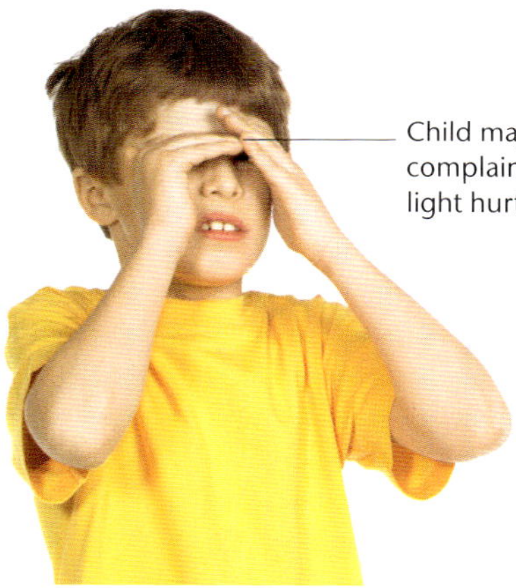

Child may complain that light hurts his eyes

1 If your child has a high fever and a flulike illness, monitor him carefully. If light hurts his eyes and he has a stiff neck, he needs immediate medical attention.

CALL 911 OR YOUR LOCAL EMS

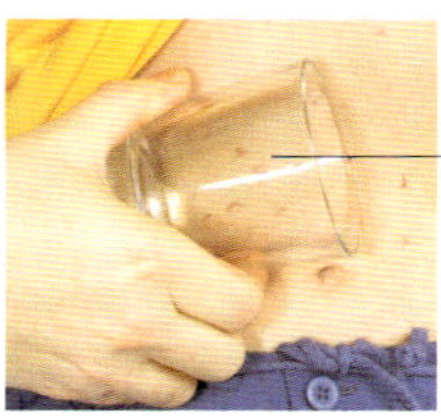

Meningitis rash will remain visible if you press a glass against it

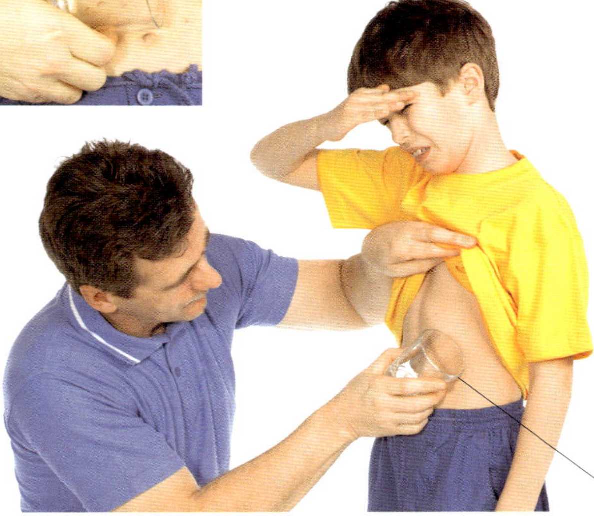

Press side of a glass against the rash

2 Treat fever. Give him plenty of fluids to drink and the recommended dose of acetaminophen or ibuprofen syrup (not aspirin). Check your child's body for signs of a rash. If you see any spots, press a glass gently against them. If you can still see the spots through the glass,

SEEK MEDICAL ADVICE

IMPORTANT

- If there is any delay contacting medical advice, or if you are concerned about your child's condition, TAKE YOUR CHILD TO THE HOSPITAL or CALL 911 even if you have already seen a doctor.
- In some cases, the rash may not develop, or if it does, it will be one of the last symptoms to appear.

see also

- Febrile seizures, *p.96*
- Fever, *opposite*

Febrile seizures

Young children may develop these seizures when they have a high temperature. Suspect a febrile seizure if your child has a fever and is having a seizure: she is shaking vigorously; flushed and sweating with a very hot forehead; eyes are rolled upward, fixed, or squinting; she is holding her breath and her face looks blue; she is clenching her fists.

IMPORTANT

- **Do not** hold her down or try to move her during the seizure.
- **If** a child becomes unresponsive, check breathing. If breathing, place in the recovery position; if not, begin CPR immediately. CALL 911 OR YOUR LOCAL EMS.

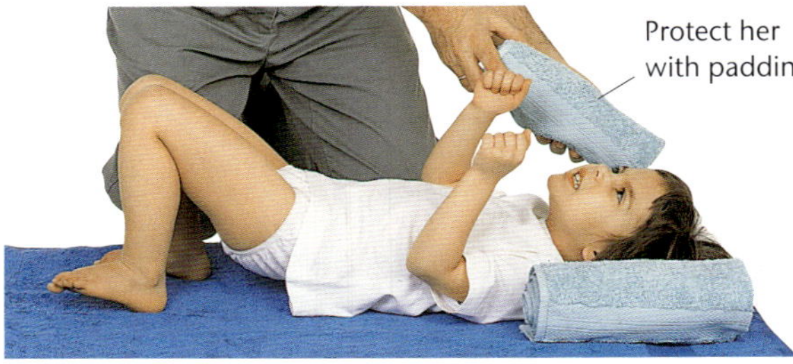

1 Place soft padding, such as towels or pillows, around your child so that even violent movement will not lead to injury.

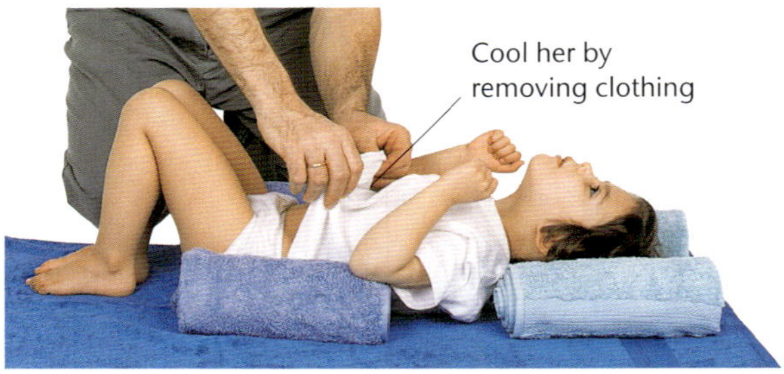

2 Undress your child to help cool her down. Make sure there is a good supply of cool fresh air, but be careful not to overcool her.

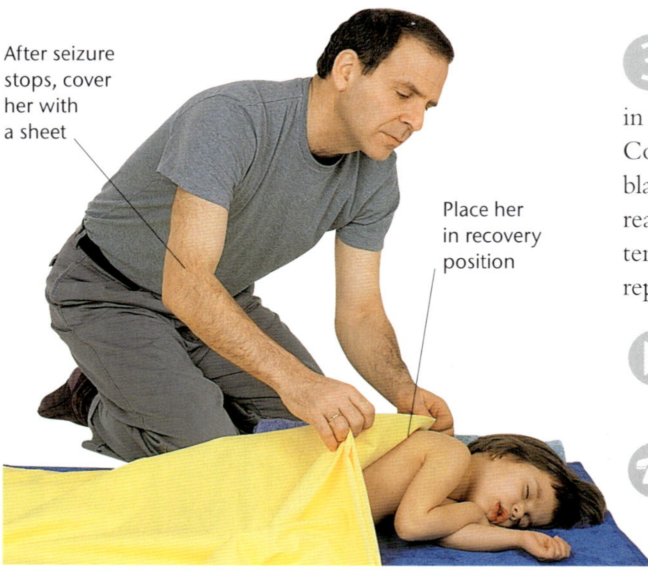

3 When the seizure stops, place her in the recovery position. Cover her with a light blanket or sheet and reassure her. If her temperature rises again, repeat steps 1 and 2.

TAKE YOUR CHILD TO THE HOSPITAL

OR

CALL 911 OR YOUR LOCAL EMS

see also

- Fever, *p.94*
- Unresponsive baby, *pp.19–21*
- Unresponsive child, *pp.22–27*

Epileptic seizures

These are caused by a disturbance in the electrical activity of the brain. A seizure may progress through stages: sudden loss of responsiveness, sometimes with a cry; rigidity and arching of back; breathing may cease; jerking or vigorous shaking movements begin; froth or bubbles appear at the mouth, possibly blood stained; loss of bladder or bowel control. The child will be responsive again within a few minutes and appear dazed. Afterward she may fall into a deep sleep.

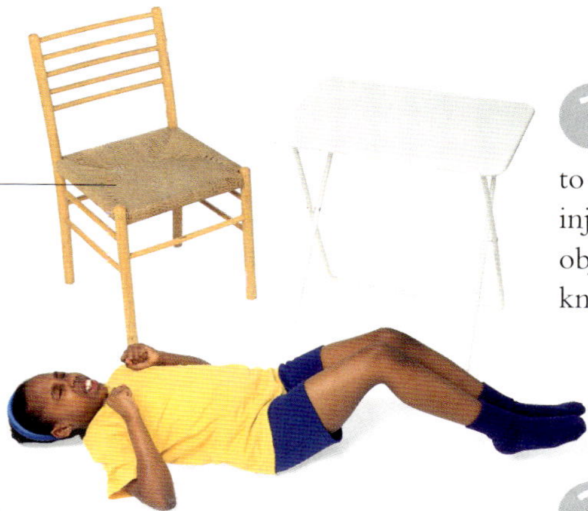

1. If your child starts to fall, help her to the floor. Prevent injury by clearing away objects that she may knock against.

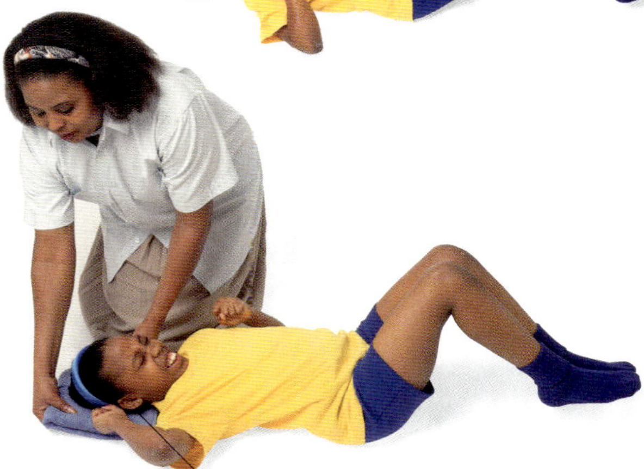

2. Place padding under or around her head to prevent injury.

3. When her seizure is over, your child may become unresponsive. Remove any padding and open her airway and check breathing.

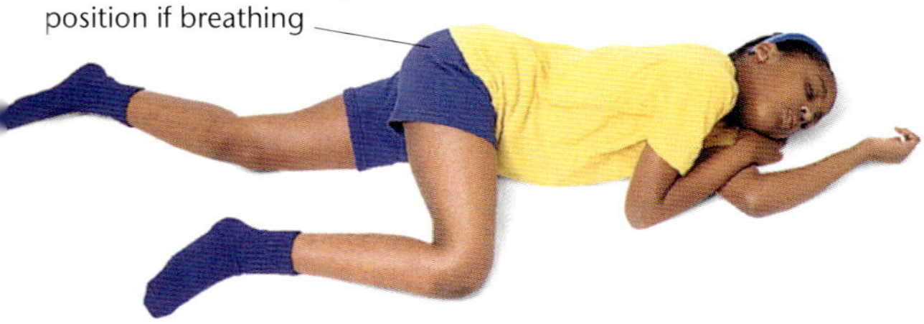

4. If she is breathing, place her in the recovery position. Stay with her until she is fully recovered. She may feel dazed and behave oddly, or sleep deeply.

SEEK MEDICAL ADVICE

IMPORTANT

- **Do not** hold her down or try to move her during the seizure.
- **Do not** put anything in her mouth or give her anything to eat or drink.
- **Look** for a card or bracelet alerting you to the fact that a child has a history of epilepsy.
- **If** your child has never had a seizure before, it lasts more than 5 minutes, she has repeated seizures, or if she is unresponsive for more than 10 minutes, CALL 911 OR YOUR LOCAL EMS.

Absence seizures

These seizures can be recognized by a momentary "switching off," some facial twitching, or distracted movements such as lip-smacking. If this happens, reassure the child and seek medical advice.

see also

- Unresponsive baby, *pp.19–21*
- Unresponsive child, *pp.22–27*

IMPORTANT

- **If** vomiting is prolonged, your child may need to be treated with oral rehydration solutions. SEEK MEDICAL ADVICE.
- **Do not** give your child antidiarrheal medication.

Vomiting and diarrhea

A baby or child who is suffering repeated vomiting and/or diarrhea can become dehydrated very quickly. It is important to replace lost fluids by giving your child sips of water. Don't give a baby or child milk unless you are breastfeeding.

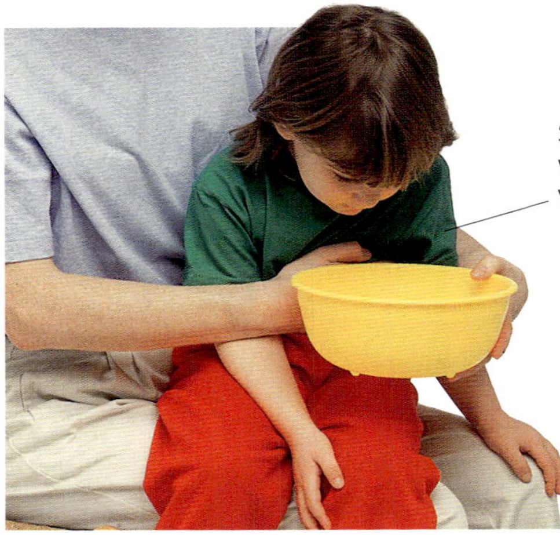
Support her while she vomits

1. If your child is vomiting, hold her over a bowl. Support her upper body with your free hand while she vomits. Reassure her.

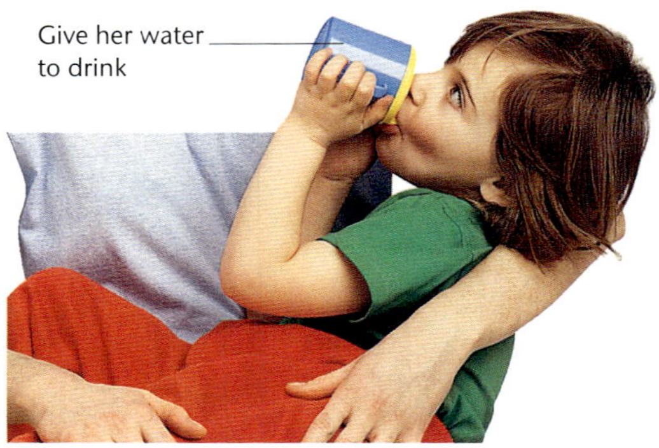
Give her water to drink

2. Give her drinks of water, juice, or oral rehydration solution to replace any fluid loss and to remove the unpleasant taste. Encourage her to sip each drink slowly.

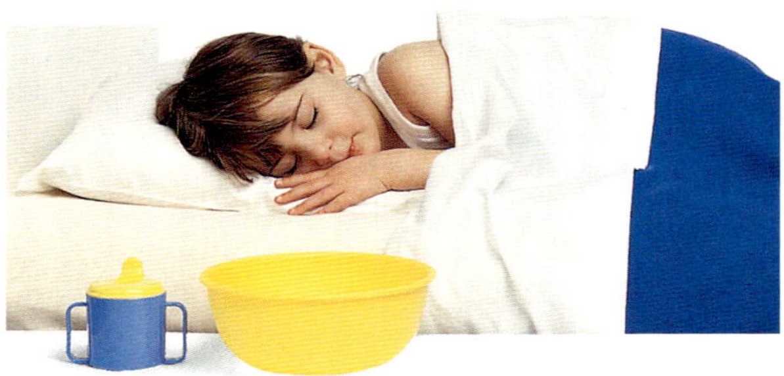

3. Let her rest quietly, in bed if she wants to. Make sure the bowl is still at hand in case she vomits again, and give a fresh drink of water. When she is hungry again, offer easily digested foods such as pasta, bread, or potatoes in the first 24 hours.

Stomachache

This is generally caused by a stomach upset, gas, constipation, or even stress.

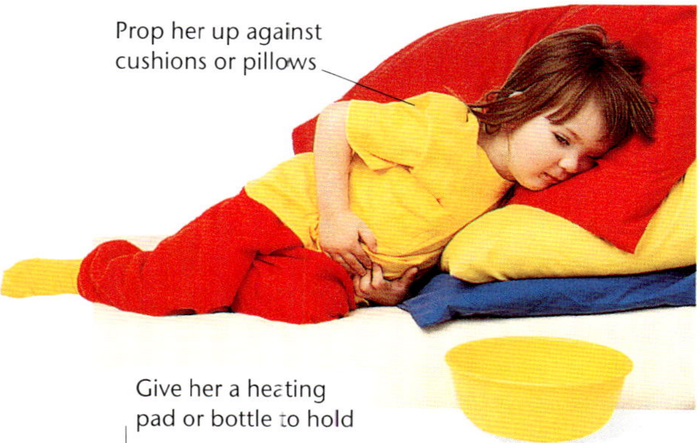

1 Make your child comfortable on a sofa or bed. Help her lie back against cushions or pillows. She may want to vomit, so leave a bowl near her.

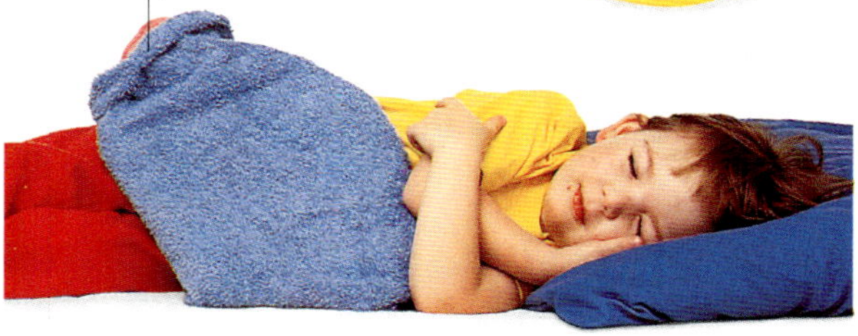

2 Warmth may help relieve the pain. Give your child a heating pad to hold against her stomach. Avoid giving her anything to eat until pain subsides.

IMPORTANT

- **If** the pain is severe, or does not subside after 30 minutes and/or is accompanied by fever and vomiting, TAKE YOUR CHILD TO THE HOSPITAL or CALL 911.
- **If** your child has been hit in the stomach, sit her down and loosen the clothing around her waist. The pain should ease quickly. If you are in any doubt, SEEK MEDICAL ADVICE.

Appendicitis

Suspect appendicitis if your child complains of pain in the middle of his abdomen or of acute pain either starting or settling in the right lower abdomen. He may also have a raised temperature, no appetite, nausea, and vomiting.

Suspected appendicitis must be treated promptly. Help your child lie down. Do not give him anything to eat or drink because he may need an anesthetic.

SEEK MEDICAL ADVICE

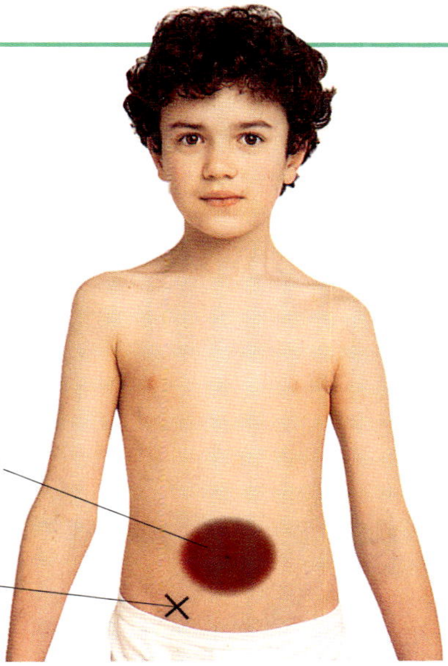

IMPORTANT

- **If** pain does not begin to subside, or if there is a discharge from the ear, fever, or hearing loss, SEEK MEDICAL ADVICE.

Pressure-change earache

This may happen on plane trips, particularly when taking off or landing, or when travelling through tunnels. To make the ears "pop" so that the pressure is relieved, an older child should be encouraged to chew gum or swallow several times. Sucking a piece of hard candy may also help.

Earache

This is most commonly caused by fluid in the ear or an ear infection following a cold or flu. Earache can also be the result of a child putting something in her ear.

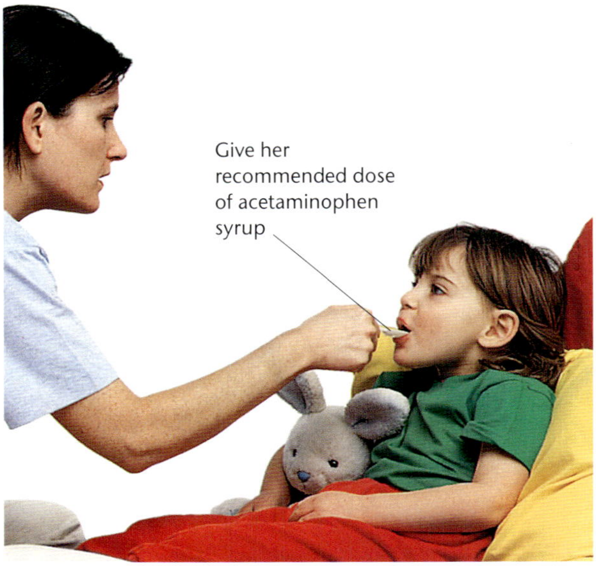

1. Make your child comfortable. Help her sit up supported by pillows or cushions if lying down makes the earache worse. You can give the recommended dose of acetaminophen syrup or ibuprofen (not aspirin). Never give aspirin to anyone under the age of 16 years.

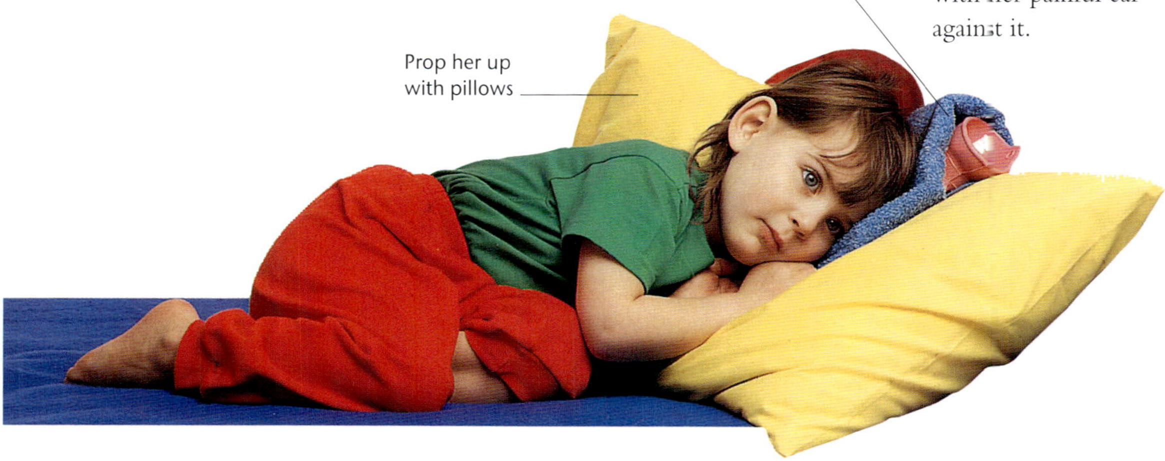
Provide a covered hot water bottle to place against her ear
Prop her up with pillows

2. Applying heat may help soothe the pain. Prepare a covered hot water bottle and tell your child to lie down with her painful ear against it.

Toothache

A toddler who complains of toothache may have a new tooth coming through. An older child may have tooth decay or an infection.

IMPORTANT

- **If** jaw is swollen and pain is severe or there is a fever, SEEK DENTAL ADVICE.

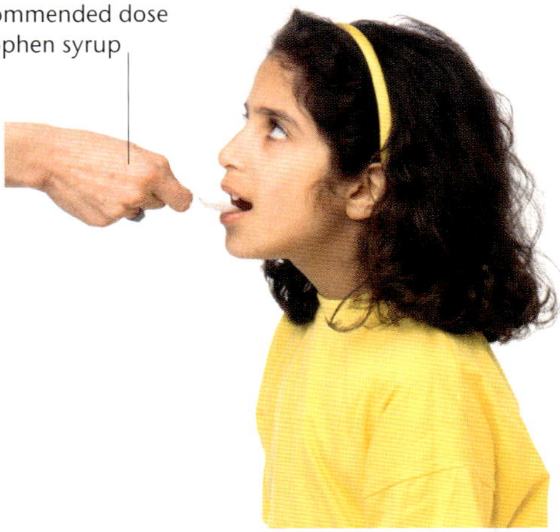

Give her recommended dose of acetaminophen syrup

1. Give your child the recommended dose of acetaminophen or ibuprofen syrup (not aspirin) to relieve the pain. Never give asprin to anyone under the age of 16 years. Arrange an early appointment with your child's dentist if pain persists.

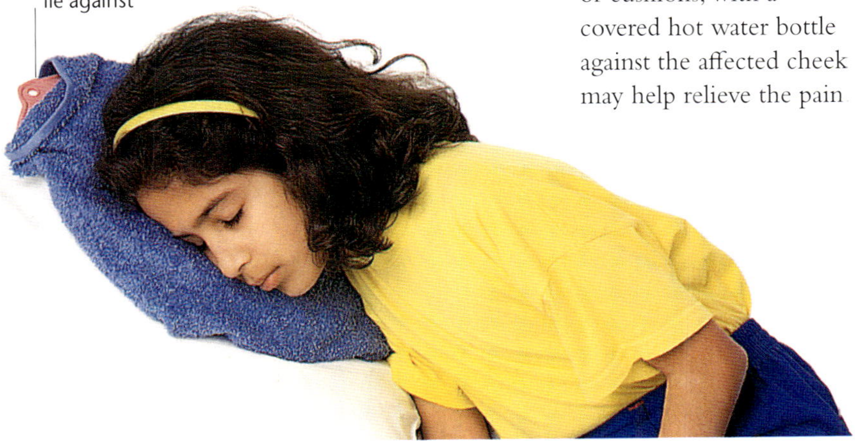

Give her a covered hot water bottle to lie against

2. Lying flat, or propped on pillows or cushions, with a covered hot water bottle against the affected cheek may help relieve the pain

A well-stocked first aid kit

- Disposable gloves (choose latex free)
- Small and large roller bandages
- Tube-gauze bandage
- Blunt-ended scissors
- Plastic tweezers
- Pack of gauze swabs
- Triangular bandages
- Tape for securing dressing pads and bandages—ideally hypoallergenic
- Sterile nonadhesive pads
- Adhesive bandages
- Sterile dressings
- Sterile or bottled water

First aid kit

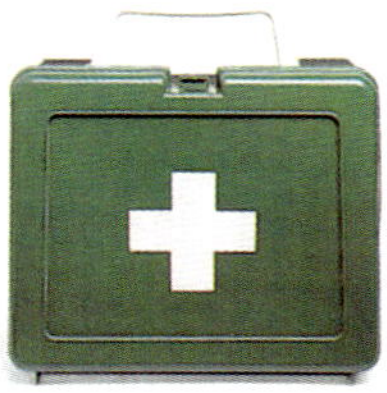

Keep first aid kits in your car and in your home. You can buy kits already made up. You may want to add extra dressings and bandages or specialized adhesive bandages—blister bandages, for example. Make sure the first aid box is readily accessible and easy to identify, and check the contents regularly. Do not keep medicines in the same box; they should be locked in a medicine cabinet. A well-stocked kit might contain the articles shown here. *See p.108* for alternative household items.

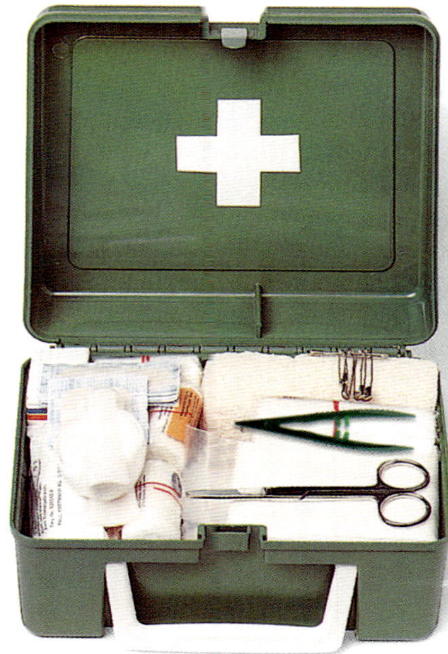

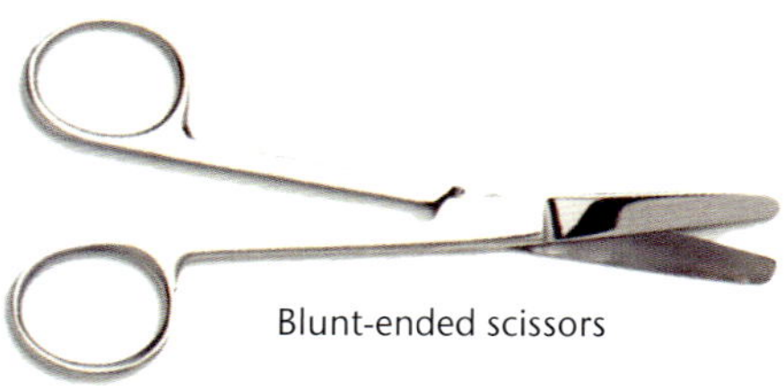

Blunt-ended scissors

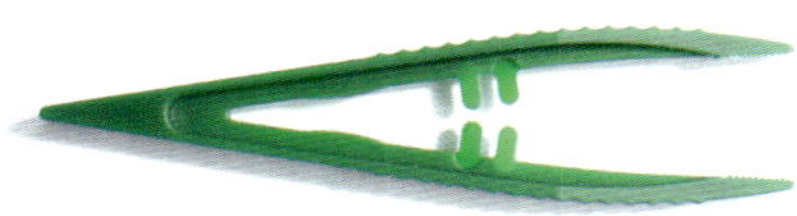

Plastic tweezers

Dressings

Adhesive bandages (dressings) are used for minor wounds. Keep several different sizes and shapes, including a selection of larger sterile dressings for more serious wounds.

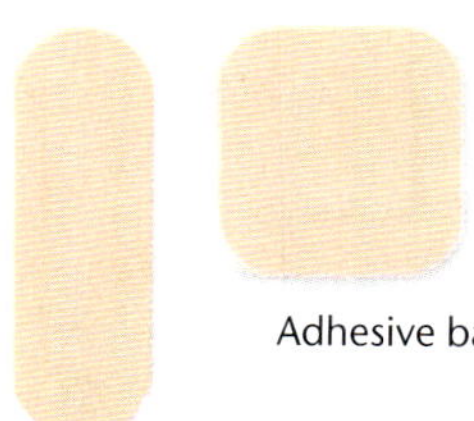

Adhesive bandages

Gauze swabs

Sterile nonadhesive pad

Sterile dressing with bandage attached

Bandages

Keep a variety of bandages to secure dressings and support injured joints. Conforming bandages shape themselves to the contours of the body and so are easy to use. Triangular bandages can be used as slings and for broad- and narrow-fold bandages.

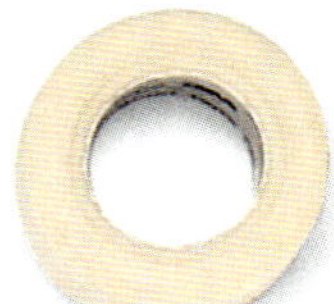

Tape for securing dressings

Large conforming bandage

Small conforming bandage

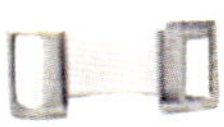

Bandage clip

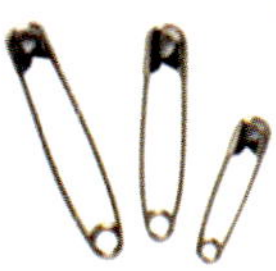

Safety pins for securing bandages

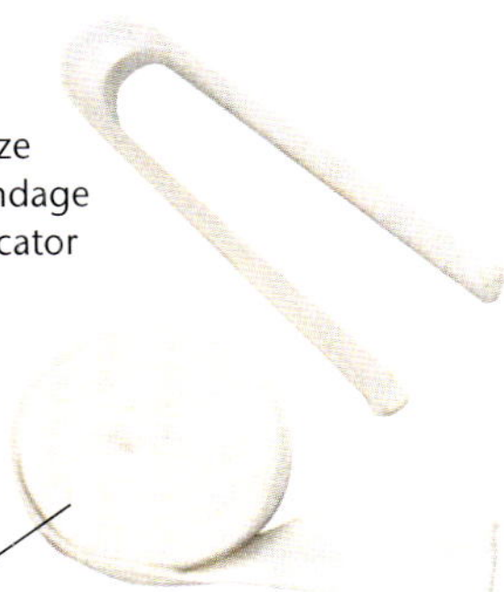

Tube-gauze finger bandage and applicator

Bandage slides over applicator

Folded triangular bandage

Additional useful equipment

- If you have a notepad and pen or pencil, you can write down important information about a child's condition to give to the emergency services personnel.
- Keep a flashlight beside your home first aid kit (for use in the event of a power failure), and in your car; check the batteries regularly.
- Plastic face shields or face masks can protect you and a child from cross-infection when you are giving rescue breaths.
- Keep a plastic or foil emergency survival blanket or bag in your car.
- Always carry a warning triangle in your car and place it in the road behind the car in the event of a breakdown or crash.

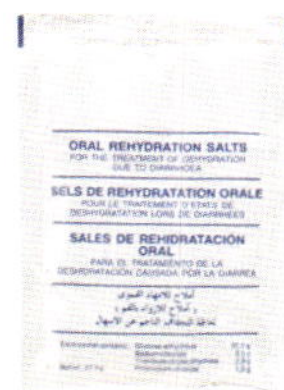

ORAL REHYDRATION SALTS

Packets of rehydration salts are added to water. Use them to treat dehydration resulting from heat exhaustion or vomiting.

INSTANT ICE PACKS

Keep a pack of these in the car—they are especially useful when you do not have access to a freezer.

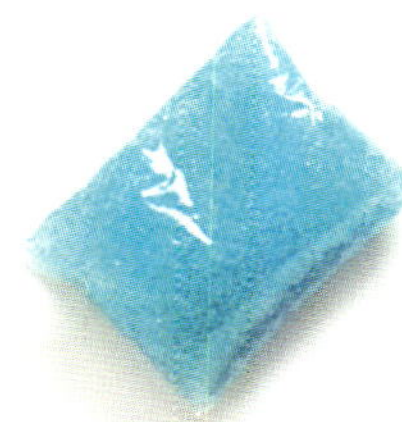

Digital thermometer

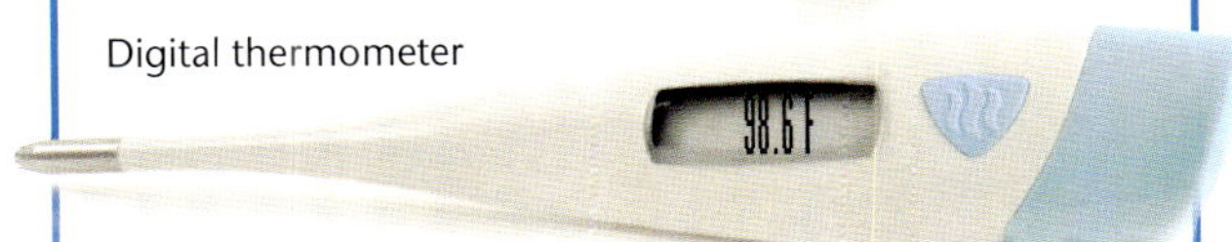

Ear thermometer

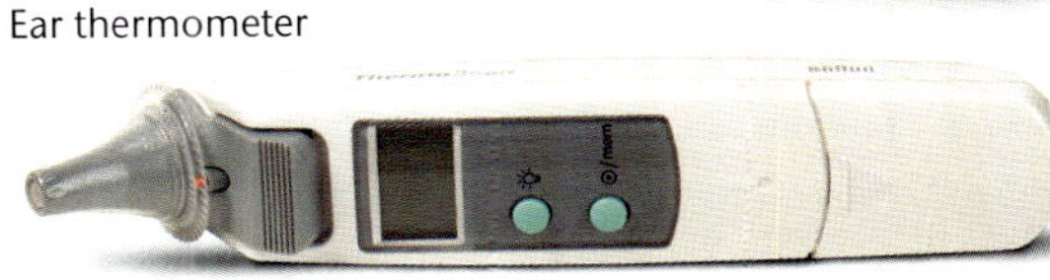

THERMOMETER

Choose one with an easy-to-read screen. Check the battery regularly.

Dressings

Covering a wound helps the blood-clotting process and prevents infection. Dressings should not be fluffy and must be large enough to cover the wound and area around it. Wash your hands before applying dressings and wear disposable gloves if possible. If blood soaks through a dressing, place another on top. Make sure bandages are not too tight (*see opposite*).

Adhesive bandages

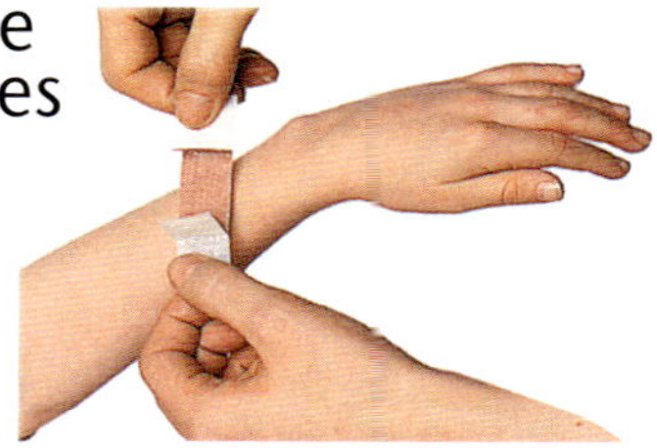

Remove wrapping and, holding the pad over the wound, peel back the protective strips. Press the ends and edges down.

Sterile pad

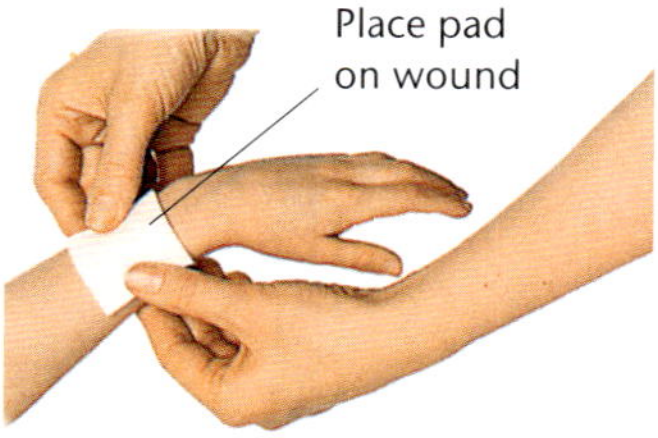

1 Place the dressing pad shiny side down directly over the child's wound.

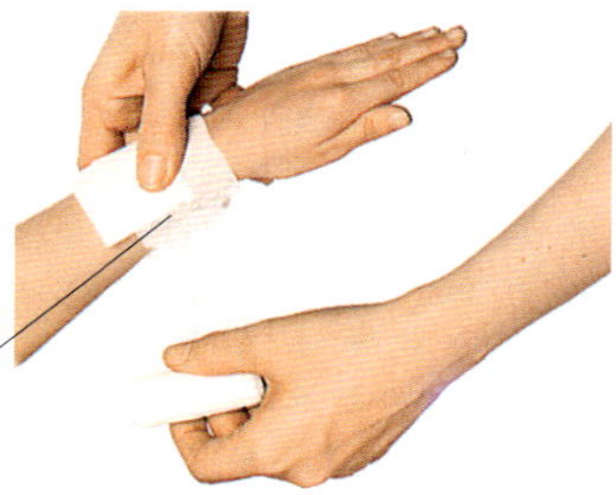

2 Secure the pad with a bandage, working from below the injury up the limb.

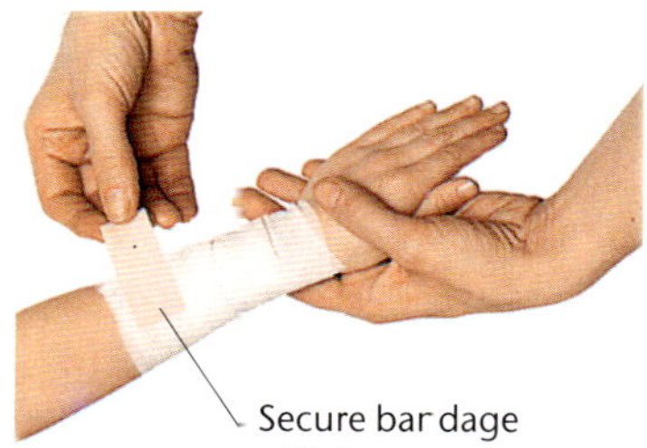

3 Secure the end of the bandage with strips of medical tape.

Sterile dressing with bandage

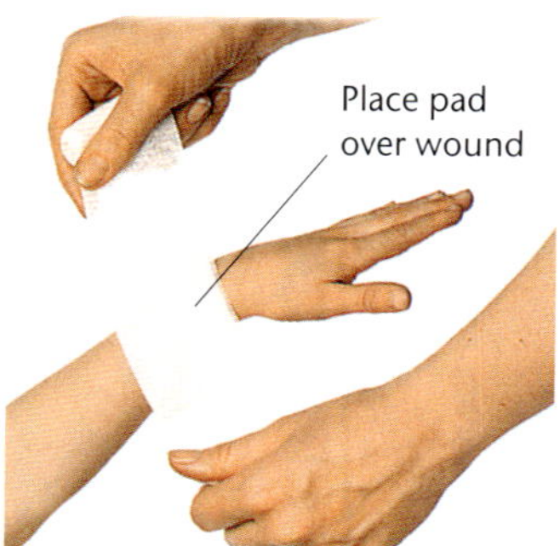

1 Hold the bandage on either side of the dressing pad and place the pad over the wound.

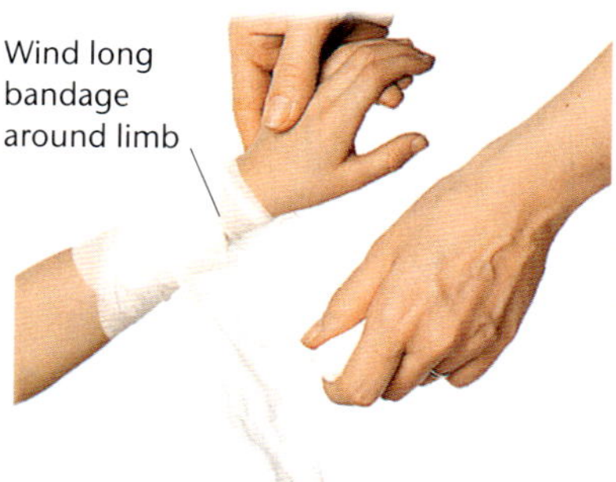

2 Leaving the short end hanging, wind the other end around the limb to cover dressing.

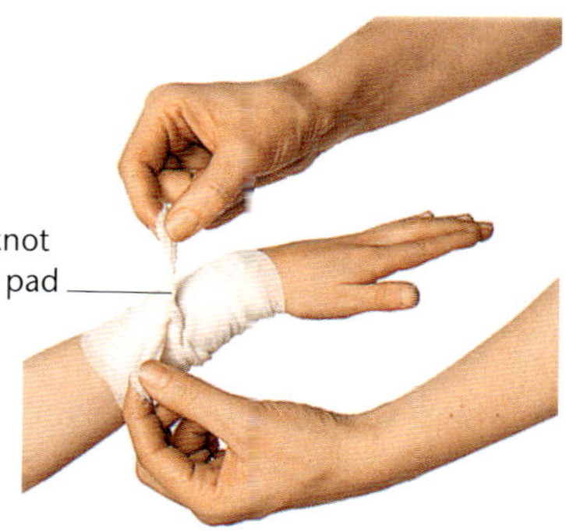

3 Tie the two ends of the bandage in a knot directly over the pad.

Bandaging

Use bandages to secure dressings, to help control bleeding, and to support injuries. Roller bandages can be used for any part of the body; conforming bandages are especially useful for bandaging joints or head wounds because they mold themselves to the shape of the body.

Check circulation

Do not apply a bandage too tightly—it will impair the circulation. To check, press on your child's nail or a patch of skin beyond the bandage, then release pressure. The colour should return rapidly. If it does not, loosen the bandages.

Roller bandage

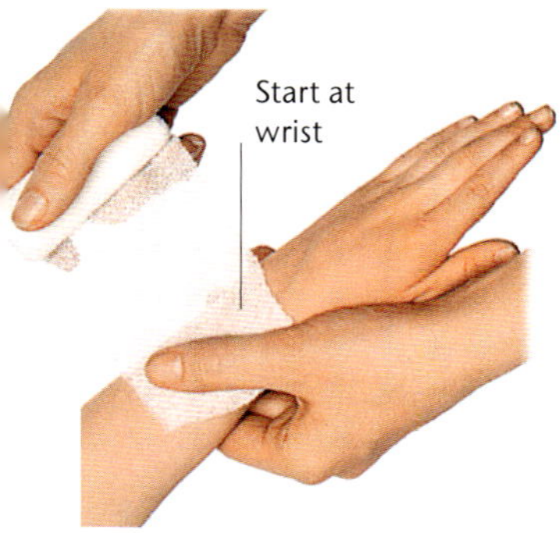

1 Place the end of the bandage on the arm below the injury and hold the bandage roll in your other hand.

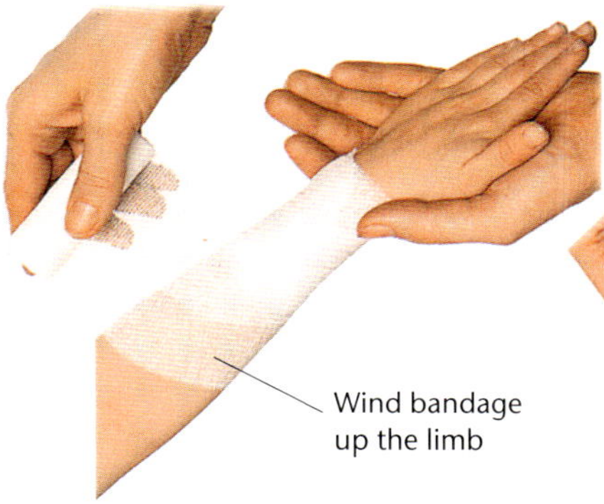

2 Still supporting the injured limb, wind the bandage around the arm, working up the limb. Stop above the injury.

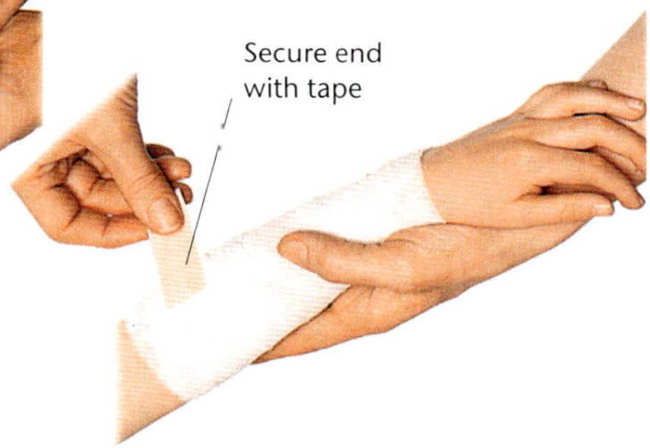

3 Wrap it around two more times to finish. Secure the end with tape. Check circulation in your child's fingers (*see above*).

Hand bandage

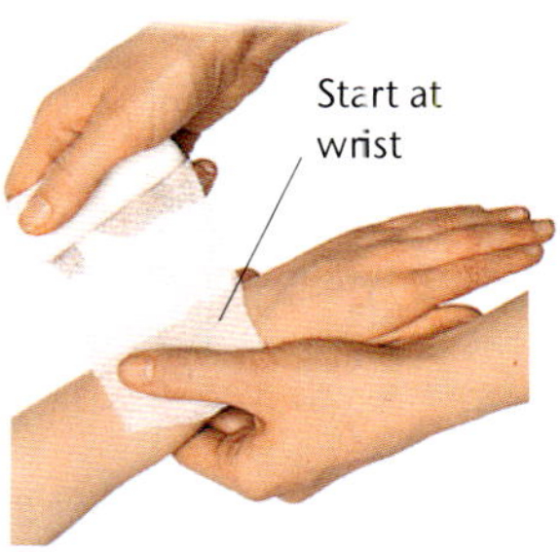

1 Supporting the injured hand, hold the end of the bandage on the wrist and make two straight turns around the wrist.

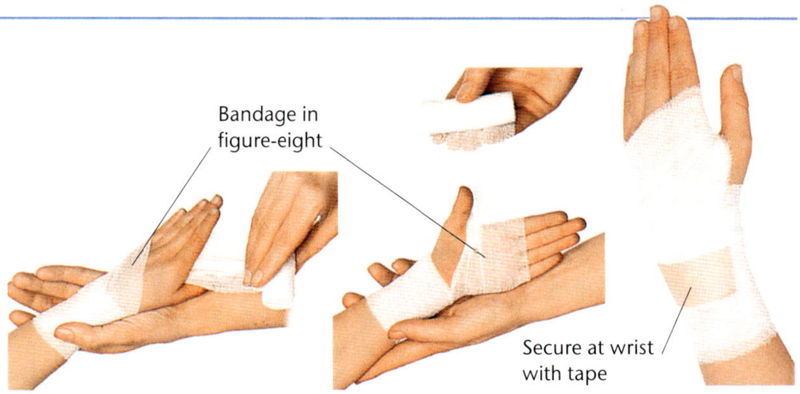

2 Take the bandage across the back of the hand to the base of the little finger. Then take it around the palm, up between the thumb and forefinger, and across the back of the hand to the wrist. Repeat the figure-eight to cover the hand. Check circulation.

Triangular bandages

These are sold singly in sterile packs or can be made from a square of strong fabric folded diagonally in half. Triangular bandages are used for broad-fold and narrow-fold bandages (*see p.65*) or slings. Arm slings support injured arms or wrists, or take weight off an injured shoulder. Elevation slings are used to support hand injuries to minimize bleeding, pain, or swelling.

Arm sling

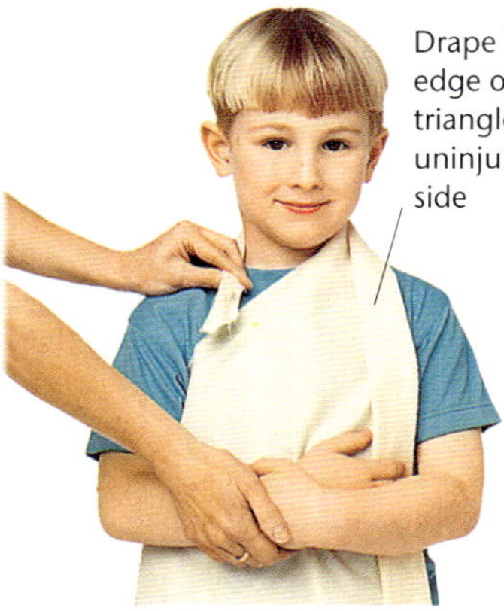

1 Place the bandage between your child's arm and chest, easing one end up around the back of his neck on the injured side.

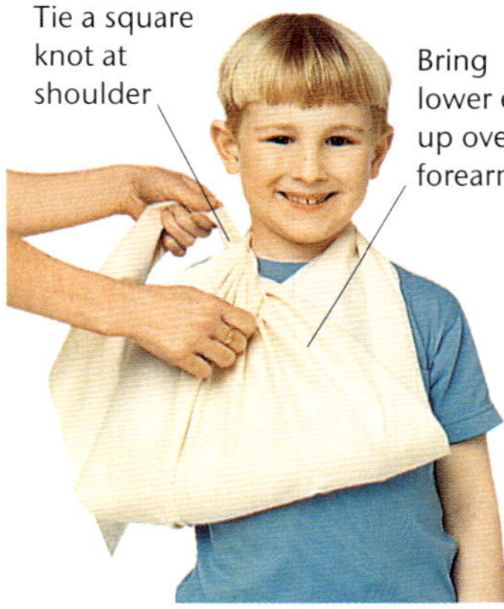

2 Take the lower end of the bandage up over your child's forearm to the end at the shoulder and tie a knot just below the shoulder.

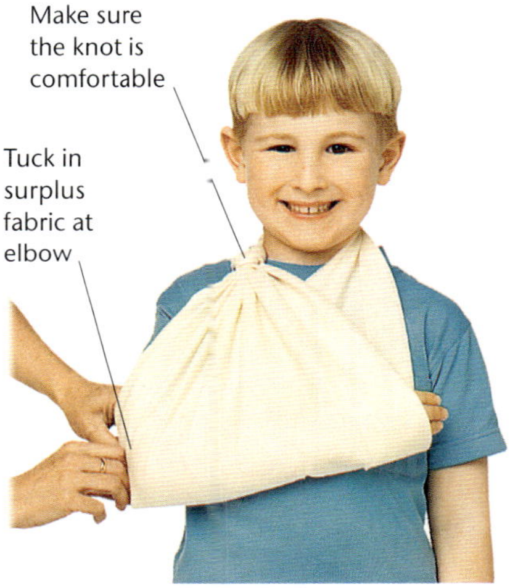

3 Fold in the surplus fabric at the corner near the elbow and pin it to the bandage.

Improvised slings

If your child injures her shoulder, arm, or hand, you can make an improvised sling to support the injury until she receives medical treatment.

- Undo a coat or shirt button and tuck the hand of the injured arm inside the fastening, but don't use this method if the child's forearm or wrist is injured.
- Pin your child's sleeve up on the opposite side of his chest.

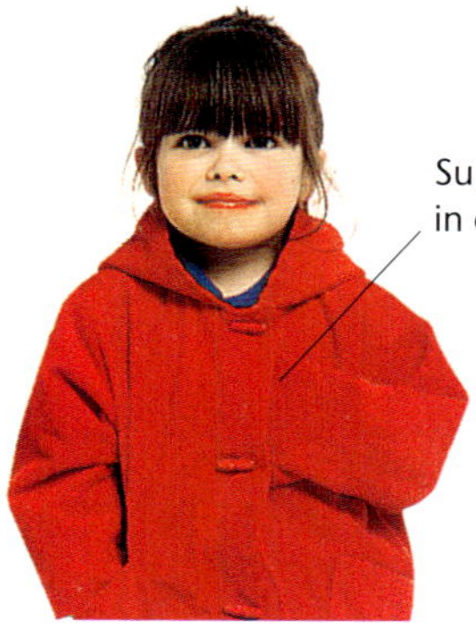

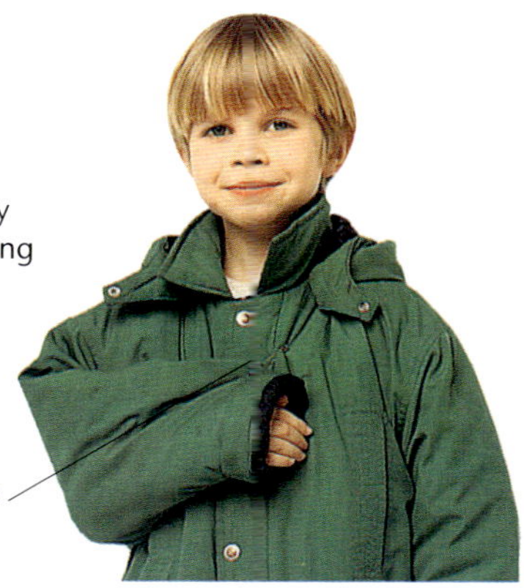

Elevation sling

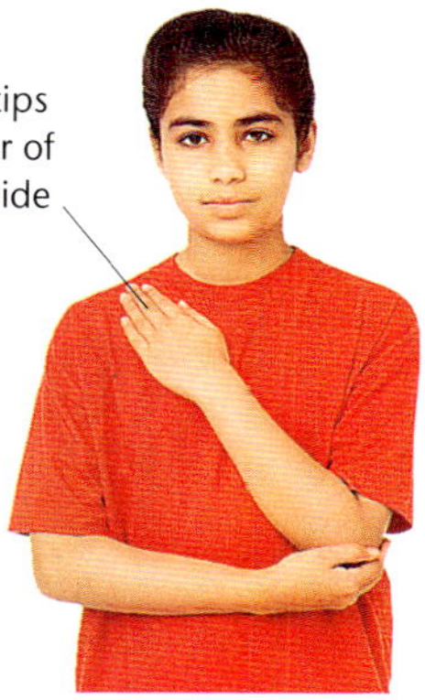

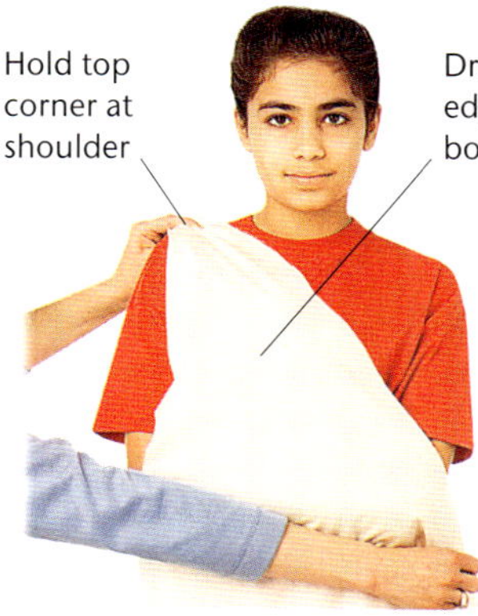

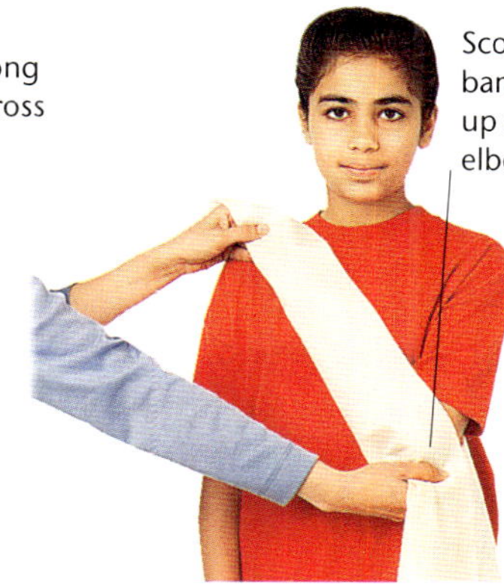

1. Bring the arm on the injured side across your child's chest. Ask her to support her elbow.

2. Lay bandage over child's arm, with longest edge on the uninjured side. Hold the top corner.

3. Support the child's arm and fold long edge of bandage in under injured arm.

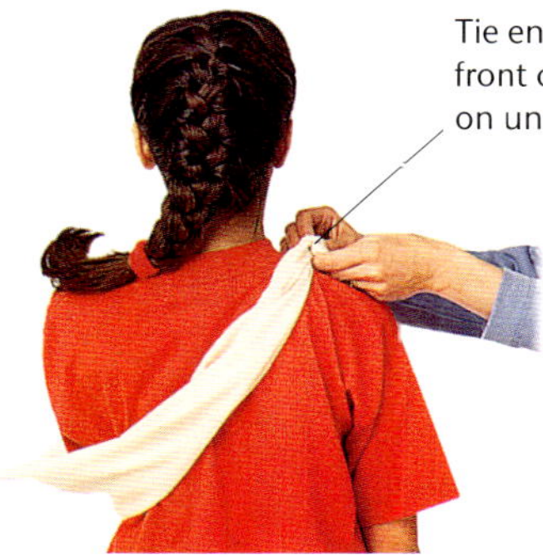

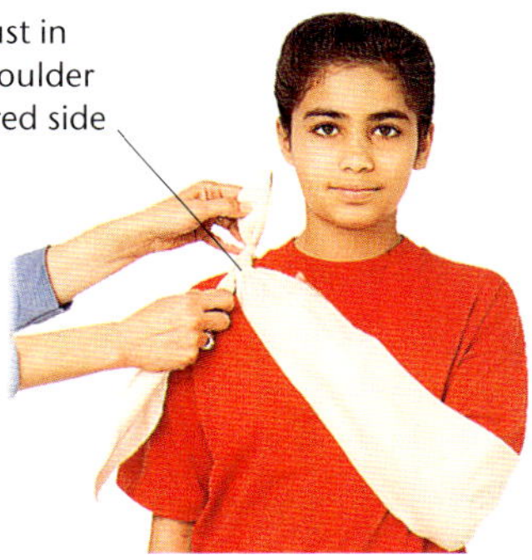

4. Bring the lower end up around her back, holding the elbow securely in the fabric. Tie a knot just below the shoulder and tuck the ends in.

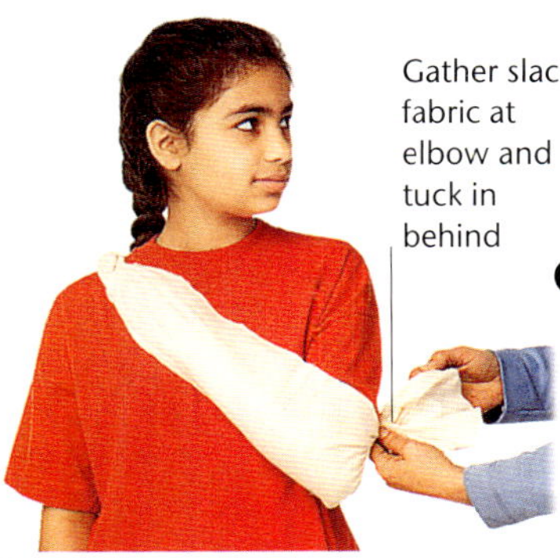

OR

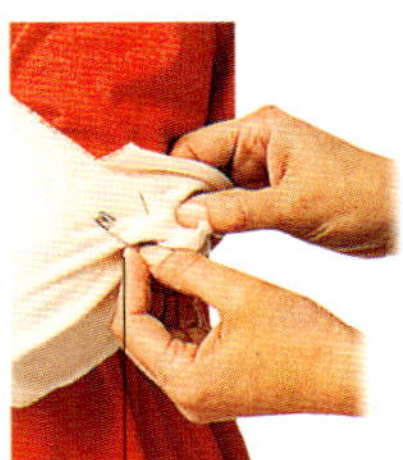

5. Secure the sling by twisting the excess fabric and tucking it in at the elbow or fold and pin in place.

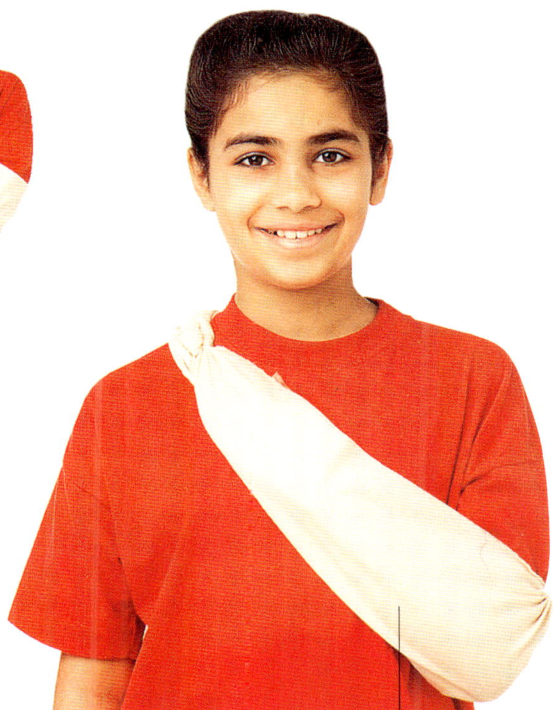

Finished sling raises, immobilizes, and supports the injury.

Useful household items

You should keep a well-stocked first aid kit (*see p.102*) both at home and in the car. However, there are many everyday items around the home that are invaluable for first aid emergencies.

- Plastic credit cards can be used to scrape off an insect stinger (*see p.80*).
- A dish towel can be used as a pad to control bleeding or as an improvised dressing or to secure a dressing.
- Use vinegar to treat a jellyfish sting (*see p.82*)—it prevents the envenomation from getting worse and prevents pain from worsening.
- Cool or lukewarm water can be used to cool a burn if running water is not available (*see p.52*).
- Milk stops a knocked-out permanent tooth from drying out while you get the child to a dentist (*see p.47*).
- Use a thick book or wooden box as insulation when dealing with electrical injury (*see p.12*).

Making a cold pack

- Bags of frozen vegetables or fruit such as peas, corn, or blueberries make ideal ice packs because the bags mold to the shape of the body and stay cool for a long time. Wrap it in cloth before putting on your child for up to 20 minutes.
- Fill a sandwich or freezer bag two-thirds full of ice, then seal the bag; wrap it in cloth before putting on your child for 20 minutes.
- Soak a washcloth in cold water, wring out excess water, then place it over the injury for 20 minutes.

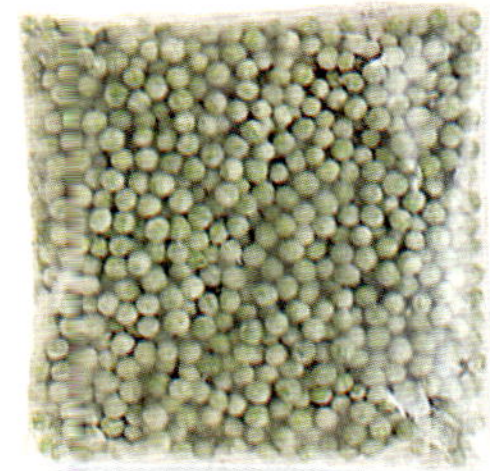

Frozen peas in a plastic bag

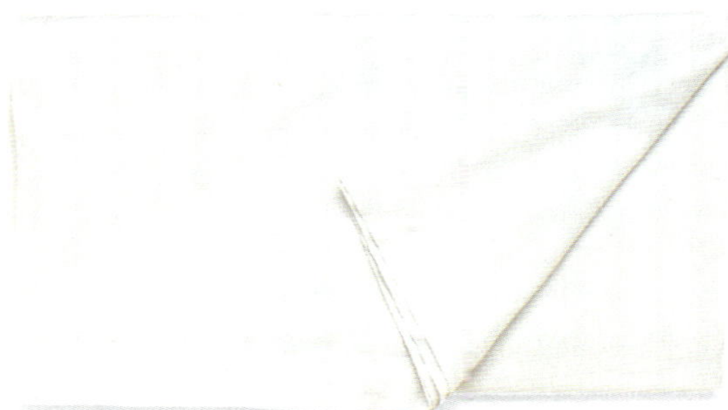

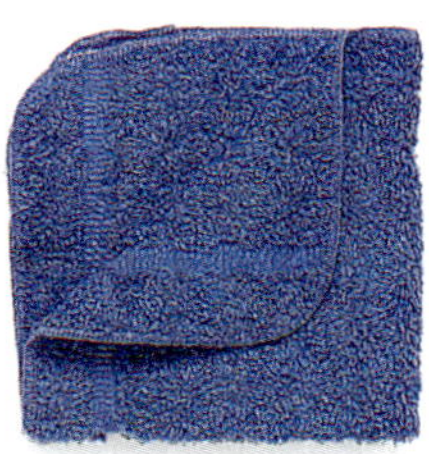

WASHCLOTH

Use a washcloth soaked in cold water to make a cold pack as well as to clean up a child after an incident.

SHEETS AND PILLOWCASES

A clean cotton sheet or pillowcase makes an excellent loose protective covering for burns.

PLASTIC BAGS

A clean plastic bag can be put over a burned foot or hand and lightly secured with bandages or tape. Always cool the burn first.

PLASTIC WRAP

Cover cooled burns with plastic wrap to protect from infection.

Safety at home

Most incidents occur at home; many are preventable if you:

- Plan the layout and position of objects and furniture at home with child safety in mind.
- Make sure that all windows are closed or inaccessible (don't leave chairs beside them).
- Never confuse containers by putting a dangerous substance, such as paint thinner, in a bottle that used to contain a harmless drink.
- Install smoke alarms, carbon monoxide alarms, fire guards, and safety gates in your home.
- Never pretend that medicines and pills are special candies to encourage a child to take medication. Keep all medicines locked away.
- Check for hazards when visiting friends and ask if you can move sharp or breakable objects.
- Teach your child basic safety rules.
- List important numbers, such as your doctor, local EMS, and Poison Control Centre, beside every phone.

Fire

If fire breaks out at home, it could be a matter of minutes before smoke overcomes you.

- Install smoke alarms throughout your home. If your home is on one level, install a detector between the living room and the bedrooms. If your house has two or more levels, install detectors at the foot of the stairs and on every floor outside the bedrooms; ideally they should be linked. If you live in an apartment building, there should be detectors in all communal areas too.
- Test smoke alarms regularly; replace batteries if they have them.
- Have an escape plan (*see p. 11*). Make sure the whole family knows what to do if there is a fire, especially at night. Practise the fire drill with your children: shout "fire"; tell everyone to drop to the floor if there is smoke and crawl to the nearest exit from the rooms; shut each door behind you; arrange a meeting point outside where everyone should wait together. Don't go back for pets or treasured possessions.

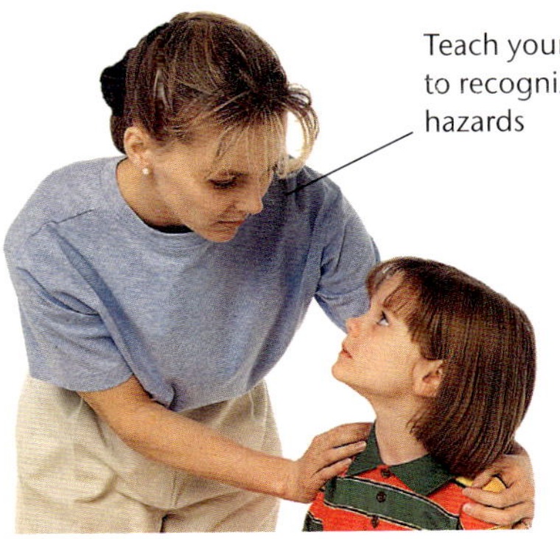

Teach your child to recognize hazards

Electricity

Protect your child from electric shock (*see p. 12*) or fire caused by electric shorts.

- Cover outlets—put heavy furniture in front of them and cover unused outlets with plastic safety plugs.
- Use bar-type fused adaptors with surge protectors on extension cords instead of block-type socket adaptors.
- Know where your electrical panel/fuse box is located, and how to reset breakers/change fuses in case one blows.
- Replace worn or damaged electrical cords.
- Coil trailing wires to prevent tripping hazards.
- Unplug electrical appliances at night, particularly heaters and hairdryers.
- Keep power tools out of the reach of children.

Gas

Fit carbon monoxide alarms and have all boilers and gas appliances serviced regularly. Find out where your main gas valve is in case there is a leak. If you smell gas, call 911 or the utility company:

- Don't turn lights or electric switches on or off—there may be a spark, which can cause an explosion.
- Don't light matches or cigarettes.
- Turn off the main gas valve and open the windows.

Hall and stairs

The staircase is not a safe place for your child to play (*see below*).

- Make sure that toys are not left on the stairs for you to trip over.
- Put a light in your hall or on the landing so that your child can see if he gets up at night. If you don't want the area too light, use a low-watt bulb. Never cover a lamp with a cloth because the cloth can easily catch fire.
- Don't let your child play on the landings or stairs of communal areas because the banisters may have large gaps between them.

Front and back doors

- Never leave your front door open.
- Don't let your child answer the door.
- Put the door latch out of reach of small children. If your toddler can reach the latch, install an additional bolt higher up the door and keep the door bolted.
- If the door has a dead-bolt that needs a key to open, make sure that the key is accessible to adults and older children so that they can escape if there's a fire.
- Install tempered or laminated glass in doors that have glass within 80 cm (2ft 8in) of the floor. If this is not possible, put plastic safety film over it to prevent the glass from splintering if it is broken. Put stickers over the glass to make it more noticeable, especially for young children.

Floors

Tiled, polished, laminated, or rug-covered floors can be very slippery for toddlers and running children.

- Put nonslip liners under rugs.
- Keep hall floors free of toys and clutter.
- Check carpeting regularly for holes or loose carpet that might trip you or your toddler.

Stairs

A child is not coordinated enough to be able to walk downstairs safely until he is at least three years old.

- Fit safety gates at the foot of the stairs and across the upper landing or across your child's bedroom doorway (safety gates at the top of the stairs can be a trip hazard). The bars must be no more than 5.5 cm (2⅜in) apart, and avoid stair gates that open leaving a bar across the base because they are a trip hazard. Always open the gate; never climb over it; your child will copy you.
- Check your banisters regularly: the handrail and posts should be secured. Posts should not be too far apart—anything wider than 6.5 cm (2½in) apart should be boarded up. Don't let your child climb banisters. If the stairs or landing has horizontal rails (so-called ranch-type banisters), they should be boarded up because it is very easy for a child to climb them.
- Replace loose or worn carpet on steps. They are trip hazards.

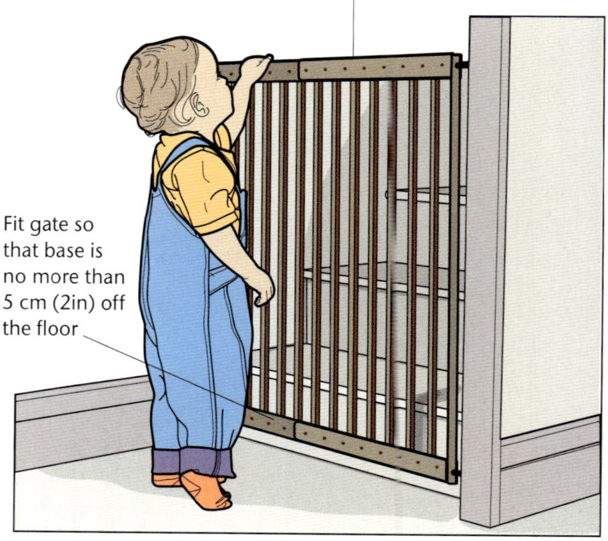
Keep the safety gate closed at all times
Fit gate so that base is no more than 5 cm (2in) off the floor

Living room or family room

While your children are very young, try to arrange the room so that both children and your valuables are kept out of harm's way.

- If you have a balcony, ensure that the railing is too high for your child to climb. Block gaps in the railings with high-density fibreboard.
- Install safety glass in patio doors if the glass is within 80 cm (2ft 8in) of the floor.

Carpets and curtains

- Check that there are no areas of carpet or rug that have holes or turned-up edges; either you or your child could trip.
- Wind up and tuck away all curtain ties and pull cords for blinds. Children can be strangled if they get caught in dangling cords.

Fireplaces and heaters

- Don't leave matches or lighters where your child can reach them.
- Cover all fires with a fireplace screen. Attach it to the wall to prevent your child from pulling it over. Also consider surrounding the hearth with a baby gate.
- Use a spark guard as well as a screen for open solid-fuel fires as an additional precaution.

Electrical equipment

- Attach wiring to the baseboards.
- Run long electrical cords behind furniture so that your child can't trip or pull on them.
- Replace items with worn wires.
- If your TV is on a stand, ensure that it is secure and cannot be pulled over. Ideally attach the TV to the wall.

Surfaces and furniture

- Place houseplants out of reach of young children. Dispose of any poisonous plants. Some can scratch or produce allergic reactions if touched.
- Do not place breakable or heavy objects on low tables. Set them well back from the edges of surfaces such as windowsills or mantelpieces.
- Put protectors on all sharp table corners, especially glass ones.
- Don't leave hot drinks, alcohol, glasses, cigarettes, matches, or lighters on low surfaces, such as coffee tables, where your child can reach them.
- Never leave a cigarette burning in an ashtray.
- Make sure all sofas and armchairs have a fire safety label; old foam furniture is lethal in a fire.
- Keep alcohol, firearms, and ammunition in a locked cabinet or safe.

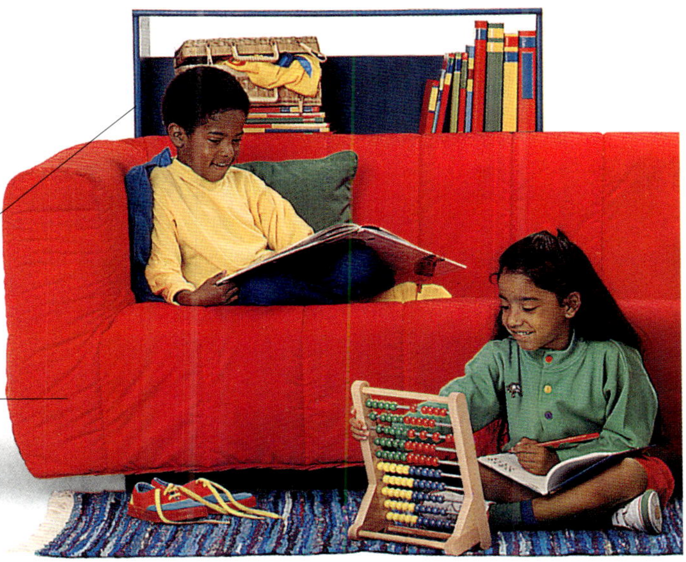

Ensure bookcases are secured to the wall

Sofas and armchairs must have fire-resistant fillings and coverings

Kitchen

This is the busiest part of your house, where you spend a lot of time with your children.

- Never hold a baby or child in your arms when you are cooking or carrying a hot drink.

Doors

- Fit safety glass to any glass panels. Cover glass panels within 80 cm (2ft 6in) of the floor with safety film, to keep glass from shattering or splintering if broken.
- Put some colourful stickers on the glass door panels to alert your child.

Floors

- Create a safe play area away from where you work. Don't let your child play between you and the work surface or anywhere you could trip over him.
- Avoid bumps and falls by wiping up spills immediately.
- Remove pet food bowls after use and keep that part of the floor scrupulously clean.
- Keep a box for storing toys and neatening clutter.

Garbage cans

- Discourage toddlers from rummaging in the garbage.
- Put sharp-edged cans and lids or broken glass straight into the outside garbage can.
- Keep the garbage can in a cabinet with a child-resistant safety catch.

IMPORTANT

- Keep a fire blanket in the kitchen for smothering flare-ups. If you want to buy a fire extinguisher, consult your local fire department to find out which is the most appropriate type. Check the fire extinguisher regularly. For more on fires, *see p.77* and *p.109*.

Babies in the kitchen

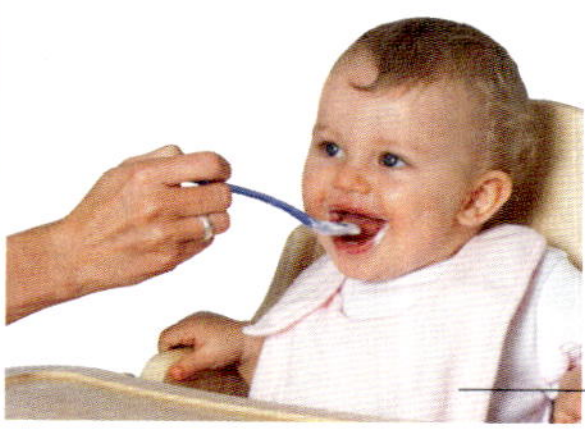

Stay with your child when he is eating in case he chokes

BOTTLES AND FOOD

- If your water is not safe due to microbes, sterilize all feeding equipment, or put it in a dishwasher.
- Don't leave a prepared feeding standing at room temperature, and don't keep the remains of the last feeding. Warmed and reheated feeds are breeding grounds for bacteria.
- Make fresh bottles for each feeding. Check the temperature before you feed your baby.

HIGHCHAIRS

- Always use the safety harness.
- Never leave the highchair where your baby can reach out and pull objects down from a surface.
- Never leave your child unattended in a highchair.

PLAY

- Put your baby in a playpen away from the cooking area, or put a gate across the doorway.
- Keep him out of range of any spills from the stovetop.

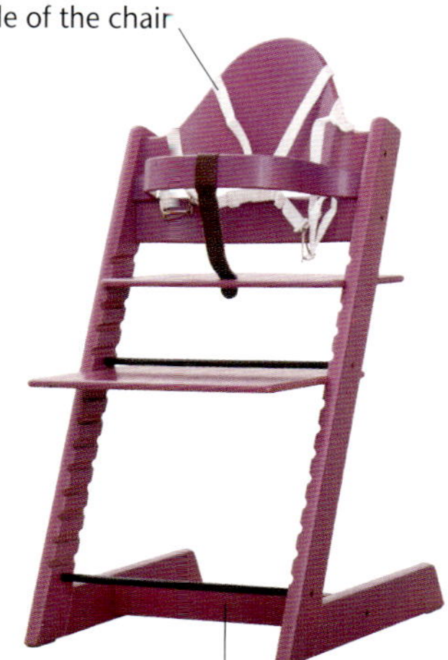

Attach a safety harness to the clips on either side of the chair

Choose a stable highchair with widely spaced legs

Tables and kitchen work surfaces

- Always be aware of your child's reach and keep all heavy, breakable, or sharp objects, or objects that could burn, well back from the edges of work surfaces.
- Keep stools or chairs away from tables and work surfaces so that a young child cannot climb up.
- Tuck cords of electric food processors, toasters, blenders, and irons out of reach. Choose appliances with short or retractable cords if possible. It is not only the electricity from these appliances that poses a hazard; they can also cause deep cuts, burns, and crush injuries if a child pulls them off the counter.
- Leave all electrical appliances unplugged when they are not in use.
- Avoid using a tablecloth. It is tempting for a crawling baby or toddler to use it to pull himself up, bringing anything on the table down upon his head. Use placemats instead, or secure the cloth.
- Do not put your baby on a table or work surface when he is in a car seat—he could easily bounce himself off.

Cabinets and drawers

- Put safety catches on cabinets and drawers, particularly those containing matches, lighters, knives, scissors, and utensils; heavy pots, pans, or china; dried food, such as lentils or pasta, which may be a choking hazard; bottles containing alcohol; medicines; cleaning materials, such as laundry soap or dishwasher detergent, even if fitted with "child-resistant" lids.

Refrigerators

Food poisoning can be caused by poor food storage. Take precautions to minimize risks:

- Keep cooked meat and poultry on a separate shelf from uncooked meat. Cover uncooked meat with plastic wrap.
- Don't store food in open cans; put leftovers into a clean container, cover, and put in the refrigerator.
- Check food regularly to see that nothing is kept beyond the "use-by" date.

Stovetops

Your child is obviously at risk of burns and scalds from hot oil or boiling water when you are preparing food.

- You can buy safety guards but remember that a child can still poke fingers through some types and be burned by hot burners.
- Always keep your child away from oven doors; they can get very hot while the oven is in use and will stay hot for some time afterward. A crawling baby or toddler is particularly at risk. Try to teach your child what "hot" means so that he understands a warning.
- Keep ignition devices, matches, and lighters well out of reach in a cabinet fitted with a safety catch.

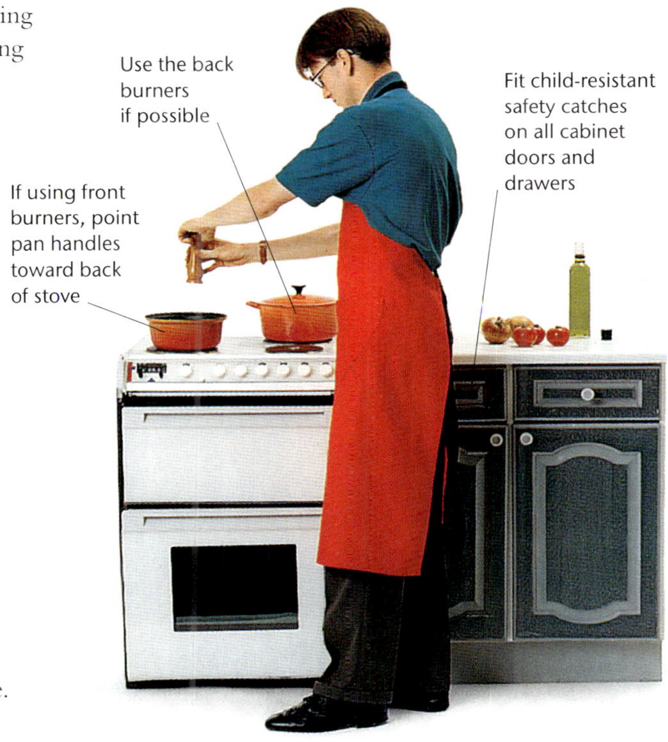
Use the back burners if possible
Fit child-resistant safety catches on all cabinet doors and drawers
If using front burners, point pan handles toward back of stove

Washers and dryers

- Keep small hands away from the glass door; it may get hot while the machine is on.
- Ensure that the door is closed when the machines are not in use. Your toddler may try to climb inside or even fill it with toys.

Bedrooms

The cabinets and drawers in bedrooms are always exciting places for toddlers and young children. Make sure any potentially hazardous items are out of reach because you may not always know when your child will decide to go exploring on his own.

Baby's cribs

- Make sure the crib is deep enough to prevent your baby from climbing out—at least 50 cm (1ft 8in) from the top of the mattress to the top of the crib.

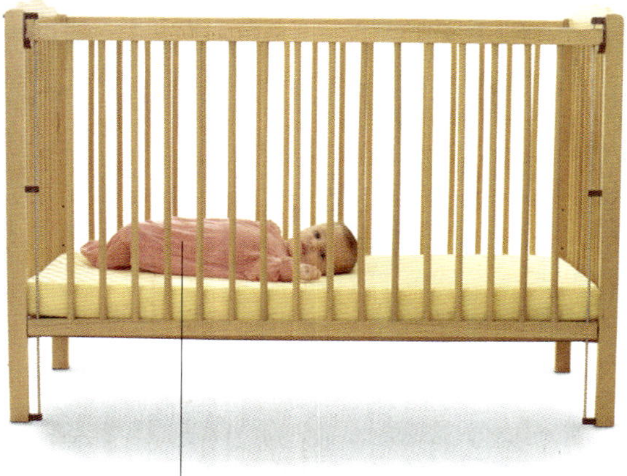

Put your baby down to sleep with her feet at the base of the crib

- Bar spaces must be no more than 6 cm (2½in) wide to prevent your baby's head from being trapped.
- The mattress must fit the crib with a gap of less than 3 cm (1½in) around the side or the baby's head could become trapped between the crib side and the mattress.
- Don't use a pillow for a baby under one year: it could suffocate him. If you need to raise his head, put a pillow under the mattress or raise one end of the crib.
- Use a sheet and cotton knit blankets rather than a quilt until your baby is one year old. Your baby could overheat or suffocate under a quilt.
- Don't put the crib near a heater or in a very sunny part of the room. Don't use a crib bumper.
- Put your baby to sleep on his back with his feet at the foot of the crib to lessen the risk of crib death; babies under 6 months should sleep in their parents' room.
- Remove toys from the crib as soon as your baby can sit up because he could use them to climb out.
- Once your child starts trying to climb out of the crib, transfer him to a bed.

Changing areas

- Keep all changing equipment in one place so that you never have to leave your baby alone on the changing mat. He will be safest on the floor, but if you have a changing table, remember that he might roll off if left even for a moment.
- Store diaper bags well out of the reach of babies because these present a suffocation risk.
- Do not have shelves above the changing area in case something falls off onto your child.
- Keep dangling mobiles out of his reach.
- Use a towel rather than talcum powder to dry your baby's skin because the fine particles can be harmful if your baby breathes in lots of them at once.

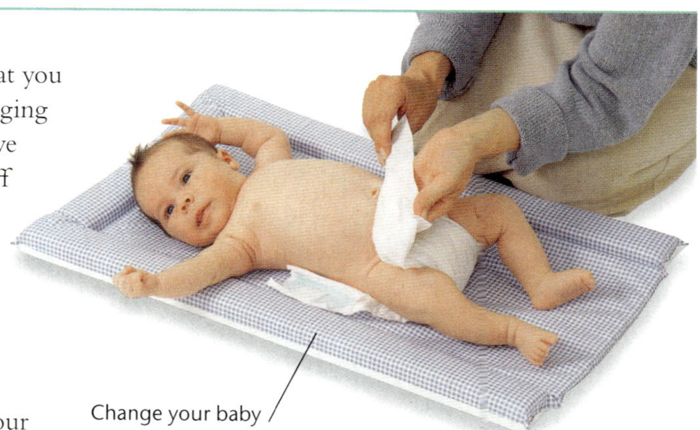

Change your baby on the floor on a changing mat so that he cannot fall

Children's bedrooms

This is a room where children are likely to be unsupervised, so it has to be as safe as possible.

- Ideally choose blinds without a loop mechanism, but if there is one attached to the blind, it must have a safety release that breaks under pressure. Stow curtain ties well out of reach of children.
- Don't use a bed guard when your toddler first moves to a bed; if you think he may fall out, put cushions on the floor beside the bed.
- A top bunk bed is not recommended for children under the age of six.
- Top bunk beds must have safety rails on both sides and any gaps in the railings or between the top of the mattress and the bottom of the safety rail should be no more than 6–7.5 cm (2½–3in).
- Never let young children play on the top bunk.
- Remove toys from the floor by the bed at night.
- Make sure there are no wires near a child's bed.

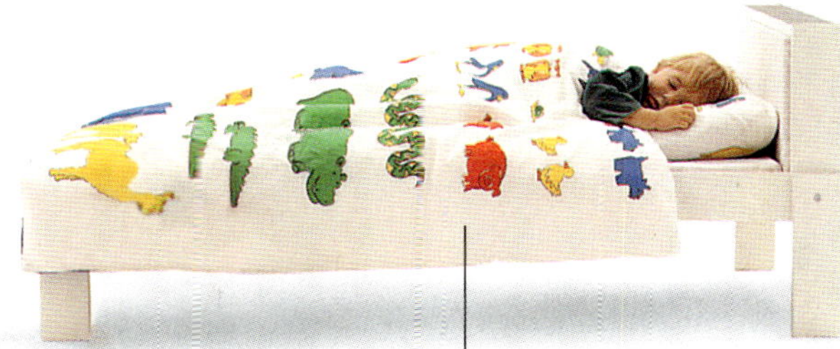

Avoid feather pillows and quilts because they can provoke allergies

WINDOWS

Make sure your child can't climb out of the window. In some areas, window guards are legally required for apartments with windows located a certain distance from the ground.

- Install a safety catch, but make sure the window can be opened easily in the event of a fire.
- Don't place a piece of furniture below a window because it may encourage your child to climb up.

TOYS *(see also p.117)*

- Keep toys that are unsuitable for very young children separate from others. This way you can easily put them out of reach if your child is sharing a room with a younger child, or if you have young visitors.

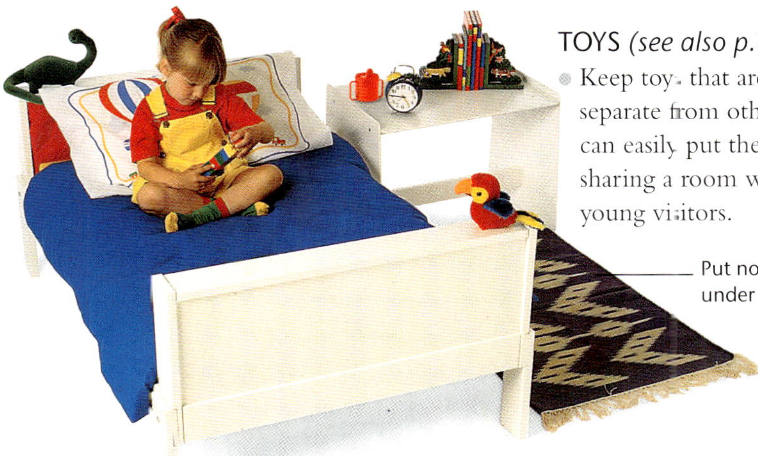

Put nonslip liners under rugs

Your bedroom

Babies under 6 months should sleep in a crib in their parent's room—but not in a parent's bed.

- Perfume, hairspray, and makeup can be harmful if sprayed or rubbed in the eyes or swallowed, so keep them out of reach or in a drawer with a safety latch.
- Medicines and pills should never be left beside your bed, or on a dressing table. Put them out of sight and out of a child's reach, preferably in a locked cabinet.
- Scissors and sewing equipment should be kept in a drawer or cabinet with a safety latch.
- Never leave a mug, teacup, or a glass on the floor by your bed, especially at night. If your child happened to be in your bed, he could roll out onto the cup, mug, or glass.

Bathroom

Your child may be at risk from falls, drowning, scalding, or poisoning in the bathroom. Keep the door shut at all times to discourage him from going in. If you install a bolt on the door, attach it near the top of the door to prevent a young child from locking himself in.

Baths

- Check the temperature of the water before your child gets into the bath. Put your elbow in the water; if it is too hot for your elbow, it is too hot for your child. A child can be badly scalded by hot bathwater.
- Install an anti-scald device to regulate water temperature, ideally set to no more than 49°C (120°F) to prevent scalds.
- Place nonslip mats in the tub and on the floor beside it.
- Keep babies and toddlers away from the tub faucets.
- Never leave a young child or baby alone in the bath (or in the care of another child). A baby can drown in just 2.5 cm (1in) of water. If you need to answer the door or telephone, take your baby with you.

Showers

- Keep a constant check on the temperature of the water.
- Use nonslip mats in the shower and on the bathroom floor.
- Put safety film on a glass shower door so that glass is held in place in case of an incident.

Cabinets

- Store bathroom chemicals and other potential poisons, such as toilet cleaners and bleach, out of reach in a cabinet with a safety lock.
- Keep other hazards, such as makeup, aftershave, razors, nail scissors, and any medicines or glass containers, out of reach in a locked medicine cabinet.

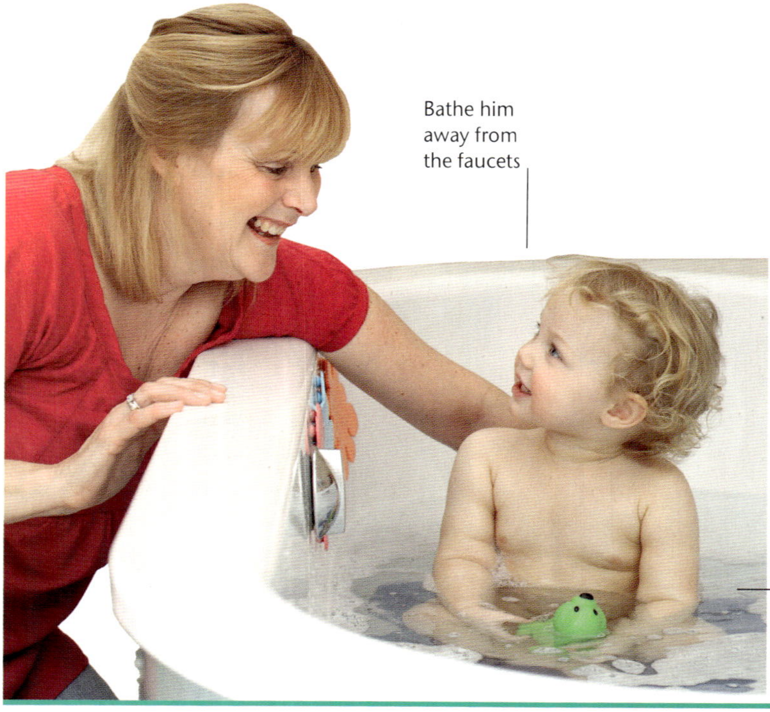

Bathe him away from the faucets

Use a nonslip mat in the bathtub

Toilets

- Use a special child toilet seat adaptor and step for toddlers so that they can keep their balance more easily and feel more secure.
- Keep the toilet seat closed when not in use.
- Don't use block toilet cleaners that a young child could pull out and chew.
- Never use both toilet cleaners and bleach because the combination will produce toxic fumes.
- If your toddler uses a potty, keep it clean, but never leave bleach or cleaning agents inside it.

Toys and playthings

If you have children of different ages in your home, keep their toys in separate boxes. In particular, keep toys with small parts away from younger children.

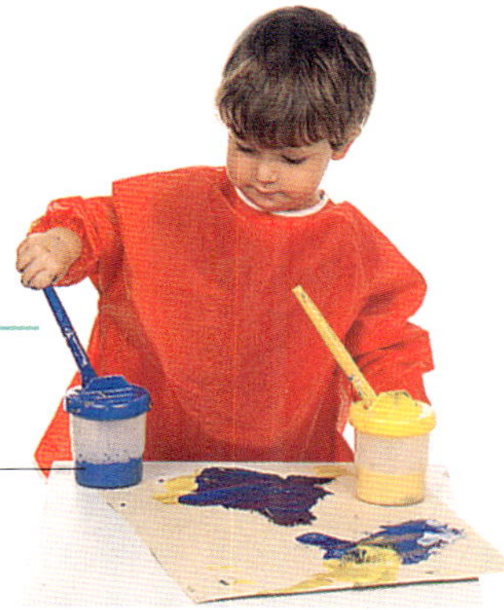

Give your child nontoxic paints to play with

Choosing toys

- Buy toys that are appropriate for the age of your child, and buy from a reputable source.
- Don't give your child anything to play with that has sharp edges, or is made of thin, rigid plastic.
- Give him nontoxic paints or crayons.
- Don't buy your child old toys: they may be broken or covered in paint containing lead.
- Avoid novelty toys that are not designed to be played with by young children: look out for warnings on the packaging.

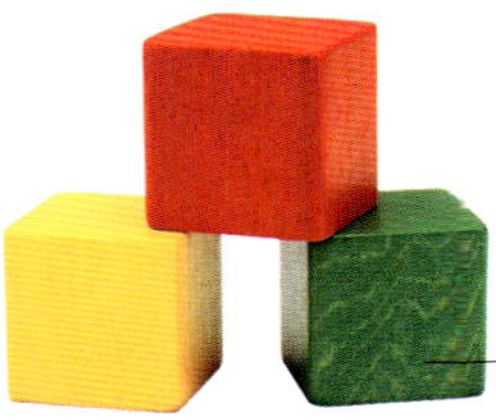

Check sets of building blocks for small pieces that could be a choking hazard for a younger child

Caring for toys

- Check toys regularly and always throw away any broken ones.
- Don't mix old and new batteries. Change them all at the same time; otherwise, the strong batteries will make the weak ones very hot.
- Keep toys in a toy box. Toys can bring about accidents or injuries if left on the floor.

Babies and toddlers

- Remove ribbons from a baby's soft toys.
- Check that the eyes, noses, ears, or bells on soft toys and dolls are well secured.
- Attach crib toys with a very short string and remove them as soon as your baby can sit up.
- Remove activity centres or bulky toys from a crib as soon as your child can stand because they provide a foothold for climbing out of the crib.
- Don't let babies chew on furry toys: the fur is a choking hazard.
- Never let a young child play with a toy that is not recommended for his age group: it may contain small pieces on which he could choke.
- Don't leave a baby or toddler to play in a room on his own.
- Baby push toys can help mobility and balance, but avoid "baby walkers," which are dangerous, banned in Canada, and may actually interfere with proper development and delay walking.

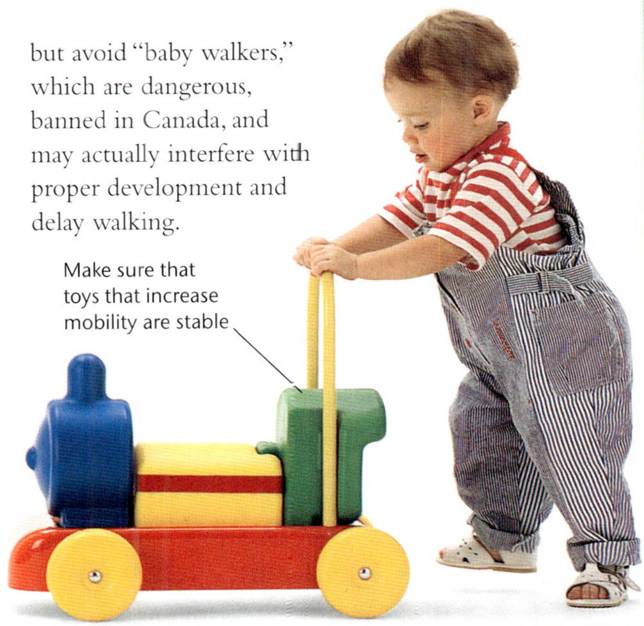

Make sure that toys that increase mobility are stable

Yard

Your yard can be a safe and interesting place for your children to play. Children will find their own corners to play in, but you must clear away trash and remove obvious hazards:

- Lock gates that lead out of the yard and make sure that fences are secure.
- Check garden furniture or play equipment regularly to make sure that it is safe. Place it over grass, not paving stones.
- Keep pets away from children's play areas.
- Make sure paving is even and remove moss so that neither you nor your child trip or slip.

Plants

Many plants are poisonous if eaten and digested in large quantities. Small pieces, or one or two berries, are not fatal but may cause some discomfort and stomach upset.

- Tell your child about the dangers of eating berries, and keep babies and toddlers away from them.
- Remove plants that you know to be poisonous, such as winterberry, black nightshade, and English holly.
- Cut back any prickly plants, such as roses, brambles, and holly. They can give painful scratches, especially to your or your child's eyes.

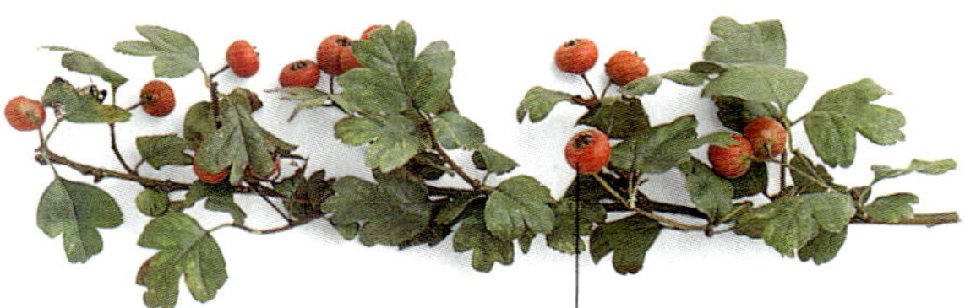

Warn your child not to eat berries or leaves

Sheds and bins

Sheds are inevitably used for storing chemicals and tools, and so are a potential hazard.

- Tell your child that the shed is out of bounds, keep it locked at all times, and hide the key.
- Put chemicals, such as weedkiller or slug pellets, out of reach in containers with child-resistant caps.
- Keep wheeled trash cans hinge side outward so that a child can't open them and climb in.

Water in the garden

Babies and toddlers are especially at risk if they slip and fall, even in shallow water. Maintain fencing to prevent children from entering a neighbour's yard where a swimming pool or pond may be a hazard.

- Never leave children unattended when they are playing in, or near, water.
- Keep ponds covered and fenced off, and cover rain barrels and empty trash cans that collect rainwater.
- Always empty out a wading pool when your children have finished playing in it and turn it upside-down in case it rains.

Gardening

- Don't put down chemicals when children will be playing in the garden.
- Don't mow the lawn while children are close by because stone chips may become dislodged and fly up into their eyes.
- Put away all garden tools when you have finished using them.

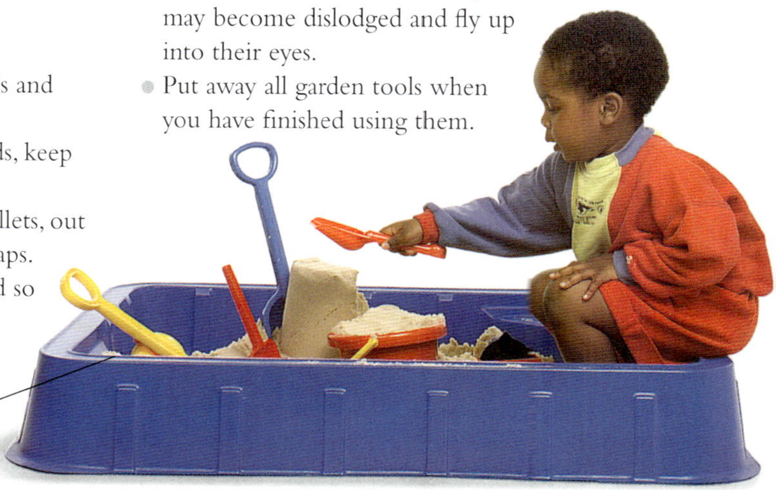

Check that he is playing in a clean, safe area with safe toys

Garage and car safety

Always leave your garage locked; likewise, keep the car locked, even if it is on a driveway off the road or in a garage. Keep the car keys where the children cannot reach them. Don't give the keys to your baby to play with because they are not clean and he could drop them.

Garages and driveways

- Keep the garage locked and discourage your child from going in there.
- Keep equipment, chemicals, or tools out of your child's reach and locked away if possible.
- Make sure you know where your child is when you are driving into, or out of, the garage or a drive.
- Chest freezers should be locked at all times.

Cars

- Never leave a young child unattended in a car, even if you can see the car. Children can overheat in minutes on a hot day.
- Don't let your child play with the car windows, whether manual or electric. Windows can trap a child's head or fingers.
- Remove the cigarette lighter from the car altogether.
- Watch out for your child's fingers when you shut the car doors.
- Use child locks on rear doors until your child is at least six years old.
- Teach your child to get out on the curb side.
- If your child is helping you wash the car, make sure you have removed the car keys from the ignition first.

Car seats

Always put your child in a special safety seat when you strap him into the car. The law requires that all children be buckled into a car seat made for their weight and height—see your provincial/territorial government guidelines for details. Never carry a baby or child on your lap even in your seatbelt—it is not only dangerous (your baby could be thrown out of the car or crushed by your body weight in a crash) but it is also illegal.

There are various types of car seats—the correct one will depend on the age and size of your baby or child and your car. Ideally when you buy a seat, go to a retailer who will show you how to use it properly. Fit the seat exactly as the instructions describe. Most cars have special Universal Anchorage System (UAS) seat fixings, which are more secure than seat belts, for child car seats. Check that your chosen seat is approved for use in your particular vehicle. Then choose the correct seat for the weight and development of your child. Check the specific child safety seat guidelines for your area, but in general:

- Babies and toddlers up to 10kg/22lbs should travel in a rear-facing car seat. The safest place for your baby to travel is in the rear seat of your car. Do not place your baby in a rear-facing car seat on the front passenger seat if there is an airbag installed that cannot be disabled—the impact of an airbag inflating could cause serious injury.
- Older toddlers up to 18kg/40lbs who have outgrown the height and weight limitations of their rear-facing seat need a front-facing car seat in the back seat of the car. Some seats have an integral harness for the child, which fits over his shoulders, across his hips, and between his legs. The seats are held in place by the UAS fixings or an adult seat belt.
- Children who weigh between 18–36kg (40–80lbs) can travel in a booster seat. Without them, adult seat belts are neither comfortable nor safe: the shoulder part cuts across the child's neck, and the lap strap lies across his stomach, which could cause internal injury in a crash. A lap strap alone is not sufficient because it does not restrain the child's upper body.

Finally, use a seat on every journey in a car, no matter how short—even in taxis.

Out and about

After the home, most childhood incidents occur in the street or in play areas. Teach your child the rules of the road from an early age, reminding him to stay alert for traffic and to cross in a safe place. It takes a long time for children to develop a true road sense.

What a child understands

- Three-year-olds can learn that the sidewalk is safe and the road is dangerous.
- Five-year-olds can learn how to cross the road, but they are still not able to put this knowledge into practice on their own.
- Eight-year-olds can cross quiet streets on their own, but they are not yet able to judge the speed and distance of traffic.
- Twelve-year-olds can judge the speed of an oncoming car, but are still easily distracted by friends.

Street and road safety

Whenever you are out with your child, show him how to be aware of his own safety.

- When out shopping or walking near a road, carry your toddler or keep him in a stroller to keep him from running off without you.
- Encourage a young child to hold your hand when you are near the road or waiting to cross a road.

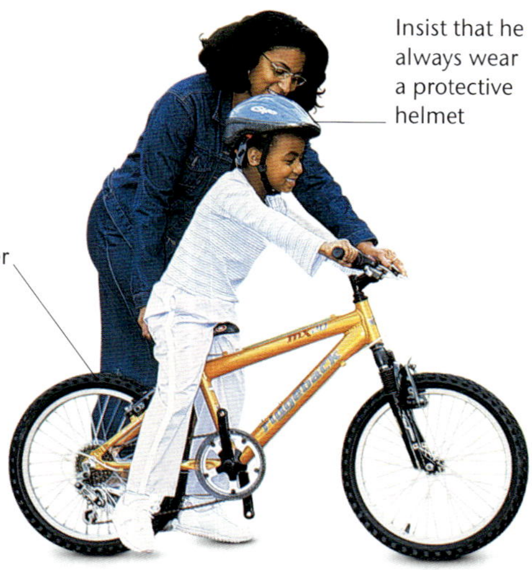

Insist that he always wear a protective helmet

Maintain the bike in good working order

Learning how to cross the road

Teach your child the rules of the road:

- Find a safe place to cross, then stop.
- Stand on the sidewalk, near the curb.
- Look both ways for traffic, and listen.
- If traffic is coming, let it pass.
- When there is no traffic near, walk straight across the road.
- Look and listen for traffic while you cross.

- Teach your child by example and always find a safe place to cross a road. This may be a crosswalk, a pedestrian crossing with lights, an underpass, or a footbridge. If there is no designated crossing point, aim for a large gap between parked cars, where you and your child can see a long way in both directions.
- At a crosswalk, teach your child to stop and wait until all the traffic has stopped and to stop at the island halfway across, if there is one.
- When using a pedestrian crossing with traffic lights, encourage your child to press the button and always wait until the traffic has stopped before crossing.

Bikes

- All children should wear a helmet when riding a bike.
- Children under 10 years old should not bicycle on roads in traffic without an adult, and all children should have training before going on the road.
- Make sure your child can be seen when he's riding his bike—with bright fluorescent colours by day and reflectors on his clothes and bike by night.

Where to play

What may seem common sense to you is not obvious to children.

- Show your child where it is safe to play—the playground, or local recreation area, for example—and supervise him if necessary.
- Teach your child the dangers of playing in open areas, such as roads, building sites, and quarries.
- Tell your child not to play in the street, or on pavement near the curb—even if your street is quiet.
- Tell him that he must never chase a ball, a pet, or another child into the road.

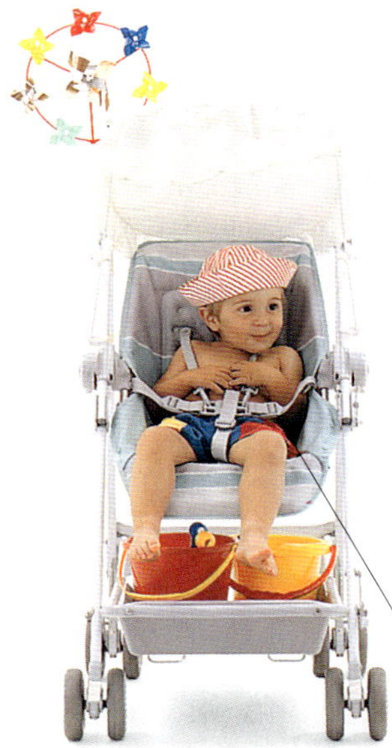

Harness your baby into his stroller

Carriages and strollers

- Never push a carriage or stroller out into the traffic to see if the road is clear to cross. Pull the stroller to one side and check whether the road is safe. Remember that a child's stroller sticks out in front of you by at least 1 metre (3ft).
- When you park a carriage or stroller, put on the brakes and point it away from traffic.
- Never tie your dog to the stroller.
- Never leave a baby unattended.
- Keep your child away from the stroller when you are assembling or folding it to keep little fingers from being trapped.

On the playground

All playgrounds should comply with safety standards; report any faulty equipment in community playgrounds to your local authority.

- The play area must be safely fenced off and away from roads.
- There should be a soft, even surface, such as mulch, wood chips, or rubber tiles, around equipment.
- Slides should be no higher than 2.4 m (8ft) and preferably constructed on an earth mound to break any falls.
- Carousels should be low, with a smooth surface, designed so that young children can't get their feet stuck underneath.
- Climbing frames should be no higher than 2.4 m (8ft), completely stable, and built over sand or a very soft surface to break falls.
- Swings should set away from main play equipment.
- There should be a clearly defined play area for toddlers and young children, set away from the more boisterous activities of older children.
- There should be someone to contact if any of the equipment is faulty.
- Dogs must not be allowed inside playgrounds.

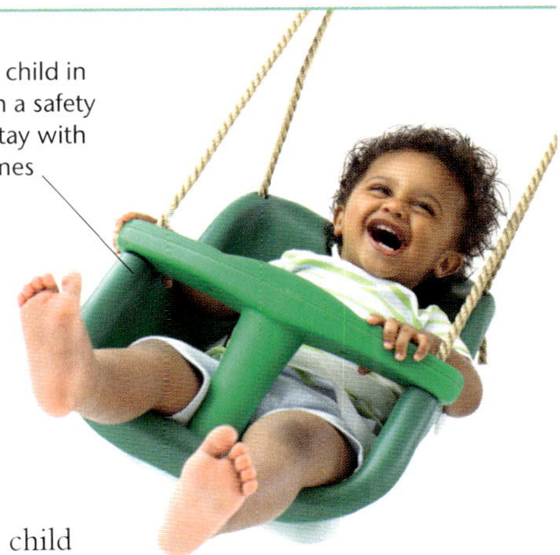

Put a young child in a swing with a safety guard and stay with him at all times

- Teach your child not to pick up any garbage from the ground.
- Look closely for any broken glass or used syringes.
- Remove from your child's clothes any drawstrings, scarves, or other items that could get caught in playground equipment

! IMPORTANT

- **Remind** your child of the dangers of talking to strangers. Have a code word that a friend can use if picking up your child. Tell your child not to go with anybody unless they use the code.

Travelling with babies and children

Away from your home all the same rules of safety apply. However, you should be aware that the place you are staying might not necessarily have been planned with young children in mind.

- If there is a swimming pool, never leave your child unattended in or near the water and, if there is a fence around it, keep the gate shut.
- Take baby milk and/or food with you; your child may not like what is available locally.

Travelling abroad

- Make sure your child's immunizations are up to date. Some countries recommend additional vaccination, or antimalaria medication; ask when booking a trip.
- Don't forget to take the necessary paperwork; babies and children need their own passports. It is a good idea to keep a photocopy of each passport (yours as well) in a separate bag.
- If you are renting a car, always ask for child safety seats, or take your child's car seat with you.
- Make sure rented cars are equipped with sufficient safety restraints and check that they are in good condition (not worn) and working properly.
- Take insect repellent suitable for babies and young children because they are particularly susceptible to insect bites. Apply the repellent in the early evening and again at bedtime, when the insects are most active.
- Use bottled water or cooled, boiled water for drinking and to wash vegetables, salads, and fruit if there is any doubt about the local water.
- Boil water used to make up baby foods or milk.

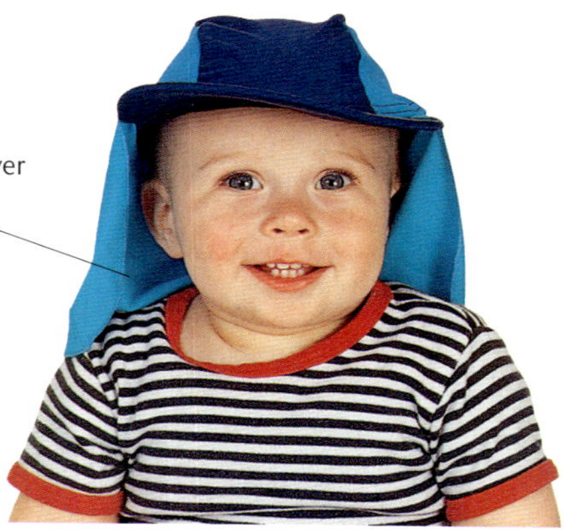

Put a sunhat on your baby whenever he is outside

Air travel

- Check with the airline to see if you can use a child safety seat for children under two. The AmSafe CARES is a child restraint device for children 10–20 kg (22–44lbs) that is approved for use on airplanes.
- Give your baby either a feeding or a pacifier to suck as the plane ascends and descends because the change in pressure can cause earache. Give an older child a piece of candy to suck, but make sure he does not choke on it.
- Take any food or milk that a baby needs on the plane trip. Airlines don't generally carry baby food, although they may be able to heat yours for you.
- Give your baby or child plenty to drink during the flight to prevent dehydration.

Sun protection

- Use sunscreen that protects your child from ultraviolet A rays (UVA) and ultraviolet B rays (UVB). The sun protection factor (SPF) numbers relate to UVB—choose SPF 30. A broad-spectrum sunscreen provides UVA protection. Reapply regularly, especially after he has been in water. Use a product that you know your child is not allergic to.
- Keep your baby or child's arms and legs covered as much as possible. Dress him in clothes made of closely woven fabric made of natural fibers.
- Make sure your child is protected by the shade in the middle of the day (from about 10am until 4pm).
- Put a wide-brimmed hat on your child's head that covers his neck and face and use a shade on a stroller.
- Give your child plenty to drink to prevent dehydration. If you are breastfeeding, offer your baby more feedings; give a bottlefed baby plain water.

Index

R

S

T

U

V

Acknowledgements

Dorling Kindersley would like to thank Phil Gamble, Anjali Sachar, and Sachin Singh for the illustrations; and Suefa Lee for editorial assisstance and indexing.

The publisher would like to thank the following for their kind permission to reproduce their photographs: (Key: a-above; b-below/bottom; c-centre; f-far; l-left; r-right; t-top)
21 Lloyd Sturdy: British Red Cross br; **81** Wikipedia: CDC/ James Gathany br; **91** Amy Kerkemeyer © 123RF.COM bl.
All other images © Dorling Kindersley
For further information see: **www.dkimages.com**
Dorling Kindersley would like to thank:
Joe Mulligan, Head of First Aid Education, Nadine Threader, Jane Keogh, and Andrew Farrar from the British Red Cross; Cardiac Science for the loan of the pediatric AED; Hilary Bird for the index; the following for modeling:
Children Aleena Awan, Navaz Awan, Max Buckingham, Madeline Cameron, Alfie Clarke, Amy Davies, Thomas Davies, James Dow, Kyla Edwards, Austin Enil, Lia Foa, Maya Foa, Jessica Forge, Kashi Gorton, Emily Gorton, Thomas Greene, Alexander Harrison, Rupert Harrison, Ben Harrison, Jessica Harris-Voss, Hannah Headam, Jake Hutton, Rosemary Kaloki, Winnie Kaloki, Ella Kaye, Maddy Kaye, Jade Lamb, Emily Leney, Harriet Lord, Daniel Lord, Crispin Lord, Ailsa McCaughrean, Fiona Maine, Tom Maine, Kincaid Malik-White, Maija Marsh, Oliver Metcalf, Eloise Morgan, Tom Razazan, Jimmy Razazan, Georgia Ritter, Rebecca Sharples, Ben Sharples, Thomas Sharples, Ben Walker, Robyn Walker, Amy Beth Walton Evans, Hanna Warren-Green, Simon Weekes, Joseph Weir, Lily Ziegler.
Adults Shaila Awan, Claire le Bas, Joanna Benwell, Angela Cameron, Georgina Davies, Marion Davies, Sophie Dow, Tina Edwards, Rachel Fitchett, Emma Foa, Emma Forge, Caroline Greene, Susan Harrison, Victoria Harrison, Julia Harris-Voss, Roy Headam, Emma Hutton, Helga Lien Evans, Sylvie Jordan, Jane Kaloki, David Kaye, Louise Kaye, Philip Lord, Geraldine McCaughrean, Diana Maine, Brian Marsh, Jonathan Metcalf, Francoise Morgan, Juliette Norsworthy, Anna Pizzi, Hossein Razazan, Angela Sharples, John Sharples, Nadine Threader, Miranda Tunbridge, Vanessa Walker, Catherine Warren-Green, Toni Weekes, Robert Ziegler.
Makeup: Wendy Holmes, Pebbles, Geoff Portas.
Additional photography Andy Crawford, Steve Gorton, Ray Mollers, Suzannah Price, Dave Rudkin, Steve Shott, Lloyd Sturdy.

Useful telephone numbers

IN AN EMERGENCY DIAL 911 OR YOUR LOCAL EMS (medical emergencies only), FIRE DEPARTMENT, OR POLICE.

FOR MEDICAL ADVICE ON POISONING, CALL YOUR PROVINCIAL POISON CONTROL CENTRE.

Telephone: ______

Pediatrician

Name: ______
Address: ______
Telephone: ______
Office hours: ______

Dentist

Name: ______
Address: ______
Telephone: ______
Office hours: ______

Hospital Emergency Department

Address: ______
Telephone: ______

Pharmacy

Address: ______
Telephone: ______
Prescriptions: ______

Specialists

Name: ______
Address: ______
Telephone: ______

Name: ______
Address: ______
Telephone: ______

Police

Address: ______
Telephone: ______

Fire Department

Telephone: ______

Gas Emergencies

Telephone: ______

Electrical Emergencies

Telephone: ______

Notes

"Richard Falk, Victor Faessel and Michael Curtin have brought together a diverse set of authors for an in-depth examination of the importance of public imagination. This is a much-needed angle into the larger debate about the decay of liberal democracy."

— *Saskia Sassen, Columbia University, author of* Expulsions

"Confronting today's public challenges demands reason and benefits from a sense of history—but neither is a substitute for imagination. We need imagination both to understand what is going on and to decide how to respond. Without imagination our public debates are inanimate and our politics mere power struggles. This book brings 30 exciting perspectives on how to renew public imagination."

— *Craig Calhoun, University Professor of Social Sciences, Arizona State University*

"Facing mounting global problems ranging from climate change to widening social inequality, our 21st-century world is in desperate need of collective action based on a pluralistic public imagination. This highly readable anthology presents the concise and innovative views of dozens of influential intellectuals on the critical role of an ethical imagination that cut across political, economic, and cultural divides. Highly recommended!"

— *Manfred B. Steger, Professor of Sociology, University of Hawai'i-Mānoa and Global Professorial Fellow, Western Sydney University*

ON PUBLIC IMAGINATION

In this wide-ranging and multidisciplinary volume, leading scholars, activists, journalists, and public figures deliberate about the creative and critical potential of public imagination in an era paradoxically marked by intensifying globalization and resurgent nationalism. Divided into five sections, these chapters explore the social, political, and cultural role of imagination and civic engagement, offering cogent, ingenious reflections that stand in stark contrast to the often grim rhetoric of our era. Short and succinct, the chapters engage with an interconnected ensemble of themes and issues while also providing insights into the specific geographical and social dynamics of each author's national or regional context.

- Part 1 introduces the reader to theoretical reflections on imagination and the public sphere;
- Part 2 illustrates dynamics of public imagination in a diverse set of cultural contexts;
- Part 3 reflects in various ways on the urgent need for a radically transformed public and civic imagination in the face of worldwide ecological crisis;
- Part 4 suggests new societal possibilities that are related to spiritual as well as politically revolutionary sources of inspiration;
- Part 5 explores characteristics of present and potentially emerging global society and the existing transnational framework that could provide resources for a more humane global order.

Erudite and thought-provoking, *On Public Imagination* makes a vital contribution to political thought, and is accessible to activists, students, and scholars alike.

Victor Faessel is Associate Director of the Mellichamp Initiative on 21st Century Global Dynamics at the University of California, Santa Barbara. He is co-editor (with Richard Falk and Manoranjan Mohanty) of *Exploring Emergent Global Thresholds: Towards 2030* (2017), and is managing editor of *The Oxford Handbook of Global Studies* (2018, Mark Juergensmeyer, Saskia Sassen, and Manfred Steger, eds.) as well as the four-volume *Encyclopedia of Global Studies* (2012, Helmut Anheier and Mark Juergensmeyer, eds.). He has been the general secretary of the Global Studies Consortium, a worldwide association of teaching programs, since its founding in 2007.

Richard Falk is Albert G. Milbank Professor of International Law and Practice, Emeritus at Princeton University, and is currently a Visiting Fellow at the Orfalea Center of Global and International Studies, University of California, Santa Barbara. He is the author or editor of numerous books, most recently *Revisiting the Vietnam War* (2017), *Power Shift: The New Global Order* (2017), *Palestine's Horizon: Toward a Just Peace* (2016), *(Re)imagining Humane Global Governance* (2014), and *The Path to Zero: Dialogues on Nuclear Dangers*, with David A. Krieger (2012). He is also the author of a book of poems, *Waiting for Rainbows* (2015).

Michael Curtin is the Duncan and Suzanne Mellichamp Chair and Distinguished Professor of Film and Media Studies at the University of California, Santa Barbara. His books include *Precarious Creativity: Global Media, Local Labor* (2016); *Distribution Revolution: Conversations about the Digital Future of Film and Television* (2014); *Reorienting Global Communication: Indian and Chinese Media Beyond Borders* (2010); and *Playing to the World's Biggest Audience: The Globalization of Chinese Film and TV* (2007).

ON PUBLIC IMAGINATION

A Political and Ethical Imperative

Edited by Victor Faessel, Richard Falk, and Michael Curtin

Routledge
Taylor & Francis Group
NEW YORK AND LONDON

First published 2020
by Routledge
52 Vanderbilt Avenue, New York, NY 10017

and by Routledge
2 Park Square, Milton Park, Abingdon, Oxon, OX14 4RN

Routledge is an imprint of the Taylor & Francis Group, an informa business

Library of Congress Cataloging-in-Publication Data
Names: Faessel, Victor, editor. | Falk, Richard A., editor. | Curtin, Michael, editor.
Title: On public imagination : a political and ethical imperative / edited by Victor Faessel, Richard Falk, Michael Curtin.
Identifiers: LCCN 2019035222 (print) | LCCN 2019035223 (ebook) |
Subjects: LCSH: Imagination (Philosophy)
Classification: LCC BH301.I53 O5 2020 (print) | LCC BH301.I53 (ebook) |
DDC 128/.3–dc23
LC record available at https://lccn.loc.gov/2019035222
LC ebook record available at https://lccn.loc.gov/2019035223

ISBN: 978-0-367-36063-4 (hbk)
ISBN: 978-0-367-36061-0 (pbk)
ISBN: 978-0-429-34359-9 (ebk)

Typeset in Bembo
by Swales & Willis, Exeter, Devon, UK

CONTENTS

ACKNOWLEDGMENTS

An anthology of this kind is only as good as its contributors. We remain overwhelmed by the outpouring of support we received from a remarkable set of respondents to our call to participate in this project, involving the very atypical assignment (at least in academic circles) of producing short, 1500-word chapters reflecting their unique perspectives on the problem and challenges of early 21st century public imagination. We are very proud of the results, and thank each of our authors for contributing to this rich and, we are convinced, important conversation.

At the University of California, Santa Barbara, we wish to express our sincere appreciation to two very talented graduate students who played significant roles in the realization of this project. In the early stages, Tymoteusz Chajdas, doctoral candidate in the Department of Global Studies, performed the herculean labor of preparing a uniform preliminary manuscript for the book proposal that led to the present volume. In the final stretch another PhD candidate, Sara Lafia of the Department of Geography, formatted the final manuscript, generated the index, performed related but invisible tasks, and—not least—produced the extraordinarily insightful set of data visualizations that appear in this volume's Appendix. The eagerness, intelligence, and responsiveness with which Tym and Sara assisted the editors, while juggling competing responsibilities under intense time pressure, remind us of the energy resources we wish we still possessed! We also gratefully acknowledge the invaluable material support of our benefactors at UCSB, including Duncan and Suzanne Mellichamp, enlightened donors to global studies initiatives on our campus, as well as Michael Stohl, director of the Orfalea Center for Global & International Studies.

Finally, we would like to thank our editors at Routledge, especially Natalja Mortensen and Charlie Baker, as well as their external reviewers of our proposal for agreeing with us about the value, in this hopefully brief and aberrant time, of this rather unusual kind of book.

CONTRIBUTORS

Celso Amorim is a Brazilian diplomat, former Foreign Minister (1993–1995 and 2003–2011) and Defense Minister (2011–2014).

Akeel Bilgrami is Sidney Morgenbesser Professor of Philosophy at Columbia University.

David Bollier is Director of the Reinventing the Commons Program at the Schumacher Center for a New Economics. He blogs at Bollier.org

Chiara Bottici is Associate Professor of Philosophy at the New School in New York.

Victoria Brittain is a journalist and former editor at *The Guardian*, and author of several books and plays.

Luis Cabrera is Associate Professor in the School of Government and International Relations at Griffith University, Australia.

Julie A. Carlson is Professor of English at the University of California, Santa Barbara.

Neera Chandhoke is Professor emerita of Political Science, University of Delhi.

Allen Chun is a Research Fellow at the Institute of Ethnology, Academia Sinica in Taipei, Taiwan.

Kevin P. Clements is Professor of Peace and Conflict Studies at the University of Otago, Dunedin, New Zealand and Director of the Toda Peace Institute, based in Tokyo Japan.

Marjorie Cohn is professor emerita at Thomas Jefferson School of Law and former president of the National Lawyers Guild.

Drucilla Cornell is Distinguished Professor of Political Science, Women's & Gender Studies, and Comparative Literature at Rutgers University.

Michael Curtin is Mellichamp Professor of Film and Media Studies and Director, 21st Century Global Dynamics, at the University of California, Santa Barbara.

Fred Dallmayr is Professor Emeritus of Political Science at the University of Notre Dame.

Ahmet Davutoğlu is a Turkish academic, former Foreign Minister, and between 2014–2016 the Prime Minister of Turkey.

Victor Faessel is Associate Director of the 21st Century Global Dynamics Initiative at the University of California, Santa Barbara.

Richard Falk is an international law scholar who taught at Princeton University for forty years. He is a Fellow of the Orfalea Center for Global & International Studies at the University of California, Santa Barbara.

Tom Farer is University Professor in the Josef Korbel School of International Studies at the University of Denver.

Johan Galtung is a sociologist, mathematician, and principal founder of the discipline of peace and conflict studies.

Behrooz Ghamari-Tabrizi is Professor of Near Eastern Studies at Princeton University.

Stephen Gill is Distinguished Research Professor of Political Science, Communications and Culture at York University.

Anna Grear is Professor of Law in the School of Law and Politics, Cardiff University.

Penny Green is Professor of Law and Globalisation at Queen Mary University of London.

Abdellah Hammoudi is a cultural anthropologist who has taught at Princeton University since 1989.

Dayan Jayatilleka is a Sri Lankan academic, diplomat, writer, politician and former UNESCO delegate.

Paul W. Kahn is Robert W. Winner Professor of Law and the Humanities and Director of the Orville H. Schell, Jr. Center for International Human Rights at Yale University.

Mary Kaldor is a Professor of Global Governance and Director of the Conflict and Civil Society Research Unit at the London School of Economics.

Catherine Keller is Professor of Constructive Theology at Drew Theological School.

Sara Lafia is a PhD candidate in the Department of Geography at the University of California, Santa Barbara.

Chandra Muzaffar is a Malaysian political scientist and President of the International Movement for a Just World (JUST).

Stephen D. Seely is a post-doctoral fellow at the University of Warwick.

Vandana Shiva is an Indian scholar, environmental activist and anti-globalization writer currently based in New Delhi.

Kamal Sinclair was recently the Director of the New Frontier Lab Program at Sundance Institute.

Elizabeth West is a freelance writer with a lifelong interest in revolution. Her political writing has appeared in *CounterPunch, Common Dreams* and *Dissident Voice.*

PUBLIC IMAGINATION

The Challenge of 21st Century Populist and Authoritarian Politics

Richard Falk and Victor Faessel

In countries across the globe including the United States, public institutions and spaces of political life are falling far short of responding to the urgent challenges facing their societies. As a result, the reasonable expectations, hopes, and demands of many citizens are not being met, causing disappointment, resentment, and alienation. This crisis of public confidence finds expression in trade wars and anti-globalization movements, as well as in the election of autocratic and demagogic leaders adhering to ultra-nationalist agendas. One consequence of this phenomenon is a decline in the quality of global leadership resulting in a dangerous failure to meet global challenges. As a response to this circumstance, we sought to stimulate a variety of articulations from scholars, activists, and political figures, covering a wide range of human and national perspectives, on the problem and potential of public imagination. Our intention was to heighten sensitivity to the wider political and historical context of our time, with the hope of engaging not only the general public but also undergraduate and (hopefully) even younger students. Our overall goal is to improve the quality of political debate and citizen participation on issues of public policy. The chapters are succinct, illuminating, and timely statements that, for all their variety of themes and perspectives produce in sum, we think, a valuable contribution to both practical and theoretical understanding of public imagination at this critical juncture in human history.

The rising populist backlash against globalization in many societies around the world has been marked by resurgent right-wing nationalism and, in many cases, authoritarianism. The series of contributions presented here aims, above all, to liberate public imagination from largely nationalist frames of reference that have fueled the surge of ultra-nationalist populisms in such countries as Russia, India, Turkey, Hungary, Egypt, Philippines, Brazil, and the United States. The Brexit vote and the rise of right wing parties in Europe point to a similar backlash against globalizing tendencies, although this brand of populism is in large part distinguished by fervent opposition to foreign policies that have generated menacing transnational migrations of people fleeing war-torn combat zones.

This regressive trend visible throughout the world signals what may be an epoch-defining abandonment of the post-1945 commitment to democratic forms of governance and advocacy of human rights. It demands in response that public engagement flourishes in modes of consciousness that transcend the national, styles of political agency committed to overcoming challenges facing humanity in common while fighting to transform specific local and national struggles.

Today's regressive politics are partly due to deficiencies of public discourse and lapses in the political and moral imagination of dominant social classes and among social movement leaders. Right-wing populism and nativism warn us that more primitive, chauvinist forms of collective political imagination are asserting themselves over what now appears to be a vanishing veneer of tolerance and political civility. The widespread lack of trust in government and governance is being intensified by disinformation, fake news, and corporatized media that have eroded allegiances among the citizenry and engendered toxic forms of polarization that give rise to savage attacks on traditional elites.

There are several systemic and structural factors that seem relevant when interpreting present trends. In part, the backlash against liberal modes of "political correctness" seems driven by a growing belief among peoples around the world that neoliberal economic globalization is both unfair to ordinary people and undermines traditional identities based on nationhood and ethnicity. Growing global inequality is a direct expression of these tendencies, whose impact on individual lives is manifested in political and social destabilization, compromised national autonomy, and feelings of diminished self-determination in many spheres of private and public life.

Furthermore, the collapse of the Soviet Union seems to have contributed to the present malaise. The loss of the binary geopolitical and ideological "other" co-determining global order in the second half of the 20th century, and the triumphalist Western response to that collapse, fed ambitions of global domination and shifted capitalism from its more compassionate Keynesian compass, inducing instead the adoption of predatory forms of economic policy. Gone are the days when foreign aid, development, and the competition for "hearts and minds" mattered. No matter how uneven the outcomes, such policies signaled an affirmation of global welfare and human well-being that no longer obtain. Capitalism unchallenged by socialism veers toward extremes, aggravates inequalities, and induces acute forms of alienation and social despair throughout civil society.

The present global atmosphere is unusual—disturbed by what exists, yet lacking any sense of a feasible alternative that extends the social democratic ethos of the West into the future. When this gap between feasibility and necessity becomes too burdensome for societies, demagogic leaders emerge who encourage denial, escapism, and extremism. Such appeals are attractive to outraged and frightened citizens. It is this sort of moral and political vacuum that Donald Trump is filling for many Americans who want enemies to blame, lethal promises to keep, and above all, entertaining spectacles to divert their attention from the complex and difficult challenges confronting humanity. "Trumpism," now manifest in diverse national forms, seems on track to capture global governance having gained control of several key national governments.

To a considerable degree, right wing populism is a response to the failures of political, economic, and cultural systems to uphold the material and psycho-political wellbeing of their respective national populations. Yet despite backlash against increasingly problematic global interconnectivities and their societal effects, public imagination needs to move beyond the narrow realm of national interests in order to respond to global realities and challenges, cognizant of all dimensions of civilizational and ecological identity, sustainability, humane values, and security. The revitalizing of public discourse to illuminate and transform present global tendencies is a matter of societal, and indeed, civilizational urgency, perhaps even species survival.

Thinking about Public Imagination

Against this background, we hope to stimulate culturally and historically informed reflection on moral/ethical imagination across borders of countries, civilizations, religions, and other relevant sources of identity. Public imagination, however diversely manifested, is closely linked with the institutions and activities of public spheres. It is engaged and shaped through cultural and religious traditions and societal norms, informal and formal politics, and diverse forms of print and electronic media. In these contexts today the channels, mechanisms, and arenas in and through which public imagination characteristically functions are being dangerously narrowed not just by demagoguery, nativist and xenophobic discourses, and moral absolutism, but also by the increasing dominance of elite interests, monetary manipulations, and media passivity in these spaces. Humane consensual political life cannot flourish in such an atmosphere.

A plurally conceived "public imagination" suggests connectivities across a cluster of interrelated ideas: a public sphere or spheres, counter-publics, public opinion, public interest, public reasoning, public space, social and spiritual imaginaries. Addressing such subject matter inevitably deals with contested domains of societal life, not least secularist worldviews. If "public" imagination is considered to be active in all societies, then its specific contours vary widely and depend on particular historical, cultural, political, religious, ecological, institutional and local configurations that must be reckoned with. For these reasons its role in shaping governance and policy also varies considerably. The idea of public imagination encompasses a variety of perspectives—philosophical, psychological, historical, affective, normative, spiritual, ecological, performative. It can be thought of as resulting from the interplay between social and private imaginaries. We are faced with the distressing question as to whether closures of public imagination can be surmounted in political spaces that are becoming more and more intolerant toward diversity and differences. To what extent are capacities of expansive public imagination foreshortened by this populist tsunami? Or alternatively, can these developments give rise to a dialectical set of responses in which imaginative visions, strategies, and tactics are articulated to discover or enlarge pathways to humane futures?

The term "public imagination" is acknowledged to be unstable, problematic if conceived monolithically, burdened by definitional, sociological, and epistemological difficulties. These include the fact that the concept of imagination as a cognitive faculty bears a long history of Western rationalist, positivist, and Romantic biases. Nevertheless, throughout the post-WWII period there are increasing recognitions of the utility of orienting inquiry around collective forms of imagination. For example, the work of Benedict Anderson, Arjun Appadurai, Donna Haraway, and Charles Taylor are indicative of this reliance on social imaginaries to interpret modern conditions. Media studies are an increasingly important resource for such investigation given the ascendance of knowledge mediation through images and the sheer ubiquity of images in a media saturated, post-Internet, digitally supercharged world in which images are viral, more of reality is becoming virtual, and more of intelligence artificial. The imagination of cultural selves *with or against* cultural "others" is being globally exploited by mainstream media for the sake of spectacle, generating a constitutive disease of the contemporary social world.

Imagining an Agenda

These phenomena encompass a wide range of vital concerns that suggest critical, aesthetic, practical and policy-oriented responses. Investigations into the failures of government policy by reference to the weakness or bias of public imagination help to explain, for example, the disappointing national and global policy responses to threats posed by climate change and the continued possession of nuclear weapons. In this respect, a multi-perspectival initiative concerned with the disappointing inability of public imagination to grasp the biopolitical historical moment, and redirect energies and attention to the currently deficient protection of human and planetary interests, is urgently called for.

An engagement with public imagination in the context of 21st-century global challenges might select a few initial priorities: 1) analyzing how to address the global and human interest in a world of sovereign states whose governments are focused on national concerns and interests, too often through either populist or elitist optics, short-term electoral cycles, special interests, and maintenance of the status quo; 2) assessing concerns of transnational and global scope, such as nuclear weapons, climate change, food security, health, economic inequality, migration, human trafficking, terror & crime networks; 3) enlarging the spheres of policy debate in democratic societies to envision alternatives that explore nonviolent and cosmopolitan paths to achieving both national and human security.

The foregoing examples underscore the need for research on the theoretical and practical dimensions of public imagination(s) toward improving discourse and policy on threats confronting every nation of the world, the biosphere, and humanity at large. Processes of public reasoning and persuasion are conditioned by particularities of time and place which affect the status and the health of public spheres and distinct "publics." Meanwhile, the limits, dangers, and potentials of imagination as a politically salient and policy-relevant variable must be explored with renewed vigor given the challenges of the 21st century. These concerns orient the explorations and conversations across borders that we hoped to stimulate within a heterogenous community of scholars, thinkers, and activists around the world who share our faith in the relevance of commentary, passion, conscience, and dialogue, and who share as well as our desire to stimulate broader debate on and deeper explorations of the vital role of humanely engaged public imagination.

PART I

Imagination

Theory and Engagement

1

RALLYING

Imagination's Political Process

Julie A. Carlson

The association of imagination with make-believe and with methodological practices that characterize the humanities and fine arts has often been said to undermine its "street cred" and contributions to public policy. This chapter argues the opposite. It puts into dialogue divergent strands of discourse on imagination to suggest why leaderless social movements such as Occupy, Black Lives Matter, and Dream Defenders are grounded in imaginative practices that are reinventing politics and why this re-orientation toward process over object is vital to the efficacy of political activity. People cannot be rallied to action if their spirits are incapable of rallying. The justice achieved by such rallying depends on the extent to which people are committed to continually reevaluating their identities, platforms, and aims.

Three of the most searching investigations of imagination come from the fields of British Romanticism, the Black radical tradition, and contemporary neuroscience. Despite their very different methods and objectives, writers in each field agree on features of imagination that specify the usefulness of its approach to reality. Imagination is a mode of perception that does not require immediate sensory input. What it perceives stems from its surrounding environment, but it is neither determined by nor invested in maintaining that environment as is. Always constructing what it perceives, imagination is a form of mentation that also blurs distinctions between thinking and doing. Brain scans show that many of the same parts of the brain are activated when one is performing or simply imagining a particular action, which is why visualizing can improve performance since both are products of the same motor program. Its primary activity is connection-making, which involves also unmaking and remaking connections that have become entrained, hegemonic, deadening. Taken together, these features explain why imagination has long been considered a visionary faculty and the prime generator of creativity. Whether writers in these traditions emphasize neuronal or aesthetic mechanisms by which absent things are present in the mind/brain or are made present to consciousness, they contend that imagination broadens sense-based approaches to interpreting reality and works to extend thought and thoughtfulness beyond the empirical and the here and now.

Imagination's circumvention of the common-sensical and reliance on unconscious processes are central to its creativity and to bringing the unforeseen into existence. This is why imagination has been deemed a revolutionary faculty and the engine of social reform. P. B. Shelley famously defends poetry—which for him encompasses all of the arts and humanities—by asserting that poets are the unacknowledged legislators of the world. They are legislators because imaginative persons reshape public sentiment as a first step to acquiring more egalitarian laws and social policies; they are unacknowledged because policy-making is the putative domain of the social sciences and because imaginative activity is nuanced and indirect.

British Romantic-era elevations of imagination as a moral as well as aesthetic faculty have rightly been censured for their possessive investment in whiteness and theoretical undergirding of a liberal subject whose alleged sympathy is tautologically self-involved. Does the fact that this white-privileging has occurred—and continues to occur—invalidate imagination's visionary potential? And should it discredit hope, as Afro-pessimists, no-future queer theorists, and Americanists averring the cruelty of optimism contend? Probing this question is why I began by outlining convergences among such an unlikely ensemble of theorist-activists. To my mind, perceiving their congruence illustrates not only the function of metaphor in forging what Shelley terms "before unapprehended connections" between things but also the reasons why artists constantly must remake a culture's figures of speaking so that they at once bespeak and focalize marginalized perspectives. This commitment to re-figuring thought is crucial to destabilizing racial regimes. As Cedric Robinson argues, because racial regimes are forgeries of memory and meaning rather than naturalized entities, the dominating connections that they have forged are vulnerable to protest. The trouble is that perceived vulnerability provokes primitive defenses, especially in those whose power is established and thereby unjustly maintained. Direct attacks on them are risky and thus require training in indirection by those whose repeated experiences of injustice have made them experts in improvisation. And thus who act in accordance with the rhythms of the "inside songs."

To the hegemonic workings of Romantic-era imaginations, then, the Black radical tradition offers some basic correctives. The subject-object binary that grounds Western conceptions of selfhood and democracy endorses slavery, treats others as things, and profits off of their objectification. To the degree that past or current imaginations strive to isolate self from other, foster zero-sum mentalities, and affirm the sovereignty and immateriality of mind, they are ignorant about the brain and are using old power tools to renovate and secure master's houses. By contrast, art in the Black radical tradition affirms collective and non-urbane renewals that prioritize process over objects. Black Radical imagination is improvisational, at play in ensembles rather than in separate and individuated individuals. Moreover, the freedom dreams that Black radicals conjure re-evoke massive resistances by no-things whose palpability in the present is the motor of whatever inspiration ensues. To say that histories of Black struggle are inseparable from histories of Black music sounds romanticized only if one hears struggle as dissonant or disconcerting and those qualities as unmusical. Here, the imaging of neuroscience is useful in registering that memory and imagination are part of the same network and that, when confronted with obstacles, neurons are resourceful at discovering new pathways. What "is," that is, cannot be entirely separated from "was" or "ought," but this does not make them an identity.

I catch something of this background in the call and responsiveness of Angela Davis's "Power to the Imagination," when she both delivered a lecture and took it to the streets as part of Occupy Philly in late October 2011. The transfer from "people" to "imagination," with its implied shift of power from rights to rites and writing, is in keeping with an aesthetics of fugitivity and conceptualization of freedom as marronage. One can, and should, hear records of defeat in this transposition of rights to rites: minimal discernible shifts of power; palpable shiftiness in the terms of order; dead bodies of color left in the streets that "the 99%" ostensibly occupy; countless projects to wall people in and out. But articulating why this occasions yet should not sanction defeatism marks another convergence among my before-unconnected ensemble.

The conclusion that "despair is criminal," reached by British Romantic-era radicals Mary Wollstonecraft and William Godwin in novels that expressly delineate the impossible obstacles that disenfranchised subjects confront in getting their stories heard, is rephrased but echoed in Fred Moten and Stefano Harney's conviction that subjects who are characteristically criminalized know that something more is going on and know just where it is happening and always has been happening—in the wild sociality of the undercommons. In such a space, folks are welcome so long as they reject a politics of recognition and its demanding uplifts. Their type of disengagement does not mean that undercommoners are, or wish to be or remain, invisible. Or that they are not preparing for a fight. They are. And how. It's that their imaginations are geared toward creativity, not identity and its reflections, and their arts co-implicate struggle and power.

In other words, radical Romantic imaginations contend that despair is "criminal" because it occasions a degree of hardening that forecloses possibility. While hardening is a reasonable response to being on the receiving end of racist projections and fire-power, Black radical improvisation keeps imaginations attuned to the sound of surprise. Staying open to surprise can be a crushing burden for subordinated peoples but it is also their lived reality, a major lesson of their histories, and their most impressive legacy. Acknowledging this skill foregrounds an aesthetic reason why Black lives matter, and why Blackness as radicals construe it remains avant-garde. Moreover, the bi-directionality between ought and is, whereby the "ought" of justice is situated in the "is" of a doubled consciousness and its un-self-conscious forms of sociality, is what new social movements like Occupy Now or Black Lives Matter embody. Their reinvention of political life, as Davis puts it, involves artful practices that stimulate imagination, evoke surprise, and are alive to the intersections among struggles as well as identity categories. Their mode of organization is prophetic by staying cognizant of the benefits of disorganization, a basic lesson of brain-based models of creativity. Relevant too is the narrowing of attention that attentiveness mandates and the habituation that neuronal efficiency dictates *unless* roadblocks are made or found to forge new connections. The evaluative standard for imaginative activists is whether whatever gets reassembled is then valued because of the exclusions its formation entails or because it provides a platform from which to conjure again the before unapprehended. Cultivating desire for the latter is what the affective power of art strengthens by ensuring that persons do not have to stare into that void alone.

References

Andreasen, Nancy C. 2006. *The Creative Brain: The Science of Genius*. New York: Penguin.

Carlson, Julie A. 2012. "Romantic Poet Legislators: An End of Torture." In *Speaking About Torture*, edited by Julie A. Carlson and Elisabeth Weber. 221–246. New York: Fordham.

Davis, Angela Y. 2016. *Freedom is a Constant Struggle: Ferguson, Palestine, and the Foundations of a Movement*. Chicago: Haymarket Books.

Doidge, Norman. 2007. *The Brain that Changes Itself*. New York: Penguin.

Godwin, William. 1794. *Things as They Are; Or, The Adventures of Caleb Williams*. London: Printed for B. Crosby. https://archive.org/details/thingsastheyare00godwgoog/.

Harney, Stefano, and Fred Moten. 2013. *The Undercommons: Fugitive Planning and Black Study*. Wivenhoe: Minor Compositions. www.minorcompositions.info/wp-content/uploads/2013/04/undercommons-web.pdf.

Howard, Charles. 2017. "Angela Davis: Power to the Imagination." Huffington Post, December 6, 2017. www.huffpost.com/entry/angela-davis-occupy-philly_b_1067740.

Kelley, Robin D. G. 2002. *Freedom Dreams: The Black Radical Imagination*. Boston: Beacon Press.

Modell, Arnold H. 2003. *Imagination and the Meaningful Brain*. Cambridge, MA: MIT Press.

Moten, Fred. 2003. *In the Break: The Aesthetics of the Black Radical Tradition*. Minneapolis and London: University of Minnesota Press.

———. 2010. "barbara lee." In *B Jenkins*, 84–87. Durham, NC: Duke University Press. https://doi.org/10.1215/9780822392675.

Roberts, Neil. 2015. *Freedom as Marronage*. Chicago: University of Chicago Press.

Robinson, Cedric J. 1983. *Black Marxism: The Making of the Black Radical Tradition*. Chapel Hill and London: The University of North Carolina Press.

———. 1980. *The Terms of Order: Political Leadership and the Myth of Leadership*. Albany: State University of New York Press.

———. 2007. *Forgeries of Memory and Meaning: Blacks and the Regimes of Race in American Theater and Film Before World War II*. Chapel Hill: The University of North Carolina Press.

Shelley, Percy Bysshe. 1821. *A Defence of Poetry*. Poetry Foundation, 2009. www.poetryfoundation.org/resources/learning/essays/detail/69388.

Wollstonecraft, Mary. 1798. *Maria; or The Wrongs of Woman*. Project Gutenberg, 2006. www.gutenberg.org/ebooks/134.

Zeki, Semir. 2009. *Splendors and Miseries of the Brain: Love, Creativity, and the Quest for Human Happiness*. West Sussex, UK: Wiley-Blackwell.

2

WHAT HAS HAPPENED TO THE PUBLIC IMAGINATION AND WHY?

Drucilla Cornell and Stephen D. Seely

What do we mean by the "public imagination"? We could look, first, to definitions of the "public." Jurgen Habermas, for example, has argued that a democratic public sphere first developed in the bourgeois revolutions where people came together in cafés and social clubs to discuss the burning political issues of their time. Crucial to this public, and to the creation of shared meaning, was the printing press, which allowed pamphlets and newspapers to be widely circulated. What is important to Habermas, however, is not the political *imagination*, but the shared meaning that grew out of these public spaces. Many social theorists have bemoaned the collapse of the public sphere in modern democracies in Europe and especially in the U.S., where only the church (and, perhaps, as queer theorists have argued, bars) seems to provide space for collective political and ethical discussion.

But we approach this question somewhat differently. Of course, we accept the insight that public spaces have diminished, especially with the collapse of the industrial unionist movement, which provided an entire edifice of public spaces, most notably workers meetings and union halls. Our approach to the public imagination, however, begins with Spinoza, the greatest thinker of the imagination in the European canon. As we argued immediately after the 2016 U.S. election, Trump's movement—as well as similar fascist, xenophobic, nationalist movements arising throughout Europe—is tied to the collapse of any ethical horizon or sense of shared meaning within neoliberal capitalism: its distorted myths of superiority are an attempt to overcome this nihilism and cultivate a sense of collective belonging (Cornell and Seely 2016). We believe that Spinoza's philosophy can help make further sense of this phenomenon, including how the left might build an effective response to it.

To put it very simply, Spinoza teaches us that the imagination is always collective. For him, mind and matter are two attributes of the same substance—two sides of the same coin, so to speak. Every material encounter produces a corresponding image in the mind (and vice versa). For Spinoza, the imagination is just as real as atoms. We live in a world in which we are constantly being affected by other people and by our own bodies as we experience them embedded in the world, and we are constantly developing images of our bodies and our relations with others. Because of our embeddedness in an affective world, there is ultimately no such thing as an isolated individual because what any one person "is" is determined by her affective encounters. As the material world is collective, so is the mind: our own imagination is inextricably tied into a collective imagination shared by those with whom we share material encounters. For Spinoza, the more we open ourselves to being affected by others, the more we allow ourselves to engage in complex situations, the richer our imagination becomes and the more we move away from our own inevitably "inadequate" ideas toward a rational commons. This is because the more complex our material engagements are the more complex our mind is.

Spinoza was therefore a proponent of democracy, defined precisely as the form of government that allows the greatest expression of different images and different material engagements. Democracy, so defined, allows us to be affected by as many people as possible, in all of their diversity, and this in turn promotes the maximal clarification of inadequate ideas. The more open we are to being affected by others who are different from what we currently imagine ourselves to be, the more our imagination is enriched and the more we are empowered in both body and mind. Given this, what we are seeing now is the dearth of collective imagination. Trump and his supporters want us literally to be walled off from Mexico, blocked off from the tragedy in Syria. He wants to keep us from interacting and creating new, enriched images of people in different religions through his grotesque Muslim ban. He wants to turn women into things whose impact on public life is as limited as possible, imagined instead as nothing other than their reproductive organs to be "grabbed" and controlled. These walls and barriers clearly block democracy in Spinoza's sense, as the widest engagement with each other.

So we wish to emphasize two points here. The first is that all of Trump's moves undermine, if not completely block, the development of a rich collective imagination—and therefore democracy itself. Secondly, shared meanings have collapsed with the death of important public spaces; in their place we have a nihilistic universe in which people are desperate to find some kind of values in their own lives. Rather than democratic engagement, which is the basis of an ever-enriched and complex commons that facilitates maximal individual and collective flourishing, we have the nihilistic hole filled in with distorted myths that provide an inadequate imaginary fueled by simple-minded fantasies that heterosexual white men are superior and should govern the world. (From Spinoza's perspective, it is telling that this form of "power" can only rule by imposing the greatest number of barriers and limits in order to restrict the collective empowerment of the commons.) Hence, the importance of feminism and movements such as Black Lives Matter: through the affirmation of the feminine within sexual difference or blackness, these movements spur collective material encounters that are otherwise proscribed. Such alternative forms of material engagement not only enable women and people of color to reimagine themselves beyond the inadequate ideas imposed on them through sexism and racism, but provide new collectively shared images of what it means to be human.

In a sense, the collective imagination can be understood as the consolidated images, symbols, stories, and histories through which groups, nations, and other institutional forms materialize themselves and imagine their place in the world. But, we argue that these must always be open to contest through democratic practices that allow us to be affectively moved and transformed through what we have called "political spirituality." Political spirituality names precisely the way in which imaginations and "regimes of truth," to use Foucault's phrase, should remain inherently open to challenge and change as we are affected differently the more we open ourselves to all others who surround us and share our world with us. As neoliberal capitalism has undermined all collectively shared horizons of ethical meaning, replacing them with the one image of the risk manager who sees others as only those who will take away from the self, it is not surprising that contact with other people becomes a frightening prospect and other humans become something that we must guard against. But as we close ourselves off to material, affective encounters with others, we close our imaginations as well, freezing the collective imagination in entrenched inadequate ideas that are impervious to democratic contestation. As we see with Spinoza, our material engagements limit our imagination and vice versa: the more we are walled off from others, the more we are unable to imagine differently (and vice versa). Trump's walls and bans therefore literally threaten the imagination with death.

We therefore want to emphasize in conclusion that a new powerful left can only create a rich collective imagination capable of confronting this crisis by opening ourselves to new forms of contact that will allow us to be affected by, and imagine, others in new ways. This in turn demands the widest forms of participatory democracy amongst ourselves. We must not limit our struggle to current forms of political engagement which accept the terms of the game—terms that, for decades, have dictated that the economy is beyond the reach of collective contestation. The rise of Bernie Sanders showed that by prominently returning the words "socialism" and "revolution" to the forefront, a new realm of the imagination was opened for millions of young people. That we may not know what a revolution or socialist economy would look like is part of the way capitalism has limited the collective imagination through the imposition of a limited range of material encounters. But the naturalization of capitalism is nothing more than a powerful collective imagination that, by preventing certain forms of collective contest, has fundamentally limited our ability to imagine other possibilities. Thus, we must continue to keep the struggle against capitalism central to any kind of struggle for a just world—but class is not separable from struggles against racism, xenophobia, sexism, and heteronormativity. This is not because of some kind of "intersection," but because these forms of systemic violence operate by distributing and regulating people in terms of consolidated narratives that limit their material encounters and their imaginations in different ways.

So if we are to be open to our responsibility for enriching the collective imagination, then we have to dare to encounter others different from ourselves, not bury them under discriminatory images. We must also challenge the reigning naturalization of capitalism that says certain things simply cannot be imagined. Trump's promise to "make America great again" plays off a lack of shared meaning, the failure of our democratic institutions, and a powerful set of limitations imposed on the kinds of encounters that we are capable of having. Too often the left has tried to bolster itself with dogmatic truths, but for us the challenge of political spirituality is to dare to risk the kind of "danger"—and it was Foucault who said that everything is dangerous, but this means we always have something to do—that our imagination of a more just world can only be opened in and through actual struggles that expand our material possibilities.

References

Cornell, Drucilla, and Stephen D. Seely. 2016. "Seven Theses on Trump." Critical Legal Thinking, November 28, 2016. http://criticallegalthinking.com/2016/11/28/seven-theses-trump/.

3

IMAGINAL POLITICS IN THE AGE OF TRUMPISM

Chiara Bottici

We often hear people saying that our politicians lack imagination. In the epoch of global governance when politics is reduced to mere administration, there seems to be little space for the free development of imagination. Yet, if we consider the spectacularization of politics that appears on our screens every day, and most recently, the upsurge of heated talk about "fake news" versus real news, we cannot but perceive an excess of imagination. How can we explain the paradox of an eclipse of imagination that goes hand in hand with its hypertrophy? In order to come to terms with such a paradox we need to rethink the link between politics and our capacity to imagine.

If one looks at the meaning of the concept of imagination, it is not difficult to perceive two quite different usages. In our everyday language, we tend to associate imagination with what is not there, with the unreal, as in common expressions such as this is "purely the fruit of your imagination." However, along with this usage of the term, there is another that goes back to the ancient Greek term *phantasia* and which is associated with the production of images in the most general sense—that is, images of both what is there and what cannot be there. It is in this second sense of the term that images are so central to our political life.

In order to recover this insight, the concept of the *imaginal* has recently come to the fore, as suggested by Cynthia Fleury.[1] Whereas imagination tends to be conceived as a faculty that individuals possess, and the social imaginary as the social context that, so to speak, possesses us, the *imaginal* is simply what is made of images and, as such, can be the product of both. Because the concept of the imaginal makes no epistemological assumptions with respect to the faculty that produces images (either the individual, as conceived in the liberal tradition, or the social imaginary, as derived from the communitarian one), it is a much better tool to theorize the politics that goes through the production and reproduction of images. Furthermore, whereas the concepts of imagination and of the imaginary are usually associated with a lack, the concept of the imaginal, as simply what is made of images, makes no assumptions as to the ontological status of images. Consequently, the imaginal is a much more open concept, and therefore is more easily adapted to diverse contexts. The imaginal thus conceived plays a crucial role in all aspects of social life, because images are what enable us to orient ourselves in the world, to disclose both what is already there and what is yet to come.

What is therefore the political role of the imaginal?[2] If we understand "politics" to mean whatever pertains to the decisions concerning the fate of a community, it patently depends on the imaginal because it depends on the possibility of making the public exist in the first place. This holds not only for large communities such as modern states, but also for small ones: even in small communities based on face to face relationships, you need to imagine a community in order to make it exist out of a simple collection of individuals. Communities exist because we imagine they exist. In other words, politics depends on the imaginal because it depends on the possibility of imagining commonalities and, thus, on the possibility of freeing oneself of one's own particularities by imagining what each of us might have in common with others. Even more crucial is the role of the imaginal in thinking of a potentially global community as an alternative to individualism and nationalism.

Given such an understanding, what then are the contemporary implications of this strict link between politics and the imaginal? Because images mediate our being in the world, they are crucial for all communication, with political communication being no exception. That images overwhelm contemporary politics is no surprise: politics today feeds on our very capacity to create images. If one thinks of what politics used to be just a few centuries ago, a huge change in its very nature quickly becomes evident. Our political experience is now inconceivable outside of the continual flow of images that appear on our myriad screens. Today, images no longer only mediate political activities; they have also become an end in themselves, thereby running the risk of doing politics in our place.

Yet, amidst this profusion of images, we find something more—a sort of hypertrophy of the imagination due to the massive diffusion of media. With its repetition of nationalistic symbols and images, contemporary politics also seems to lack the capacity to question what is given. This apparent paradox is the result of a hypertrophy of the more *passive* side of imagination, which happened at the expense of its more *active* side. We are so image-saturated that it has become increasingly difficult to create radically new images. This, in turn, is the consequence of a change in both in the *quantity* and the *quality* of the images produced in our global epoch.

In terms of quantity, we cannot but notice a decisive increase in the sheer number of images that enter our life. Indeed, the quantity of images produced by the media has reached such proportion as to effect a qualitative leap: images have become an end in themselves. Many authors, for instance, have noticed the ritual function of elections. By virtue of their mere repetitions, elections reinforce a certain model of society by providing it with visible continuity. However, the quantity of images that accompanies contemporary elections in most Western countries has become such that the spectacle completely prevails over the content. Images are too many, and they seemingly proliferate without any logic of selection. Audiences, instead, provide the filter: only those images that can capture people's attention are raised out of the stream. Hence, the predominance of spectacle. However, the battles staged on our screens during elections obscure the fact that no real battle is taking place, because the real clash is not among the official candidates (who most often have very similar programs), but instead lies beyond our screens. The real fight is between the political options that are admitted and those that are denied entry into the public arena. The decisive distance is not between candidates and elections, but between those candidates and political platforms that secure a role in the spectacle, and those left out.

In terms of quality, we find another intrinsic change in the nature of images, a change that is likely to affect the link between politics and the imagination even further. Behind the virtual revolution, there is indeed a deep change in the nature of images: not only have images become commodities, which are therefore subjected to the laws and treatment of all other commodities, but now they are also malleable in a way never before possible. In the epoch of Photoshop, images are both serially *reproducible* and fundamentally *modifiable* such that they can be completely falsified. In other words, images lose their connection to a tangible "here" and "now." Whereas with celluloid photography images were still connected to their original act of creation (a picture of something needed to be taken before being reproduced), with virtuality this tether has been overcome. There is no "here" and "now" of the original creation in a virtual image, and therefore no authenticity to be preserved. Virtual images are not objects that can be created once, but rather are ongoing processes, signalling a technological change that deeply affects the way we relate to images, and also our assumptions about knowledge and reality, since images are what mediate our experience of the world.

Although this dynamic process has great democratic potential because everybody can intervene in a virtual image, it also opens new and terrifying scenarios because we have no secure criteria to determine the authenticity of such images. Anything goes—even faked information—so long as it captures the audience's attention. When linked together with the desire to be noticed, we are invited to give up on truth and reality as the ultimate criteria for deciding what matters in politics and everyday life.

It is only in this context of a deep transformation in the phenomenology of the imaginal, that we can come to terms with phenomena such as Trumpism. The latter does not simply result from a manipulation of our capacity to imagine: it feeds on this transformation that made Trumpism possible in the first place, which it consciously seeks to affect in turn (Bottici 2016). In other words, we need to understand why people were ready to exchange "fake news" for "real news" in order to understand why the most professional politician one can imagine has lost the presidential elections to the most unprofessional one in generations, who now sits in the White House.

This imaginal transformation also explains the paradox from which we started—a political world full of images but deprived of imagination. Because we are saturated by the deluge of images and rendered even more cynical by their increasing spectacularization and virtualization, we have more difficulties creating radically alternative images of our present, and future, political life. It is in this imaginal space that appeals to revivals of nationalist sentiments proliferate. But it is also in this space that we need to operate if we want to create alternative views of our future.

Notes

1 The concept has recently been recovered from Islamic Neoplatonic thinkers by Cynthia Fleury. See in particular her edited volume (Fleury 2006).
2 I have dealt with these issues more extensively in Bottici (2014).

References

Bottici, Chiara. 2014. *Imaginal Politics: Images Beyond the Imagination and Beyond the Imaginary*. New York: Columbia University Press.

———. 2016. "The Mass Psychology of Trumpism: Old and New Myths." November 17, 2016. www.publicseminar.org/2016/11/the-mass-psychology-of-trumpism/.

Fleury, Cynthia. 2006. *Imagination, Imaginaire, Imaginal*. Paris: Presses universitaires de France.

4

PUBLIC SPACE

Thinking at the Edge of the Cave

Fred Dallmayr

What is "the public"? What do we mean by "public space" or "public sphere"? What kind of space is this, and how can we find it? Is it just an outer or external space contraposed to an inner or internal one? Is it the case that, when we leave our home, we enter a different space, a public one? And if we cannot find it, can we simply construct it, fabricate it, or imagine it (using our faculties of reason, will, and imagination)? Perhaps, the space we are talking about is more like what Martin Heidegger called "world"—which, as he told us, is neither outside nor inside, neither an external object nor an inner/subjective faculty because it is located on an entirely different (an "ontological") level. Heidegger has written much about space and spatiality, which I shall not repeat here. Late in his life, in 1969 he wrote an essay on "Art and Space" (*Die Kunst und der Raum*). There we read: "Space—does it not belong to those Ur-phenomena at whose encounter (in Goethe's words) human beings are overcome by awe and even anguish? For behind it, there is nothing to which it could be further traced."[1]

As one can see, the question of public space is not simply a matter of physical or geometrical extension; in a way, it shares the awe surrounding spatiality as such. Clearly, the "public" is not just the "others," nor is it me; it is neither their property nor mine. Differently put: it cannot be appropriated, instrumentalized or controlled by any side. In traditional languages, the public is something "in-between" or "metaxy" (as Plato called it), and even something beyond "in-between" because it involves what makes the "between" possible. To this extent, the public has an ethical quality, or perhaps an ethical-spiritual quality, because genuine ethics is always transformative, a move beyond you and me. This is why dealing with the "public" is always a demanding or challenging enterprise; it means participating in a happening or "event" (*Ereignis*) stretching us beyond ourselves.[2] In Heideggerian language, the happening is neither an external fate, nor can it be engineered. It occurs at the edge of human self-interest—or, if you will, at the edge of the Platonic "cave."

Contrary to widespread opinion, the momentous quality of the public event has not disappeared in modernity. In fact, despite secularization, commercialization, and the rise of scientism and technology, the public lives on in uncanny, subterranean ways. While in earlier times the public was anchored or instantiated in substantive institutions—like monarchy or empire—this anchor has vanished with the onset of democracy. Since that time, the center of gravity has shifted or has moved out of sight. But although out of sight, it has not vanished. In his book

Democracy and Political Theory, French philosopher Claude Lefort has clearly addressed the "out of sight" character of the democratic public space. In a chapter instructively titled "The Permanence of the Theological-Political," he speaks of the public center of democracy as an "empty place" or "empty space." To be sure, "emptiness" here does not mean a sheer vacuum, but rather something like a hidden resource or generative power. In this sense, it is close to Heidegger's view of "nothingness" (*das Nichts*) and to the Buddhist "emptiness" (*sunyata*). The main point is that this center cannot be appropriated, possessed and exploited for partisan aims. As Lefort writes: Of all the regimes we know, [democracy] is the only one to have represented [public] power in such a way as to show that it is an *empty place* … It does so by virtue of discourse which reveals that power belongs to no one; that those who exercise power do not possess it; that they do not, indeed, embody it.[3]

Unhappily, democracy in recent times has been moving precisely in the opposite direction, namely, the direction of appropriation, ownership, and embodiment. In Lefort's time, the chief danger to emptiness was totalitarianism, predicated on the identification of the public with "the people as One." In the meantime, other kinds of dangers have emerged, most prominently a predatory capitalist system (styled "neo-liberalism") bent on surrendering everything in society to individual and corporate appropriation. Political theorist Bonnie Honig recently published a remarkable book called *Public Things*, subtitled *Democracy in Disrepair*. Although, on the surface, the title "Public Things" is just a routine translation of the Latin *res publica*, Honig injects into the phrase a radical twist which exposes the "disrepair" of contemporary democratic politics. Although upholding the need for publicly shared concerns, her book also launches an indictment: namely, that increasingly such concerns are reified and objectified and thereby transformed into targets for individual or corporate appropriation. As she writes: "My focus on public 'things' is occasioned in part by the contemporary impulse to privatize everything"—where privatization involves schools, prisons, military forces and ultimately even the "White House" as the seat of American government.[4] Honig here agrees with fellow-theorist Wendy Brown who has called attention to "the stealthy work of neoliberal rationality" in our time. Although leaving the shell of democracy intact, neoliberal strategy—for both Honig and Brown—ultimately undermines democracy and "hollows it out" from within: "People are now trained to think of themselves as a resource to be invested in for future profits or earnings, not as subjects of integrity or … as stewards of shared futures."[5]

Behind the scenes, other issues are subtly stirred up in Honig's book involving the status of "thinghood." Although taking her bearing from D. W. Winnicott's "object-relations" theory, Honig's notion of "thing" may not be the same as "object" (since the latter always involves a subject-object relation, with objects serving as targets of acquisitive subjects). Maybe "thing" is closer to what I said before about "space" and "public space"; at least in the treatment of Heidegger, "thing" is a relational notion, a gathering of elements in the "fourfold" (Heidegger 1954, 37–55). From this perspective, things share in the awesome or noumenal aura surrounding spatiality. The cultivation and preservation of things are a human-transhuman challenge. Wedded to the maintenance of "public things," democracy emerges also as a human-transhuman challenge or as an ethical-spiritual task. Honig seems to be in accord on this point when she writes that her entire argument is "in favor of embracing publicness in democratic life, for the sake of democratic life, because public things constitute citizens equally as citizens, or ought to, and can be made, sometimes, by action in concert, to deliver on that promise" (Honig 2017b, 11).

Honig here throws into relief the status of democratic citizenship when she says that the public or "public things" constitute citizens as citizens (and not the other way around) Strictly interpreted this means that citizens do not actually "constitute" or engender the public space;

rather they become citizens by virtue of that space. Thus, whenever individual or corporate agents seek to seize or appropriate the public space, democratic citizenship vanishes, and with it democracy itself. This may be the meaning (or one of the meanings) of Sheldon Wolin's well-known statement about the "fugitive" character of democracy, about democracy's tendency to slip from one's grasp as soon as it is treated as a property or instrument of political control. Against this tendency, Wolin marshaled a completely different conception according to which democracy is construed not as a reified structure, but rather as "a mode of being" that derives from struggle and bitter experience but remains "a recurrent possibility" as long as the meaning of the public survives.[6]

What follows from these considerations is a lesson about public agency. As indicated before, individuals become citizens and public agents by virtue of the public space. Seen in this light, citizens are not "sovereign" masters, but participants in the multilayered "happening" of that space. To this extent, they are bound together not just by "interests," but by bonds which, in a way, point beyond the edge of the cave: toward a realm of non-possession, non-domination and freedom. In traditional language, this direction is called the "good life." Honig in this connection speaks appropriately of a "promise"—which means that "good life" refers not so much to a factual condition as to a possibility or potentiality. Moving—however haltingly—in this direction, citizens inevitably have the character of stand-ins, precursors or heralds of things "to come."[7] Richard Falk uses the term "citizen pilgrims."[8] The goal of the journey here cannot be concretely described or pinpointed because it is more in the nature of a call. But all of us, remembering keenly the despair inside the cave, are impelled by an urgent plea: the plea for what we call—almost breathlessly—the city of justice and peace.

Notes

1 (Heidegger 1969, 7). For Heidegger's more extensive discussion of space and spatiality see (Heidegger 1962, 135–148). His view of space is in many ways akin to the notion of "topos" as articulated by the Japanese philosopher Kitaro Nishida.

2 On Heidegger's notion of "*Ereignis*" see especially his book (2009).

3 See (Lefort 1988, 225). On Heidegger's notion of "*das Nichts*" see (Heidegger 1977, 95–112). See also (Dallmayr 1996, 175–199).

4 See (Honig 2017b, 3). Compare also her (1993, 2013, 59–76); and her stirring (2017a).

5 (Honig 2017b, 13–14). See also (Brown 2015, 18; 200) and (Dean 2015).

6 See (Wolin 1996, 31–45); also (Dallmayr 2001, 71–89). Compare in this context also (Elshtain 1995), a text which sees democracy today chiefly threatened by the onslaught of boundless individual and corporate self-aggrandisement.

7 Honig seems to be open to the spiritual or noumenal quality of the public trajectory. Referring specifically to Franz Rosenzweig's *The Star of Redemption*, she writes (2017b, 106, n. 14) that the book "may be read as a kind of education to miracle" because it "presupposes and teaches attentiveness, receptivity, preparation, orientation." As she adds: "Democratic theorists may learn from Rosenzweig. Receptivity to miracle has its secular political analogues, one example of which is the power of public things to gather us together."

8 See (Falk 2002, 27–28). Compare also (Dallmayr 2017, 2010).

References

Brown, Wendy. 2015. *Undoing the Demos: Neoliberalism's Stealth Revolution*. New York: Zone Books.

Dallmayr, Fred R. 1996. "*Sunyata* East and West: Emptiness and Global Democracy." In *Beyond Orientalism: Essays on Cross-Cultural Encounter*, New York: SUNY Press, pp. 175–200.

———. 2001. "Beyond Fugitive Democracy." In *Achieving Our World: Toward a Global and Plural Democracy*, Lanham, MD: Rowman & Littlefield, pp. 71–90.

———. 2010. *The Promise of Democracy: Political Agency and Transformation*. New York: SUNY Press.

———. 2017. *Democracy to Come: Politics as Relational Praxis*. New York: Oxford University Press.

Dean, Jodi. 2015. "Neoliberalism's Defeat of Democracy." Review of *Undoing the Demos: Neoliberalism's Stealth Revolution* by Wendy Brown. *Critical Inquiry*, October 27, 2015. https://criticalinquiry.uchicago.edu/neoliberalisms_defeat_of_democracy/.

Elshtain, Jean Bethke. 1995. *Democracy on Trial*. New York: Basic Books.

Falk, Richard. 2002. "An Emergent Matrix of Citizenship: Complex, Uneven, and Fluid." In *Global Citizenship: A Critical Introduction*, edited by Nigel Dower and John Williams. New York: Routledge, pp. 15–29.

Heidegger, Martin. 1954. "Das Ding." In *Vorträge und Aufsätze*, Vol. 2. Pfullingen, Germany: Neske, pp. 37–55.

———. 1962. *Being and Time*. Translated by John Macquarric and Edward Robinson. New York: Harper & Row.

———. 1969. *Die Kunst und der Raum; L'Art et l'Espace*. St. Gallen: Erker Verlag.

———. 1977. "What is Metaphysics?" In *Martin Heidegger: Basic Writings*, edited by David F. Krell. New York: Harper & Row, pp. 89–110.

———. 2009. *Das Ereignis Gesamtausgabe*. Vol. 71. Frankfurt am Main: Vittorio Klostermann.

Honig, Bonnie. 1993. *Political Theory and the Displacement of Politics*. Ithaca, NY: Cornell University Press.

———. 2013. "The Politics of Public Things: Neoliberalism and the Routine of Privatization." *No Foundations* no. 10.

———. 2017a. "The President's House is Empty." Boston Review, January 19, 2017. http://bostonreview.net/politics/bonnie-honig-president%E2%80%99s-house-empty.

———. 2017b. *Public Things: Democracy in Disrepair*. New York: Fordham University Press.

Lefort, Claude. 1988. *Democracy and Political Theory*. Translated by David Macey. Minneapolis, MN: University of Minnesota Press.

Wolin, Sheldon S. 1996. "Fugitive Democracy." In *Democracy and Difference: Contesting the Boundaries of the Political*, edited by Seyla Benhabib. Princeton, NJ: Princeton University Press, pp. 31–45.

Bibliography

Rosenzweig, Franz. 2014. *The Star of Redemption*. Notre Dame, IN: Notre Dame Press.

5

SCALING IMAGINATION

The Political Implications of Popular Media

Michael Curtin

At the dawn of the 21st century, cultural homogenization was widely considered one of the most threatening aspects of globalization. Following a decade of deregulation, financialization, and technological innovation, powerful media conglomerates were plying their way across national frontiers, hailing new audiences that seemed to transcend culture, gender, and generation. Disney, Fox, and Time Warner led the way, soon joined by new media titans, such as Facebook, Netflix, and Activision Blizzard. Yet even as American media seemed to be growing ever more influential, new transnational competitors began emerge as well: Rotana from Dubai, Reliance from Bombay, and CJ Entertainment from Seoul. They were complemented by digital, gaming, and social media companies such as China's Tencent, France's Ubisoft, and Russia's Yandex.

Arguably, these conglomerates have saturated the world with images that participate in the spectacularization of politics, which in turn favors the interests of neo-liberal capitalism and squeezes out alternative visions (Bottici, Chapter 3). This cultural environment has also been conducive to the rise of authoritarian leaders like Trump, Modi, Putin, and Xi (Falk and Faessel, Introduction). Training their sights on enemies foreign and domestic, these leaders deploy divisive imagery and rhetoric aimed at "walling off" meaningful encounters across frontiers of difference (Cornell and Seeley, Chapter 2). Paradoxically, nationalism and authoritarianism seem to be gaining traction because of, and in spite of, the globalization of contemporary media.

And yet the implications of this media revolution are more complicated and perhaps less dire than some critics would suggest. For at the same time that media conglomerates have commodified many domains of culture and sought to shape modalities of cultural expression, they have also unexpectedly fostered new forms of social affinity and public imagination, many of which transcend social differences and index fresh prospects for progressive politics.

If, as Richard Falk and Victor Faessel argue, "public imagination" is a plural concept that invites connections between diverse modalities and processes, both formal and informal, it should encourage us to use popular culture as a lens for exploring these new topographies of imagination (de Certeau 1984). A first step may be to set aside explicitly political considerations and reflect instead on the dynamics of popular culture within and across localities. By popular culture, I'm referring here to what some might call entertainment media—such as film, television, music, gaming, sports, and social media—those forms of culture that focus on pleasure and performance as opposed to expressly political forms of journalism and information media. Although the two domains are inevitably intertwined, popular culture is generally considered distracting, derivative, and commodified. It is rarely a touchstone for analysis of, for example, resurgent nationalist authoritarianism. Instead, critics point to neo-liberalism, jihadism, and mass migrations of the dispossessed as fueling the wave of resentment against globalization.

For most people, however, these phenomena are highly mediated and it's important to understand that many who embrace the political right are exceptionally concerned about their eroding status as tastemakers and cultural arbiters. This unease plays out most conspicuously across gender and generation. Husbands are concerned about their wives' media use; parents are bewildered by their children's expansive access to popular culture; and older citizens are nostalgic for the days of collective spectatorship in the living room rather than personalized media use via smartphones, tablets, and laptops. Even if only intuitively, people are aware that new media configurations, flows, and practices are re-scaling social connections and imaginaries in ways that may jeopardize patriarchal notions of family, community, and self. Conversely, women, children, immigrants, minorities, and LGBTQ communities commonly turn to popular culture for resources to help them narrate their experiences outside dominant frames by sharing fantasies or making themselves more publicly visible. In many cases, their media use isn't explicitly political. They are making do and getting by. Theirs are the "footsteps in the city," tactical maneuvers by which they negotiate terrains that are structured by dominant elites.[1] Yet it is their cumulative engagement with media from near and far that generates new affinities and topographies of imagination.

Popular Media

Therefore, if it seems a particularly dark moment in the realm of explicit politics, the tacit politics of popular culture offer perhaps a more hopeful if contradictory blend. For media globalization has engendered a complex play of integration and differentiation, of dominance and resistance, and of nationalist authoritarianism and post-national solidarities. Popular media are therefore central resources for imagining the diverse publics of today and tomorrow.

What are the characteristics of this new era of media globalization? How do 21st century media differ from their predecessors?

First of all, as mention above, modes of finance and circuits of distribution have changed dramatically since the 1990s. Not only are Hollywood films conceived, financed, and circulated transnationally, so too are Arab television shows, Korean pop songs, and French video games. Of course, many other cultural products still serve local and national audiences, but transnational media distribution has escalated dramatically, driven by competitive pressures and facilitated by new technologies.

Secondly, modes of media production and creativity have stretched across space, initiated primarily by the pursuit of cost economies among the worlds most prosperous and prolific producers, the Hollywood studios. As the budgets for film, television, and video game productions ballooned into the hundreds of millions of dollars, producers began to develop relations with studio facilities and government entities around the world. Today, cities such as Vancouver, Prague, and Hyderabad compete to offer "world class" infrastructure, labor, and government subsidies that facilitate a geographically mobile and protean mode of production.

Thirdly, this transnational production apparatus is made possible by a convergence of professional practices that have emerged via knowledge exchanges that take place in offices and production studios, as well as in the international markets for content exchange (e.g., MIPCOM). Workers at these sites share techniques as well as insider tips, gossip, and industry folklore. Film festivals (Busan) and awards ceremonies (African Movie Academy Awards) also provide contexts for deliberations about aesthetic and professional practices.

Fourthly, as media professionals interact in these transnational venues, much of what they learn and observe filters back to national and local contexts where textual features and production techniques are imitated or adapted, resulting in hybrid content that is reimagined for different publics. Remarkably, adaptations move "up" and "down" as well as "across." That is, content and aesthetics not only circulate widely, they are also refigured in order to address different topographies of imagination. And they create new topographies. What was once a Latin American regional media market has recently become interwoven with the very substantial and prosperous Latinx market in the United States, resulting in a new hemispheric scale of popular imagination, creation, and circulation. A foundational genre of this media sphere is the telenovela, which has changed dramatically as a result of globalizing forces, and has moreover become an agent of change by influencing producers in distant locales, such as Istanbul, Lagos, and Beijing.

Finally, we are witnessing new patterns of interaction between media users and producers, as well as among users themselves. Once seen primarily as consumers, today's viewers and fans amply express themselves in a variety of ways and media producers systematically monitor this discourse, creating feedback loops that shape story lines and characters. Moreover, online commentary and recommendations have become fundamental factors in the popularity of media texts and in the expansion of media options (Jenkins 2018).

In China, for example, social media sites like Weixin and Weibo have stimulated an explosion of awareness about foreign titles as well as local niche offerings, which used to be unavailable in mainland mass media. Netizens also volunteer for subtitling teams that each year make thousands of foreign films and television shows almost instantly available. Moreover, user-generated content has mushroomed, again blurring the distinctions between media creators and consumers, and blurring distinctions between cultural points of origin. Setting aside debates over piracy, one finds that peer-to-peer sharing of media content has exponentially increased the transnational availability of media content.

Politics of the Popular

Consequently, we now live in an era of transnational media scapes, spheres, regions, and zones. These are protean spaces of imagination that are constituted and reconstituted from top to bottom, spaces that would have been unimaginable during the 1980s when it cost $3.20 per minute to place a phone call across the Pacific, when blockbuster cinema was the proprietary province of Hollywood, and when government regulations and technical standards prevented TV viewers in Singapore and Senegal from watching the same program.

Researchers have historically focused on media's capacity, or putative mission, to reinforce local and national ties, but we're now seeing the ways in which media worlds emerge, scale, and diminish in response to a relentless tug of actors and forces. Importantly, these creative dynamics provide groups and individuals with resources for negotiating everyday life and imagining new futures.[2]

Still, this analysis should not be mistaken for a utopian embrace of the autonomous power of electronic media to bring about beneficial social change. Mobile phones have come to rural

India, but in many places they are in the hands of men who use them to obtain market prices and job postings when they're not viewing movies and music videos. Women are barred from using phones for fear they will be distracted from their chores or seduced by online suitors. In some ways, the affordances of the mobile phone make men both more inquisitive and more guarded about their status and authority. These are the sorts of complex dynamics that play out in the everyday world where media globalization generates friction, and this friction helps to explain why some people find nostalgic authoritarianism appealing while others see it opening up the landscape of personal and political opportunity (Tsing 2005).

Media globalization has therefore engendered a complicated cultural geography that is characterized by what John Tomlinson describes as complex connectivity, a product of novel interconnections and interdependencies that have emerged despite the enduring realities of physical distance (Tomlinson 1999). This connectivity fosters social experiences and relations that change one's perspective in place and allow new interactions across space, but it also may accentuate differences and new forms of social conflict. Authoritarian nationalism is therefore one response to these conditions, but so too are the new progressive sensibilities that are circulating in unexpected ways via today's popular media and culture.

Notes

1 See in this regard Dallmayr (Chapter 4).

2 Athique (2016). They also can provide the basis for more politically engaged forms of media activity, see Carlson (Chapter 1) and Sinclair (Chapter 6).

References

Athique, Adrian. 2016. *Transnational Audiences: Media Reception on a Global Scale*. Cambridge: Polity Press.

de Certeau, Michel. 1984. *The practice of everyday life*. Berkeley and Los Angeles: University of California Press.

Jenkins, Henry. 2018. "What 'Black Panther' Can Teach Us About the Civic Imagination." *global-e* 11, no. 27.

Tomlinson, John. 1999. *Globalization and Culture*. Cambridge: Polity Press.

Tsing, Anna Lowenhaupt. 2005. *Friction: An Ethnography of Global Connection*. Princeton, NJ: Princeton University Press.

Bibliography

Bottici, Chaira. "Imaginal Politics in the Age of Trumpism." Chapter 3, this volume.

Carlson, Julie A. "Rallying: Imagination's Political Process." Chapter 1, this volume.

Cornell, Drucilla, and Seely, Stephen D. "What Has Happened to the Public Imagination, and Why?" Chapter 2, this volume.

Dallmayr, Fred. "Public Space: Thinking at the Edge of the Cave." Chapter 4, this volume.

Falk, Richard, and Victor Faessel. "Public Imagination: The Challenge of Populist and Authoritarian Politics." Introduction, this volume.

Sinclair, Kamal. "A New Operating System For Humanity: The Power of Narrative." Chapter 6, this volume.

6

A NEW OPERATING SYSTEM FOR HUMANITY

The Power of Narrative

Kamal Sinclair

Since humankind's earliest days, we have used stories to communicate knowledge, to form our understanding of the world, prescribe behavior, and imagine our futures. Therefore, the stories we tell and the identities we construct about our future are literally writing the next operating system for humanity.

Over the last few decades we've experienced a rapid expansion of our communication architecture that mediamakers have leveraged to give audiences new experiences of story. They are now able to transport audiences into parallel human-scale environments, where they can traverse space and "be" in another part of the world instantly and break them out of a pedestrian reality to have non-human-scale experiences. These new technologies allow audiences to embody another person's perspective; to connect story to place and have live interactions through their devices; to perceive humanity from a macro scale through smart algorithms sculpting beauty from our data. They can even preserve a persona for future generations through AI enabled holograms and use audience members' own biometrics as input for interactive experiences.

These emerging media are projected to be worth trillions of dollars in the coming decade. They form part the Fourth Industrial Revolution, which is ushering in sweeping changes with enormous promise for advancing civilization. However, we know from history that industrial revolutions can bring great injustice as well as great value.

Why should economists and business leaders care? Because repeating patterns of exclusion and injustice in this industrial revolution will worsen the climate change bill we are already struggling to pay from past innovation cycles, and will fail to fully optimize our new capabilities for global prosperity.

The technologies coming with the current paradigm shift are arguably more powerful than those developed in past industrial revolutions, yet are we repeating the same mistakes of having a narrow group of people decide their value for humanity, as well as lining up only a small number of people to benefit economically from their implementation? What viruses will emerge as a result? What are the consequences of repeating this pattern of exclusion?

It is imperative that we include people in this emerging media landscape from a broad set of communities, identity groups, value systems, and fields of knowledge, in all roles and levels of power. This will mitigate the pitfalls of disruption. Right now, we could have a window of opportunity that allows us to create an inclusive process for designing our future. Frankly, this time the stakes are too high to have a small fraction of our global community define the values and features of our next operating system.

Late last year, I interviewed Skawennati, a Mohawk woman from Canada who is also a machinima artist, who facilitates game design workshops with indigenous youth. She shared her experience of a long-standing struggle to reconcile the values of her indigenous and technologist cultures. The former centers on family time, community, nature, and a sometimes non-analytical process to generate inspiration and creativity. The latter centers on fast-fail, rapid iteration, bottom-line ROI, and an often highly analytical process for sparking new ideas.

During the course of our conversation about new gains in artificial intelligence, we imagined the possibility of a future that achieved a true integration of these value systems. What if, instead of just replacing jobs and leaving many people in an outmoded class, AI allowed us time to focus more on our families, on our communities, on philosophy and creativity? Diverse story coders might generate shared imaginations of our future, where AI is used for inclusion, rather than exclusion.

Let's assess this democratized imagination framework with the hindsight of past industrial revolutions. What if this process had been in place when manufacturing jobs went overseas, or became automated, during the 20th Century in the United States? What if those people "left behind" were prompted to imagine a future they wanted to live in and to imagine their role in it? Could such an imaginative process have mitigated 50 years of economic downturn? Could it have helped us better mitigate the unethical disruptions we experienced? Perhaps this transition approach might have allowed a greater diversity of ideas to bubble up and uncover the full potential of new human capabilities in the computer age. At the same time, it might have mitigated the deep resentments created by the top-down or prescriptive-transition approaches of the time.

Alas, we may not have been able to achieve this in the past, not only because of the ideological challenges, but also the limited technologies. Now, however, for the first time in history, humanity is equipped with the tools and social-media culture to collectively imagine our future on a global scale.

What if, instead of the majority of the world being marginalized from the process that is defining our future, we used the new interactive tools, data science, smart algorithms and immersive platforms to include a broad scope of people? What if this fuller representation of humanity collaborated on defining the value and purpose of our new and extraordinary technological capabilities through the stories they make about the world we will be living in? What kind of human-centered uses would we imagine for artificial intelligence, synthetic biology, supercomputing, and immersive media? What bugs in our operating system might be circumvented? This is the opportunity offered to us by emerging media.

For example, new capabilities in machine learning can exacerbate inequality; or, depending on the value systems we create in the AI infrastructure, they can end inequalities, such as hunger and homelessness. We also know that a robust machine-learning infrastructure will require a greater interdependence between companies, institutions and governments than previous technologies, as indicated by DeepMind's experiment with competing AIs.

How would a truly diverse set of storytellers imagine this interdependence working? What aspects of our traditional economic models—individualistic, free-market capitalism, communism, or socialism—will endure, what will we shed, and how will this impact culture? What identity frameworks will we imagine for our future? What will the future role of, say, a farmer look like? These are just a few of the bold calls upon our imagination that media makers could answer through story.

We already have proofs of this concept in the work of initiatives like The Detroit Narrative Agency, which is changing the potential future of Detroit, by supporting community members who are excavating and creating stories that shift the overall narrative within the city towards the value of justice. The Agency uses science fiction, futurism, and healing narratives to tackle inferiority complexes created by biased media representation and other factors of the past, while also fostering innovation.

The Illustrating the Future Imaginary program in Canada is another example. It asks indigenous artists to enter the territory of science fiction and illustrate themselves or their communities seven, 10 or 20 generations from now. It even challenges the youth to experiment with creating new indigenous inspired computer languages, in solidarity with the movement to recover lost indigenous languages. Similarly, the Iyapo Repository, in Brooklyn, New York City, co-creates a resource library that houses a collection of digital and physical artifacts created to affirm and project the future of people of African descent.

The World Building Institute (WBI) established a process that empowered communities in economically depressed parts of the United States, Middle East, and Africa to build a vision of themselves in 20 to 50 years. Then, using immersive media, interactive design and methods of storytelling, the WBI supports the community to create media that represents their shared vision. The result of this project has been that these communities have been able to introduce practical innovations and develop infrastructure that are charting pathways to economic prosperity. Examples include the development of new water-management systems for drought-stricken areas, and new water-transportation systems for water-logged areas.

The JustFilms initiative at the Ford Foundation, which commissioned this research, is supporting some of these models, asking what an engaged and inclusive moving image storytelling practice could be in emerging media—one that according to Cara Mertes, JustFilms' Director, "places the creativity, imagination and narratives of those closest to the experience of exclusion and marginalization at the center."

In the past, we wielded awesome power and rushed into exponential "advancement," while instigating numerous intentional and unintentional atrocities. Building a system of inclusion through emerging media that allow a diversity of people to write the code of this next operating system, is a critical part of how we mitigate our blind spots and optimize our future.

For the first time in history, we have the tools and the connected social cultures to catalyze hyperlocal and global participation in imagination. We also have decades of storyworld-building practice that can articulate our shared imagination with great fidelity, while allowing individuals to contribute and navigate their own pathways into the future. With the right strategic actions, we just might be able to do something that has yet to be achieved in our 500-year history of mass media—the making of a new reality, where justice and equality are truly central values.

Bibliography

Sinclair, Kamal. 2017. "We have the power to code a new operating system for humanity." World Economic Forum, June 26, 2017. www.weforum.org/agenda/2017/06/artificial-intelligence-code-better-world/.

PART II

Imagining Communities and Rights

7

LIVING TOGETHER

Secularism and the Making of an Indian Public Sphere

Neera Chandhoke

The important introductory chapter by Richard Falk and Victor Faessel in this volume lays out clearly and cogently the dangers that stalk our world today: rabid intolerance, fear of the stranger, and the closing down of minds. Across the world, people seem to inhabit frighteningly blinkered worlds, and time-tested projects of living together have been breaking down. In some measure this breakdown has been propelled by the emergence of religion from the closet to which it had been consigned by Western Enlightenment philosophers. Since the end of the twentieth century religious identities have made more strident demands and engaged in state-breaking and state-making endeavors.

The increasing role of religion as politics in the public domain has unnerved western political philosophers. The boundary between the public and the private has simply evaporated, and there are new political forms and vocabularies in the public domain. Some scholars have proclaimed an end to the age of secularization and the collapse of secularism.[1] In some quarters, the dismissal of secularism as an attribute of a democratic state is part of a generic rejection of Enlightenment rationality. For Habermas, however, we have to "go beyond" secularism to accommodate religious identities. In an October 2001 speech titled "Faith and Knowledge," Habermas piloted the concept of post-secularism to the center stage of political theory. A post-secular society, he argued, is one that acknowledges the salience of religious identities. Conversely the religious minded must accept the authority of secular knowledge. However, the burden Habermas places on secular citizens is far less than the one borne by the religiously inclined. Since he does not allow religious vocabularies into the domain of policy making, these have to be translated into secular languages.

Habermas does not seem to appreciate the difficulty of translating religious into secular languages. Nor does he recognize the problems, the paradoxes, and the irresolvable dilemmas that are integral to the project of the co-existence of religion and the secular. He should have looked at India, a country that has learnt to live with both, not very well, but not too badly either.

India had no choice in this matter. In the early nineteenth century, the colonial state embarked on a project of understanding, translating, codifying, and freezing the plural and decentered religion of Hinduism into the mold of Judeo-Christian notions of what religion is, and what it should be. These attempts provoked sometimes anxious, sometimes assertive responses by Indian intellectuals and political leaders.

Colonial interpretations, rationalist reformulations and orthodox defenses of Hinduism shaped an emerging Indian public sphere in which religion was debated, discussed, and ultimately made the anchor of a nationalist project. Reeling under a barrage of criticism from Christian missionaries, influential western philosophers, and colonial officialdom, Indian leaders and social reformers set out to refashion Hinduism along the doctrinal lines found in sacred texts. Indians were swept up in and swamped by discussions on religion—new interpretations, new modes of measuring and critiquing received wisdom, and anxious defenses by orthodoxy—in a newly constructed public sphere. In India, modernity arrives through processes of intense public reflection on and critique of religious identities and their politicization, not through the privatization of religion as in Europe.

Religion was of course not the only obsession of participants in the public sphere. Public intellectuals were concerned with the intricacies of imperial rule, the economics of exploitation and domination, and modes of cultural control through education, language policies, translations, and interpretations of history and tradition. But interpretations and reinterpretations of Hinduism occupied a dominant place in public debate. Ultimately the country was partitioned in the name of religion. But nationalist leaders held fast to the cherished value of secularism, freedom of religion, and rights of minorities. This commitment was made in 1928, when amidst heightened religious conflict between Hindus and Muslims, the Motilal Nehru Constitutional Draft authored by leading nationalists offered to the minority Muslim community protection of its religion and culture. In 1931 the Karachi Resolution on Fundamental Rights authored by the Indian National Congress emphasized that a post-independent state would be neutral to all religions.

However, the concept of secularism was elaborated neither by the leaders of the freedom struggle nor by the members of the Constituent Assembly. In the Assembly, discussions on secularism were a by-product of discussions on minority rights, personal codes, and the insistence by B. R. Ambedkar (representing the lower castes) that religion, which is the source of injustice, should be regulated by the state.

It was in 1951 that Jawaharlal Nehru, India's first Prime Minister, spelled out the implications of secularism. Secularism, he said, did not mean a state in which religion is discouraged. It means freedom of religion and conscience, including freedom for those who may have no religion. It is perhaps not very easy to find a good word for secular, he said. Some people think that it means something opposed to religion, but this is not correct. For Nehru secularism means freedom of religion or irreligion; it means equality before the law and a state that honors all faiths equally and gives them equal opportunities.

Strictly speaking, we do not need secularism to ensure freedom of religion or the right not to be religious. Nor do we need secularism to mandate equality. Both these rights are protected by democracy. Secularism holds that the state shall not be aligned to one religion, which thereby becomes an official religion. This is fundamental to the right of equality, even in the weaker form of non-discrimination. It is precisely this interpretation that has been upheld by the Supreme Court of India.

Living Together

The coexistence of religion and secularism in India has been uneasy, unpredictable, and contingent. That the two can coexist at all is not surprising, given the capacity of Indian philosophy to contain contradictory phenomena, unlike Western philosophy that subscribes to neatness and to hierarchy of principles. In fact it is possible to trace three legally protected modes of coexistence between religion and the secular.

In some cases, the Indian Supreme Court has subordinated religious practices to democracy and social reform: gender justice, reforming the caste system, enabling the lower castes to enter temples, and banning untouchability. In 1996, the Supreme Court stipulated that the constitutional right to religion is not an absolute or an unfettered right. It is subject to reform for social welfare by appropriate State legislation. In other cases, the court has tried to ward off conflict through inaction. It still has to decide the Ayodhya case, whether a temple can be built on the site at which the sixteenth century Babri Masjid, which was demolished by the religious right in 1992, had stood.

In a third instance, anachronistic practices have been allowed to exist side by side. For example, according to the Jain practice of Santhara, persons are allowed to fast unto death in specific circumstances and under supervision. So even though suicide is, according to the Indian Penal Code, a criminal offence, the Supreme Court lifted a ban on Santhara in 2015. Jain philosophy, which sees the body as a prison of the soul, is completely different from the Christian view that the body is a creation of God and therefore suicide is a crime. The two philosophies are simply incommensurate, but the legal system has found a way to accommodate both.

India teaches us that although we have little choice but to accommodate religion in the public sphere, the outcome of the coexistence of secularism and religious politics is extremely untidy, unwieldy, and generates unexpected outcomes. It cannot be otherwise. Religion gives to us thick conceptions of the good, which enables us to understand our worlds. Political secularism as an attribute of a democratic state is a procedural norm that protects equality between all religious groups. Secularism in India not only recognizes the significance of religion in public life, it commits to equality between religious groups. In 1994, the Supreme Court ruled in the Bommai case that the Indian version of secularism stands for equality of all religions. Considering the specific circumstances in which state governments can be dismissed by the federal or the central government, the Court opined that the central government has the right to impose central rule upon a state government if the latter violates the principle of secularism, which is part of the basic structure of the constitution. These definitions have not only given a new meaning to secularism in a multi-religious society, they have protected pluralism.

Conclusion

In India, secularism has contributed to the construction of a normative structure whereby people can pursue their faith unburdened by discrimination. Yet in many cases, secularism has not been able to overrule religious belief, for example the personal laws of minorities. This is perhaps natural, for the world of politics is shot through with discrepancies and irreconcilable paradoxes, and does not lend itself to neat ordering of principles. Attempts to bring neatness into either explanation or prescription for understanding contradictory practices can therefore prove flawed.

In such situations, we have to employ the resources of political imagination to make choices between different sorts of options that minimize harm. The dilemmas we find ourselves in might well prove intractable, but there is no reason why we cannot negotiate them with some degree of resourcefulness and ingenuity.

Note

1 The term secular refers to non-religious practices, political secularism is used interchangeably with secularism as an attribute of the state.

Bibliography

Dillon, Michelle. 2010. "Can Post-Secular Society Tolerate Religious Differences?" *Sociology of Religion* 71, no. 2 (Summer): 139–156. https://doi.org/10.1093/socrel/srq024.

Habermas, Jurgen. (2006). "Religion in the Public Sphere: Cognitive Presuppositions for the 'Public Use of Reason' by Religious and Secular Citizens." In *Between Naturalism and Religion*, Translated by Ciaran Cronin. Cambridge, UK: Polity Press, pp. 114–147.

Jacobsohn, Gary Jeffrey 2003. *The Wheel Of Law: India's Secularism in Comparative Constitutional Context.* New Delhi: Oxford University Press.

Madan, Triloki Nath. 1997. "Secularism in its Place." In *Secularism and its Critics*, edited by Rajeev Bhargava, 297–315. New Delhi: Oxford University Press.

Nehru, Jawaharlal. 1949. *Jawaharlal Nehru Speeches: Volume One*. September 1946 to May 1949. Calcutta: Publications Division: Ministry of Information and Broadcasting.

Sen, Ronojoy. 2007. "Legalizing Religion: The Indian Supreme Court and Secularism." *Policy Studies*. Washington, D.C.: East-West Center.

8

HOW TO THINK ABOUT POPULISM

Akeel Bilgrami

A report in the *Financial Times* (2017) on President Trump's inaugural compared it to President Obama's first inaugural and declared: "Obama radiated hope. Trump channeled rage." This is factually correct. But if so, the fact needs diagnosis. Why hope in 2013 and rage only four years later? An obvious answer is because the hope was not fulfilled and so roughly half the electorate refused to believe that Obama's anointed successor in the Democratic party—nor even the orthodox core of the Republican party—would fulfill it either. Brexit seems to be channeling the same rage against Britain's political establishment. But the political establishment is not a self-standing class. Even a glance at the lineup of support for the Remain vote and for Clinton (both in the primaries against Sanders and in the presidential elections) shows the extent to which what underlies this political class is a parade of corporate and banking elites, ranging from the IMF, Wall Street, OECD, and Soros, to the Governor of the Bank of England.

That leads into the subject of how to understand the meaning of "populism" as a term of opprobrium. The term is defined as "ordinary people's opposition to elites." So defined, it is too under-described to be a term of opprobrium. After all, *democracy* is intended to give ordinary people a chance to counter elites through representative politics. What populism today seems to add to democracy is that it also opposes the power of *un*elected officials with specific economic interests who dominate the formation of policies—with the general acquiescence of elected representatives.

But this still does not capture what we instinctively recoil from in populism. How can it be wrong to oppose the voluntary implicit surrender of sovereignty by elected law and policy makers to unelected wielders of elite financial interests?

Suppose, then, for a moment, that a working or workless person in Nottingham or Crete or Seville were to ponder the humane policies that some nations in Europe came to embrace since the Second World War, policies that provided safety nets (whether of health or education or housing) for people like him. He might ask: what was the site where these safety nets were administered and implemented? And he would answer: well, the site of the nation. He might scratch his head and wonder: Has there ever been a supra-national site at which welfare was ever administered? What would a mechanism that dispensed it at a supra-national level even look like?

Now, of course, such a person might go beyond these shrewd questions to associate supra-national affiliation with immigrant hordes who not only deprive him of economic opportunities, but dilute the centuries long national culture of which he is so proud. But there is no logical link between those excellent former questions and these latter trumped up anxieties. One may rightly ask the questions without having these anxieties. And so here at last we have what is the defining element of populism from which we recoil. The term stands for precisely the assumption of such a link, a link that is not compulsory.

So a question arises: whence the compulsion to make this *un*compulsory link? And here we must resist the temptation to blame the people themselves. The assumption they make of such a link is not due to their feebleness of mind but to a wide variety of distortions not only by the media they read and watch, but by the political class, and not just the extreme elements of that class but the political establishment. We cannot forget that the British Prime Minister's Remain campaign ratcheted up the immigration theme to prevent its being owned by his more extreme Right opposition, just as Obama in his first campaign was far worse on immigration than John McCain, again with a view to gaining ownership of a Republican platform, for electoral gains.

So the lesson is this. Even if we identify what we recoil from in populism as the uncompulsory linking of sound questions with unsound anxieties, this cannot simply be attributed to an *intrinsic incapacity* in the judgment of ordinary people, but must be attributed to the failure of public education provided by the media and the political class. One cannot believe in democracy and dismiss the electorate as vile or stupid. For the electorate is shaped by what *knowledge* it possesses.

For two millennia, philosophers have said that the central ethical question is: What ought we to do? Or, How ought we to live? But in our own complex time, the more crucial prior question has become: What ought we to know?

And the question of what we ought to know is a matter of public imagination and education by public institutions that have failed, whether they be the media or the universities. In a sense, these institutions always did produce and sustain the ruling class, so it is perhaps wrong to expect them to be the sites of public imagination. Where the public got educated on the fundamental issues that shape our societies have tended to be movements, from the Left labor movements of Europe and the United States (now ebbing to the point of non-existence) to the civil rights and anti-war and women's movements of some decades later. In countries of the South this learning happened in the prolonged and highly creative movements of struggle against colonial rule during which millions of people were mobilized and were educated into the possibilities of a progressive future after gaining independence. But all of these examples seem now like a distant past.

So on the question of contemporary populism, I would conclude by saying that (to put it in the most general terms) the two underlying causes of this phenomenon are 1) a chronic crisis of capitalism and 2) the failure of the Left to find an adequate response to it. It is a reaction to capitalism in its neo-liberal mode of the last few decades: its inability to create sufficient employment, its seemingly irreversible inequalities, its systematic destruction of the bargaining power of labor, its undermining of national economic sovereignties, and its making immigration—which could be a source of strength for national economies—into a deep source of anxiety and complaint among working people. The failure of the Left to mobilize an adequate response to these crisis conditions creates what we might call a "movement vacuum." Just as there can be a power vacuum, there can be a movement vacuum. And so extreme right wing nationalist movements, that is to say "populism" in the bad sense of the term, step into the vacuum. Such a vacuum may represent a failure of public imagination on the part of the Left, but to be fair, Left movements today are increasingly constrained by the turn that capitalism has taken in the last few decades.

First of all the old style movements based on trade union activism are hardly possible because ever since the dominant nature of capital itself changed from industrial capital to finance capital, trade unions in the traditional sense have only a residual agency; and, in any case, such unions as are still in place have been beaten down by neo-liberal economic policies that generate chronic unemployment and the informalization and impermanence of employment in many parts of the world, which undermines the bargaining power of unions (for the obvious reason that corporations can hire and fire as they please, knowing that there is what Marx called a "reserve army of the unemployed" from which labor can be recruited if unions bargain too hard for the employed and organized workers). And even more crucially, ever since the tremendous increase in the mobility of capital after the dismantling (or remantling) of the Bretton Woods institutions, even if a working class movement throws up the possibility of progressive policies, those possibilities for the most part can't really be implemented because of the fear of capital flight. Thus, for example, Lula, as a result of a working class movement, got elected on a very progressive platform in Brazil but was not really able to implement it for fear of capital flight. If such platforms were to be implemented and capital flight ensued (quite apart from the hardship caused by that to working people), *oppositional movements would have to be waiting at the place to which capital flies*. And that form of international solidarity in the global labor force is not a realistic possibility. One needs more than public imagination, one would need a magic wand to forge such solidarities. The mind boggles at the idea of a serious possibility of *global* labor movements to oppose global finance capital. I myself think that that is just fantasy, a fantasy expressed by some political theorists such as Hardt and Negri (2004) with such terms as "multitude."

What, I believe, is more plausibly within our public imagination—at least for countries of the South, where I come from, which are suffering from the oppressiveness of these neo-liberal policies in our period of financial globalization—is that they would be better off de-linking (at least partially) from the global economy and getting sovereignty over their own nations' political economies. Such ideas need to be explored in serious detail. They may require partial South-South relinking so as to protect some of the smaller economies of the South, and they may require creating alternative credit agencies—alternative, that is, to the IMF and World Bank. These are all under-explored ideas worth considering, and it would take a great deal of public imagination on the part of the Left to do so.

References

Financial Times. 2017. "President Trump's speech puts the world on notice." January 20, 2017. www.ft.com/content/b5859136-df3f-11e6-86ac-f253db7791c6.

Hardt, Michael, and Antonio Negri. 2004. *Multitude: War and Democracy in the Age of Empire*. New York: Penguin Press.

9

MAGIC OF PUBLIC IMAGINATION

Transcending Public Evil

Victoria Brittain

There was a moment on July 7, 2015 in the Mother Emmanuel African Episcopal Church in Charleston, South Carolina, when Barack Obama seized his people's political imagination as he had done in his early days in politics. He stood tall at the lectern, surrounded by black religious leaders in robes, to give the eulogy for the Reverend Clementa Pinckney and the seven others gunned down during a bible study at their church. The President took a long pause, leaned forward, and began to sing alone, the 18th century Christian hymn, *Amazing Grace,* written by the slave-trader turned Christian minister John Newton. Visibly stunned, then smiling broadly, the priests in unison began to sing along. Obama then named each victim, following each name with the words, "XX … found that grace, through the example of his/her life."

Obama himself is a man of grace. But in these distracted political times he has often struggled for his hold on public imagination—the foundation of people's political empowerment. On that July day he reminded me of another powerful moment caught forever on film, when another great American leader sang on another continent, and seized the imagination of another world.

Half a century ago, in the radical political days after World War II, the black actor and singer Paul Robeson visited Scotland, invited by the Scottish branch of the National Union of Mineworkers to give a concert in a large hall in Edinburgh. (Robeson's history with the NUM dated back to the late 1920s when he visited Welsh miners and went on their hunger marches in 1927 and 1928.) Before the official Scottish event Robeson visited a colliery, lunched in the miners' canteen, and then, impromptu, he rose to his feet and began to sing *The Ballad of Joe Hill* in the middle of a rapt room of white working class men. Hill was a legendary Swedish/American union organizer, who was executed in 1915 on a framed murder charge. In a parting telegram to a fellow union leader he wrote, "Goodbye, Bill, I die like a true blue rebel. Don't waste any time mourning. Organize!"

In those postwar years Robeson became the mentor to another American whose art and whose words have fired political imagination across the world for decades, and still do. Harry Belafonte was a janitor's assistant, a high school dropout in New York feeling a sense of loss. Wartime service in the Pacific had shown him a different life, but the post-war US showed him only white oppression. A chance meeting with Robeson during Belafonte's first ever visit to a theatre changed his life. "Paul Robeson set my course, by his intellect and courage, gave me a purpose in life, showed me the value of profound thought, showed me global commonality."

Robeson, a victim of McCarthyism in 1950s America, was blacklisted and his artistic career shattered. But Belafonte went on to become the most articulate of global citizens, fired by the power of art and words to feed imagination. He has plunged forward with fearless resistance to oppression wherever it is found. He was a luminary of the anti-apartheid struggle in South Africa, and at home in the most dangerous years of the US civil rights movement. Inevitably, he was one of the sponsors of the Washington women's protest march on Donald Trump's first day as president.

A decade earlier Belafonte had protested another president's political choices and referred to George W. Bush as "the greatest terrorist in the world" for launching the war in Iraq. He went on to criticize the powerful African-American members of the Bush administration, General Colin Powell and National Security Advisor Condoleezza Rice, referring to them as "house slaves." Belafonte resisted intense media pressure and steadfastly refused to apologize. To Powell and Rice, he said, "you are serving those who continue to design our oppression."

Obama in that church in Charleston was a man at home, and he seized the moment of raw emotion to speak from his heart about his people's "systematic oppression and racial subjugation," and of how the killer's action had been "a means of control, a way to terrorize and oppress," and "an act that he presumed would deepen divisions that trace back to our nation's original sin."

These were wonderful powerful words, and words that Obama could have spoken about the dark anti-Muslim world of torture, dehumanization and fear which he inherited from his two Bush predecessors, and associates such as Donald Rumsfeld and Dick Cheney. President Obama thought he could close Guantanamo and end a shameful episode. But his early decision to be a president who looked forward, not back, was a failure of his own political imagination. His Justice Department knew well that the law had been broken in the Bush years, but was itself on the same trajectory in arguing before the courts in cases involving prisoners and torture. Obama did not see then (though surely he should have as the years passed) that Guantanamo was not an episode but an era. And the lack of accountability for Guantanamo and the tortures, renditions and secret prisons which grew up around it, changed Americans themselves, changed much of the world's attitude to America, and allowed the unraveling of the post-World War II international architecture of idealism in the Geneva Conventions and other United Nations conventions.

"Humankind cannot bear very much reality," T. S. Eliot wrote so memorably. In these torture years many thousands of Americans including politicians, doctors, psychologists, lawyers, soldiers, guards, interrogators have been witnesses, participants, and instigators of unspeakable cruelty and degradation on Muslim men. How did they live with their reality? Denial, lies, false justifications, military and institutional discipline, and media complacency kept most of these people inside the web of numbed acceptance. (The whistle blowers—from Thomas Drake and John Kiriakou to Chelsea Manning—fired imagination across the world, but paid a very high price, including on Obama's watch.)

The first terrible photographs from Abu Ghraib prison in Iraq showed the world indelible images of US torture, which deviated starkly from the expressed principles behind the "war on terror." The Bush administration's attempt to pin responsibility for Abu Ghraib on "a few bad apples"—junior soldiers—soon fell apart and there was initially shocked reaction from the media and others. Calls for the resignation of Secretary of Defense Donald Rumsfeld came from across the board. In May 2004 former Vice President Al Gore called also for the resignations of CIA director George Tenet, National Security Advisor Condoleezza Rice, Deputy Secretary of Defense Paul Wolfowitz, and senior Defense officials Stephen Cambone and Douglas Feith.

But, none of this shaming happened. Cynicism was fed and torture was normalized in the public mind. Two years later even more Abu Ghraib images were published. In December 2015 the long awaited Senate report on US torture in the secret CIA black sites revealed years of even more degrading practices. But the airwaves were filled with Dick Cheney assuring the US that it had all been necessary, even worthwhile, and that he would certainly do it all again.

During more than a decade of the "war on terror" there was a progressive shutdown of public imagination about the enormity of this illegal and immoral reality, in which the US had many complicit partners in Europe and the Middle East. We know now that denial won the battle of public opinion and brought to the White House a man locked in his own random certainties, and someone who shares none of the attributes that Robeson showed Belafonte: "intellect and courage … a purpose in life … the value of profound thought … global commonality.'

From Guantanamo Bay prison, of all places, came a man with just this array of qualities, a Mauretanian, Mohamadou Ould Slahi, detained without charge for 14 years. His book, *Guantanamo Diary,* was written in an isolation cell after he had been broken by torture in Donald Rumsfeld's Special Interrogation Plan. This book is the antidote to numbness, to forgetting, to cynicism, to loss of humanity. It is a gift to our public imagination. The fine editor of Slahi's book, American writer Larry Siems, describes the author, whom he was never allowed to contact in Guantanamo, as "curious, forgiving, social." Siems writes, "he has the qualities I value most in a writer: a moving sense of beauty and a sharp sense of irony. He has a fantastic sense of humor." The book is written so vividly that it is hard to believe English is Slahi's fourth language and one he mostly learned while in custody, despite so often being completely deprived of human contact by his American jailers.

Slahi's warm personality, his intelligence, and his vivid descriptions belie the grimness of his material. It took nearly a decade of battles by his tireless lawyers to get the manuscript cleared by the US authorities—albeit with 2,500 black lines of redacted names and whole passages scarring the pages. It has been published in 26 countries and 23 languages and made the *New York Times* best-seller list. There you see the power to set alight public imagination—and renew an empathy that had been dulled to the point of extinction.

One year after it was published and Slahi was known around the world, he was released home to Africa. I hope Mr. Obama has had time since to read this book and discover a man of grace who survived the worst of his presidential time. The empathetic former president must deeply regret that this innocent man is still an American prisoner, considering that the US has made it impossible for him to get his passport back and leave Mauretania for medical care abroad to treat the injuries caused him by American torturers two decades ago.

Bibliography

Shahi, Mohamedou Ould. 2005. *Guantánamo Diary*. Larry Siems, ed. New York: Little, Brown and Company. Restored Edition, Back Bay Books, 2017.

10

TRUMP, PUBLIC IMAGINATION, AND ISLAMOPHOBIA

Chandra Muzaffar

Donald Trump's crafty manipulation of Islamophobia, we are told, was one of the factors that propelled him to the presidency of the United States of America. He was very much aware of the prevalence of negative sentiments towards Islam and Muslims within segments of the American electorate. Because Islamophobia was part of the public imagination, he had no scruples about exploiting it for political gain. Even though Trump's actions have been widely criticized, the Western media have failed at a deeper level to examine and reveal the ways in which Western interventions and occupations in Muslim societies have fuelled a sense of popular frustration and hostility that has been manifested in dramatic acts of violence by a very few, which have in turn provided fodder for further interventions premised on the need for "regime change" in order to ensure the stability of a global Pax Americana. Consequently, Islamophobia is not simply a form of cynical populist politics but is rather a fundamental component of a longer cycle of geopolitical struggle. One that must be scrutinized more carefully if we are to imagine alternatives.

Taking Advantage of Islamophobia

Islamophobia has been embedded in the Western psyche—more in the European than in the American worldview—for centuries. There are a number of reasons for this: the early triumph and rapid expansion of an emerging Islam among Christian entities in WANA right up to the Iberian Peninsula from the 8th to the 12th centuries; the onslaught of the European Crusades, their re-conquest of Jerusalem and their subsequent defeat at the hands of the Muslims between the 10th and 13th centuries; the rise of Western colonialism from the 16th century onwards which led to the subjugation of most Muslim polities in Asia and Africa; and the re-assertion of these polities from the middle of the 20th century as they seek to establish their own identities within a global order that centers around US dominance. All have contributed, in different ways, to the spread of a negative attitude towards Islam and Muslims in the West.

Needless to say, this attitude has been exacerbated by a series of acts of violence and terror committed by Muslim groups and individuals themselves in the US, Europe, Africa and Asia. The association of terrorism with Muslims and Islam in the public imagination in the West has now spread to other parts of the world and constitutes a formidable barrier to inter-civilizational dialogue between Muslims and the rest. Though it is a miniscule fraction that perpetrates acts of terror, their diabolical deeds have fuelled Islamophobia as never before.

Trump's own campaign coupled with his personality was also undoubtedly a factor. He exaggerated and dramatized violence that implicated Muslims, ignoring evidence that showed that Muslim American involvement in terror attacks had decreased by 40% in 2016. By focusing upon Muslims and equating them as a religious community with terrorism—his use of the phrase, "Islamic radical terrorism" is a case in point—he has brought Islamophobia to a new low. This is reflected in the steep increase in attacks upon hijab-attired Muslim women, in the physical targeting of mosques, and in the venomous vitriol leveled against Islam and the Prophet Muhammad in the popular media.

Islamophobia: Failure to Address Root Causes

Trump's antagonistic posture towards Islam and Muslims has provoked condemnation from a significant segment of the US citizenry. It is not just liberals in the political arena who have criticized him. Christian and Jewish theologians and others who are committed to an inclusive America have also been vocal.

These public pronouncements have made an impact upon public imagination. They help to some extent to check the toxic negativity arising from the politics of hatred and distrust generated by Trump. But they do not address the underlying causes of Islamophobia.

There are two closely related dimensions to these causes. Because their lands have been occupied and their people massacred and marginalized, some of the victims of injustice have resorted to violence which in turn has reinforced Islamophobia. This is part of the explanation for the wave of terrorist acts that occurred in the sixties and seventies associated with Palestinians and those committed to their cause. At the root was Palestinian dispossession as a result of Israeli occupation and usurpation of their rights. The invasion and occupation of Iraq in 2003 by the US and Britain and the death and destruction that ensued is yet another major reason for the violence of the victims and their sympathizers in recent years, which has reinforced a negative perception of Muslims in the West.

Occupation is related to the larger politics of US hegemony and "regime change." In order to ensure that it perpetuates its global power the US has on a number of occasions sought to overthrow governments in Muslim and non-Muslim countries. Different excuses are employed to justify these violations. Fabricated threats of "weapons of mass destruction" or "mass murder of innocent civilians" easily morph into fears of Islam and Muslims in a situation where Islamophobia is already embedded in American cultural imagination.

That occupation, regime change and hegemony in general—all linked to US foreign policy—have also contributed in no small measure to Muslim anger, and that anger in some instances has expressed itself in terrorism, is something that most Americans are not conscious of. It is not part of the public consciousness. Mere criticisms of Trump's antipathy towards Muslims will not lead to a deeper understanding of the profound forces that shape Islamophobia. The media and even the intellectual community as a whole have failed to develop that sort of awareness among the public. It is partly because of their failure that Islamophobia has become such a virulent force in the hands of Machiavellian politicians like Trump. Of course, there are individuals in the media and intellectuals—few and far between though they may be—who keep reminding Americans and the world at large of the less benign face of US power and what its consequences are.

It is not just less benign. The US "deep state" has been involved in something much more hideous. Through its security network, it has been providing arms, training, and intelligence to terrorist groups in places such as Syria where it aims to achieve regime change. While not known to the general public, a handful of Western journalists and intellectuals have also played a role in exposing this nefarious activity.[2]

There are Muslim governments that are not only colluding with the deep state in Washington DC and other capitals but are also in the forefront of terrorist operations. The role of the Saudi elite in such operations is well established.[3] It is ironic that an elite that is perceived in the Muslim world as the protector of the sanctity of the religion is also guilty of tarnishing its image. This may be because of ideological bigotry and power. More specifically, Wahabism associated with the influential stratum in Saudi society justifies the elimination of those who do not subscribe to its puritanical view of Islam. The Saudi elite's Wahabi ideology is also one of the main reasons why it is opposed to Shiism and Iran, which it perceives as a challenge to its regional power and status.

Countering Islamophobia; Transforming the Public Imagination

It is obvious that countering Islamophobia in the US will have to set as its priority the interrogation of power. How the US elite uses and abuses power in its relations with other countries, especially Muslim states, should be subjected to intensive scrutiny. The overt and covert manifestations of power should be analyzed in an honest and transparent manner. The media, specifically the alternative media, will have to play a central role in this. Scholars and activists should utilize new communication technologies to the fullest extent and explore how attitudes towards Islam and Muslims have been moulded over time by the hegemonic thrust of US foreign policy. In a nutshell, it would be an attempt to discover how the desire for global dominance and power has undermined the potential for amity and empathy between the American people and the Muslim world.

If responsible media together with the strong, explicit support of civic and cultural leaders of high moral standing in the society undertake this mission with sincere conviction, there is a possibility of a significant transformation of public consciousness in which Islamophobia yields to empathy for Muslims and with Islamic civilization. Such an effort might even herald respect and affection for other civilizations.

This is the kind of public imagination—in the US and around the world—that should set the tone and tenor for a new era in international relations in the 21st century.

Notes

1 "Muslim American involvement in terror attacks decreased by 40% in 2016, report says" (Schladebeck 2017).
2 I have in mind well-known journalists such as John Pilger and Eric Margolis and intellectuals like Tim Anderson and Michel Chossoduvsky. See for instance Margolis (2017a and 2017b). See also Anderson (2015).
3 For details of Saudi involvement in terrorism see Wight (2017) and Cockburn (2014).

References

Anderson, Tim. "Who Supports the Islamic State (ISIS)? Saudi Arabia, Turkey, Qatar, Israel, UK, France, USA." *Global Research*, November 20, 2015.

Cockburn, Patrick. "Saudi Arabia, 9/11 and the Rise of ISIS." *Counterpunch*, September 15, 2014. www.counterpunch.org/2014/09/15/saudi-arabia-911-and-the-rise-of-isis/.

Margolis, Eric S. "Hail to the Chief – fingers crossed." *The Sun* (Malaysia), January 24, 2017a.

———. "Not so fast, crusader Trump." *The Sun* (Malaysia), February 1, 2017b.

Schladebeck, Jessica. 2017. "Muslim American involvement in terror attacks decreased by 40% in 2016, report says." *New York Daily News*, January 28, 2017. www.nydailynews.com/news/world/muslim-american-involvement-terror-attacks-decreased-2016-article-1.2958125.

Wight, John. "Trump Is Wrong — Saudi Arabia, Not Iran Is the World's Number One Terrorist State." *Transcend Media Service*, February 13, 2017. www.transcend.org/tms/2017/02/trump-is-wrong-saudi-arabia-not-iran-is-the-worlds-number-one-terrorist-state/.

11

AMERICA'S DIVIDED POLITICAL IMAGINARY

Paul W. Kahn

The polarization of the American electorate has been attributed to racism, sexism, greed, resentment, and a host of other social pathologies. It has also been attributed to globalization, automation, urbanization, and other economic and structural changes. There is some truth in all of these efforts to plot the causes of our political discontent. Different theorists will identify the causes in the context that they know best. This search for causes tends to see politics as a secondary phenomenon, as if politics is only the working out of interests and values formed elsewhere. Of course, politics does not stand alone, but neither is political identity reducible to these social and economic factors.

Politics in America has been a deep source of individual and collective identity. Americans have practiced a civil religion since before the Civil War. Lincoln spoke of a "reverence for law." More broadly, the sovereign people have been imagined as a transhistorical collective subject that stands to our ordinary concerns as the sacred to the mundane. "We the people" has carried a claim on citizens that was deep and rich enough to support generations of sacrifice. Americans have revered their history of Revolution, Civil War, and the great wars of the 20th century. Pilgrimages are made to these markers of citizen identity: Valley Forge, Gettysburg, and even Omaha Beach. The saints of this civil religion include Washington, as the paradigmatic founder, and Lincoln, the sacrificial son.

The beliefs and practices of this civil religion are strained today. Vietnam remains a site of trauma to our political identity. Was it a war of sacrifice or a politics of senseless killings? Despite the sacrificial construction of 9/11, the wars in Iraq and Afghanistan are a long way from entering the mythical space of the sacrificial imagination. The foundation of American politics was, for a long time, sacrifice as practice and belief. Every town square is decorated with memorials to those who sacrificed. This is hardly surprising in a nation that traces so much of its traditions of belief and practice to Christianity. But where is the idea of sacrifice in today's politics?

The American civil religion combined two distinct ideas: popular sovereignty and the rule of law. The manner of that union gave Americans a distinct way of imagining themselves. They imagined law—particularly the Constitution—as the product of their own authorship. The people gave the law to themselves. Apart from revolution, the sovereign people can do just one thing: author law. For this reason, there is no space for a legitimate, extra-legal politics in our national history. Law is everywhere for the simple reason that "We the People" is everywhere and always. The imagined relationship of popular sovereignty to law is captured in that of Revolution to Constitution. Revolution was the direct presence of the popular sovereign; constitution was the remnant and marker of that presence, which was left behind once the sovereign retreated.

Because America has always defined itself as a nation of self-government through law, we don't notice the tension between "self-government" and "law." These two elements point to distinctly different moral grounds at the foundation of our political enterprise. Self-government appeals to an idea of autonomy: we the people must rule ourselves without interference or direction from outside. The rule of law appeals to an idea of justice. The promise of law is that it will treat each person equally and fairly. There is not one law for the rich another for the poor; not one for the powerful and another for the weak.

Looking at the experience of other nations, we recognize that self-government and the rule of law do not necessarily coincide. We see nations voting autocrats into office. Elections provide them legitimacy, even as they exercise rule without law. Elsewhere, we see that the rule of law does not necessarily rest on self-government. This is the story of the European Union, which strives for equal and fair laws but suffers a democracy deficit. Everywhere, the courts claim responsibility for the rule of law, and almost everywhere the courts are accused of not being democratic.

In the long history of the West, democratic self-government and the rule of law have more often been in conflict than they have been aligned. That is why Socrates famously disapproved of democracy. He thought the people would inevitably turn to authoritarians, who would claim to rule in their name. He might have been describing modern Turkey, Hungary, or Russia. The rule of law, in contrast, was thought to require elites with special expertise—that is, lawyers and courts. At the time of the American Revolution, the British claimed the virtue of the rule of law. This did not satisfy the revolutionaries, who wanted self-government. Their plea was "no taxation without representation." It was not "just taxes only."

The American political narrative has been uniquely powerful because it has combined these two distinct threads. Rule by law *is* rule by the people as long as the people believe they are the authors of the laws by which they are governed. Laws may be drafted by our representatives, but we must understand ourselves as the authors of those laws. Our representatives do not rule us by imposing laws upon us—just or otherwise. We rule ourselves by taking responsibility for the law. We want those laws to be just, but we also want them to be our own.

The idea that rule by the people and the rule of law can coexist was a radical idea at the time of the founding. It remains a radical idea today. It is always a challenge to keep the two pole stars of our political life in alignment. It is, after all, not a matter of fact that can be proven, but a matter of faith: we must believe ourselves to be the collective author of our law. That is the fundamental American myth upon which the belief in the legitimacy of our enterprise depends.

Arguably, this myth is failing today, for our polarized politics represents the splitting apart of these two ideas. At stake is the very meaning of citizenship and the nature of our political order. This division is what makes the polarization so intractable. Each side feels that it stands for something that goes to the very heart of what it means to be an American.

On one side, some citizens look at American laws and no longer recognize their own authorship. They believe that they are being governed by elites or experts who do not share their identity. Government has become something done to them, rather than something we are doing together. They would "take back" their government. For a long time, those who thought of themselves as excluded from the authorship of law were women and minorities. They campaigned for the right to be included in "We the People." Those who would "take back" today are refighting this battle of who belongs.

On the other side, some citizens focus less on authorship and more on injustice. These citizens do not believe that the rule of law has realized a just order. They want to reform and to extend the law. Their agenda is one of progressive reform for which they rely upon lawyers and courts. Their rallying cry is not self-government, but justice.

Of course, neither side ignores completely the virtues claimed by the other: everyone is for self-government and just laws, rightly understood. Yet each finds a unique power in one side of our double narrative. Similarly, each criticizes the other for the choices made. One side criticizes the turn to courts as an effort to bypass democratic politics, while the other side criticizes the populist efforts of their opponents as lawless.

Is our national faith in self-government or the rule of law? If we have to choose between them, we have already lost ourselves, for we long imagined ourselves as a people who gave the law to ourselves. If we are to recover from our current political pathologies, we will have to figure out how we can again come to see the rule of law as the expression of popular sovereignty.

Bibliography

Ackerman, Bruce A. 1993. *We the People, Volume 1: Foundations*. Cambridge, Mass: Belknap Press of Harvard University Press.

Kahn, Paul W. 1992. *Legitimacy and History: Self-Government in American Constitutional Theory*. New Haven and London: Yale University Press.

———. 2005. *Putting Liberalism in its Place*. Princeton, NJ: Princeton University Press.

———. 2008. *Sacred Violence: Torture Terror, and Sovereignty*. Ann Arbor, MI: University of Michigan Press.

———. 2011. *Political Theology: Four New Chapters on the Concept of Sovereignty*. New York: Columbia University Press.

———. 2016. *Making the Case: The Art of the Judicial Opinion*. New Haven and London: Yale University Press.

Morgan, Edmund Sears. 1989. *Inventing the People: The Rise of Popular Sovereignty in England and America*. New York: W.W. Norton.

Schmitt, Carl. 1932. *Political Theology: Four Chapters on the Concept of Sovereignty*. Translated by George Schwab, 2005. Chicago: University of Chicago.

Taylor, Charles. 2004. *Modern Social Imaginaries*. Durham and London: Duke University Press.

12

MIGRATION, TERRORISM, AND THE SURVIVAL OF THE LIBERAL PROJECT

Tom Farer

Liberal,[1] equal-opportunity democracy is not the default reflex of most societies or of a majority of the peoples constituting them. Even rarer is empathic concern for persons, other than ethnic or religious kin, living beyond national frontiers.

Only in recent decades has Western Europe become an exception to those two truths. In its constitutions, courts and ministries it has institutionalized respect for human rights while displaying through foreign assistance programs a sustained measure of concern for the wretched victims of war, greed, ineptitude, autocracy, and natural disasters in the Global South. Civil society in the form of non-profit organizations has reinforced and extended the reach of official manifestations of cosmopolitan sympathy.

The liberal project is not the unique possession of people living in affluent democratic states. It finds supporters in every corner of the globe, though in many corners it is a distinctly minority faith. But with very few exceptions the West is the place where it has become embedded in law and powerful public institutions and has deeply influenced popular discourse.

Proliferating instances of terrorism, growing inequality among social classes, rising tension between multi-generational citizens and culturally-distinctive groups of relatively recent settlement, and a looming intensification of migration pressures from Africa and the Middle East now threaten the liberal consensus in Western Europe, the site of its greatest strength. The threat is manifest in such phenomena as a multiplication of violent attacks by right-wing vigilantes on people of color, mosques, and migrant shelters (Germany), the entry of xenophobic parties into governing coalitions (Denmark), France's prolonged state of emergency, and the negotiation of agreements with point-of-departure countries like Turkey intended to keep prospective asylum claimants from reaching European shores.

If anything in our volatile world can be predicted with confidence it is that pressure on Europe's borders will continue to grow. In the Middle East and North Africa, a population which rose from 93 to 347 million between 1950 and 2000 is projected to reach by 2050 nearly 680 closely packed millions of people for whom employment prospects are dismal (Clawson 2009). War and repression are certain to join grim economic forces in driving migration.

The electorates of West European countries, like those in the United States, do not oppose all forms of additional migration. Welcoming the bearers of wealth or persons with special skills in short supply locally poses no difficult political problem and they arrive under criteria for admission which became narrowly drawn beginning in the 1970s when the great post-war surge of growth slowed drastically. The main focus of popular hostility has been migrant families from the Global South, above all people from Muslim-majority countries.

The Muslim presence became an issue with bristling political resonance in different countries at different times, often propelled by a single catalytic event. In the UK it was the 1988 Rushdie Affair. In Denmark, already uneasy after the 9/11 2001 terror attacks in the US, it was the 2005 affair of the Mohammed cartoons and the role Danish imams played in arousing a furious response around the Muslim world which included mob attacks on identifiably Danish buildings and a boycott of Danish goods. In Germany it came much later, the end of 2015, when hundreds of young men apparently of largely North African origin harassed, groped, forcibly undressed and robbed young women during the traditional New Year's Eve celebrations occurring in the center of Cologne and a number of other German cities. The French watershed was the 2005 Banlieue riots.

Looming over the events specific to each country has been the threat of mass-casualty terrorism perpetrated in the name of Islam. That threat, together with the perception of elites and ordinary citizens, varying in time and intensity, that a not inconsequential (but hugely exaggerated) proportion of new arrivals and of second generation Muslims are deeply alienated, have conspired to reduce both the admission of asylum applicants and levels of economic support for them when they are able to pass through the door. In addition, the accumulation of highly publicized instances of cultural clash and terrorist attacks have led political leaders in countries that once supported the so-called multi-cultural approach to integration to declare it a failure which could imply some movement toward the French assimilationist ideal.

Collectively these developments have led to deep ambivalence and agonizing uncertainty among people of cosmopolitan sympathies including myself as a vicarious participant in Europe's struggles. Liberal cosmopolitans face painful choices with respect to three related but analytically distinct questions. One is who should be admitted and on what terms? The second is the twinned dilemma: How to define integration and how to advance the integration of Muslims into secular societies with a Christian background? The third is what anti-terrorist measures to support? My searching for answers begins with the conviction that the first duty of persons concerned with human rights is the preservation of liberal regimes against authoritarian competitors and recognition that preservation may require recourse to a certain measure of illiberal means.

What more than anything else makes the migration question peculiarly troubling are two core liberal principles. One is that the state should not use violence against persons who pose no threat to the security or health or exercise of rights by others. Yet violence of some degree is a condition of maintaining borders that are more than nominal.

The second background norm is that a gross unearned disparity in life chances is fundamentally unfair. Being born in Lagos rather than Louisville is a matter of chance that results in just such a disparity. In individual cases it can be corrected simply by allowing people from Lagos to settle in Louisville assuming they can pass individualized determinations that they do not pose threats to public order, public health, or national security. We do not know how many would exercise that choice if they had it; however, in a Gallup poll of Nigerian sentiment with respect to migration, 40 percent said they would migrate to the West if they could, a result which suggests orders of magnitude for Africa as a whole where the population is projected to increase by one and one-half billion people by 2050 (Porter 2015).

Since advocacy of open borders spells suicide for politicians everywhere in the West, the real policy questions are: How many should be admitted annually? Should asylum claimants be able to jump the queue? Should family reunification trump skills? And should countries apply cultural as well as economic tests for admission?

Family reunification can be sold to Western electorates both on moral grounds and on the security-oriented ground that young men without wives or parents are the most volatile group in any society. It is likely that Western voters would also be receptive to immigration policies that screened prospective migrants for their willingness to accept—although not necessarily to endorse—contemporary European norms regarding sexual orientation, gender rights, and free speech.

A related but contentious question is whether governments should accommodate cultural practices that clash with those of the secular majority, such as hostility to exogenous marriage, polygamy, veiling, refusal to shake hands with members of the opposite sex, patriarchy in its various manifestations, separation of the sexes in school. Both conservatives and a number of liberal public intellectuals, feminists prominent among them, have—in the name of liberalism—called for intolerance of illiberal practices. For them liberalism is more than a recipe for social peace achieved though tolerance of different world views; it is a crusading faith.

Because illiberal practices are frequently associated with fundamentalist tendencies within the world of Sunni Islam, often referred to as Salafism or Wahabism, polemicists concerned primarily with national security rather than morality are divided over immigration policy as well. What divides them are differing convictions about the relationship between Salafist religious views and the leap to jihad. Some have argued that Salafism's emphasis on a sharp separation between Muslims and non-Muslims, with the latter seen as intrinsically hostile and debased, makes young Western Muslims susceptible to jihadi recruitment. Others like Olivier Roy reject the grooming hypothesis and argue that manifestations of respect for the Muslim religion in all of its forms other than jihad will foster a more benign relationship between minority and majority to their mutual benefit (Roy 2007).

Also potentially dividing people who identify with the liberal creed are the complex of issues stemming from the use of security services and criminal law to mitigate the ongoing risk of mass-casualty terrorism. One thing that both sides of the security debate agree on is the prison system's role in recruitment. Does it follow that convicted terrorists should be isolated either within national prisons or abroad? A second issue is whether to treat them as presumptively incorrigible and therefore subject to imprisonment for life, measures forbidden by the European Convention on Human Rights and most national constitutions? A third is whether persons who leave the country to join a terrorist organization like ISIS or Al Qaeda should be deemed to have committed treason or to have voluntarily relinquished their citizenship. And a fourth, to some degree encompassing the others, is whether certain measures of prevention—for instance detention or at least limits on mobility and extended periods of interrogation without the presence of counsel, both justified only on the basis of reasonable suspicion—should be normalized. Populists of the Right will undoubtedly support such measures, especially in light of attacks like those that struck Manchester, London, Paris, Nice, and Barcelona. Far less certain, however, is the future course of the liberal project in Western Europe, which as outlined above will be sorely tested as migration pressures intensify over the next thirty years.

Note

1 For purposes of this brief chapter, I define liberalism as a commitment to fostering equal opportunities for individuals to pursue their dreams as architects of themselves, but subject to the conditions that in shaping their own lives, they do not intrude on the equal life-shaping rights of others and they assume the civic duties necessary for the survival and continuing refinement of a system of government dedicated to the defense of the human rights first enumerated in the Universal Declaration.

References

Clawson, Patrick. 2009. "Demography in the Middle East." The Washington Institute for Near East Policy. www.washingtoninstitute.org/policy-analysis/view/demography-in-the-middle-east-population-growth-slowing-womens-situation-un.

Porter, Eduardo. 2015. "A Migration Juggernaut is Headed for Europe." *The New York Times*, September 15, 2015. www.nytimes.com/2015/09/16/business/international/europe-must-plan-for-immigration-juggernaut.html.

Roy, Olivier. 2007. *Secularism Confronts Islam*. New York: Columbia University Press.

Further Readings

Collier, Paul. 2013. *Exodus: How Migration is Changing Our World*. Oxford: Oxford University Press.

Kelly, Paul Joseph. 2002. *Multiculturalism Reconsidered: 'Culture and Equality' and its Critics*. Cambridge: Polity Press.

Kepel, Giles. 2015. *Terror in France*. Princeton, N.J: Princeton University Press.

Okin, Susan Moller, Joshua Cohen, Martha Craven Nussbaum, and Matthew Howard. 1999. *Is Multiculturalism Bad for Women?* Princeton, N.J.: Princeton University Press.

Parekh, Bhikhu C. 2006. *Rethinking Multiculturalism: Cultural Diversity and Political Theory*. Basingstoke: Palgrave Macmillan.

Wellman, Christopher Heath, and Phillip Cole. 2011. *Debating the Ethics of Immigration: Is there a Right to Exclude?* Oxford: Oxford University Press.

13

BUILDING A MOVEMENT AGAINST GENOCIDE IN MYANMAR

Recovering Democracy's Promise

Penny Green

In this short piece I want to explore the nature, limits and possibilities of a post-genocide Myanmar. My own view is that Myanmar's civil society, and its capacity to publicly imagine a free, equal and peaceful future, will remain stifled until it acknowledges the state's genocide against the Rohingya. The public imagination in Myanmar is at present deeply fractured and tainted with bigotry, exclusion, and fear. Even for the most progressive and previously oppressed sections of that society the prospect of a truly multi-cultural, democratic Myanmar is one in which the Rohingya are absent.

In November 2010 following her release from house arrest, Aung San Suu Kyi and the party she led promised the hope of a new Myanmar—free from the confinement, cruelty and repression of military rule. This new Myanmar would respect human rights, hold out the possibility of an end to civil war, end the persecution of minority groups and opposition activists, and introduce a new era of free speech, civil rights and democracy.

But it is Myanmar's genocide against the Rohingya ethnic minority that now globally defines Aung San Suu Kyi and the character of human rights in the country. We know about the genocide, not because the government has acknowledged it as a crime of past military regimes that it now urgently seeks to redress—on the contrary Suu Kyi's government has not only continued the legacy of genocidal persecution but has escalated it. We know about the genocide because of the critical work of a small group of organized Rohingya, regional and international civil society organizations, academic research, and investigative journalism.

Daw Aung San Suu Kyi presides over a genocide, a range of civil wars, most viciously against the Kachin, lends succor to the ugliest forms of racist nationalism, and inscribes that racism with her own hegemonic Buddhist Bamar ambitions. After decades of economic, political, and social isolation, Myanmar's return to the international stage is smeared in blood.

The state's long persecution of its Rohingya ethnic minority entered a new phase when we at the International State Crime Initiative began a 12-month study, investigating the nature of that persecution[1] (Green, MacManus, and de la Cour Venning 2015). Our research, and the work of regional NGOs (*Al Jazeera* 2015; Human Rights Watch 2012, 2013; Lindblom, Marsh, Motala and Munyan 2015; Zarni and Cowley 2014) confirmed systematic, widespread, and ongoing violations, including institutional discrimination, torture, sexual violence, arbitrary detention, destruction of communities, apartheid structures of segregation, targeted population control, mass killings, land confiscation, forced labor, denial of citizenship and identity, severe restrictions on freedom of movement and access to healthcare, food, education, and livelihood opportunities, and last but not least, state-sanctioned campaigns of religious hatred. Our evidence demonstrated without any doubt that the Rohingya are currently experiencing the genocidal onslaught[2] that renders the population so physically and psychologically diminished that they are unable to engage in purposeful life.

In response the state declared: "The government and people of Myanmar do not recognize the term Rohingya as it is an invented terminology … the Government of Myanmar categorically rejects the unfounded allegations …" (Global New Light of Myanmar 2016). Sadly, much of Myanmar's progressive civil society agree.

In October 2016 repression against the Rohingya intensified, this time in the isolated Northern Rakhine State (NRS) with widespread killings (including of children and babies), arbitrary detention, disappearances, mass gang-rape, collective punishment, arson, and village clearances by Myanmar's military and security forces. On-the-ground reports supplemented by a powerful UN "Flash Report" revealed a chilling picture of a trapped, terrified, and desperate Rohingya community, with tens of thousands of Rohingya having fled across the border into Bangladesh.

In August 2017 a Myanmar government-appointed commission dismissed the UN allegations and cleared the state security forces of mass rape, ethnic cleansing and mass murder. Moreover, Aung San Suu Kyi's government has since denied visas for three UN investigators on the grounds that such an investigation would "aggravate" the situation in NRS.

The election of Suu Kyi's National League for Democracy (NLD) in 2015 elicited much global optimism. Yet in the build-up to the 2015 national elections the NLD did not stand any Muslim candidates (contrary to previous practice) and slighted the Rohingya during campaigning, dismissing them as illegal Bengali immigrants unworthy of consideration in electoral and citizenship processes. Since its election victory the NLD's "barbarism of indifference" has translated into active genocidal practice. The new government, rather than challenging the hate campaigns of ultra-nationalist Rakhine groups and Buddhist monks, has instead been complicit in advancing institutionalized anti-Muslim discrimination in both law and policy. Aung San Suu Kyi has demanded that foreign governments refrain from using the term "Rohingya," and the government's public statements continue to simultaneously demonize and deny the existence of the Rohingya identity.

Despite the fact that this is the most significant test of Suu Kyi's leadership, she has remained remarkably indifferent[3] (Funakoshi 2016). Rather than visit the scene of the violence or challenge the perpetrators of hate and violence, she and her NLD government have instead fashioned crude denials which at heart blame the Rohingya for their own persecution.

Rather than taking allegations of security force abuse seriously, Suu Kyi's government has adopted military dictatorship-era tactics of blanket denial, an absolute ban on international observation, severe limitations on humanitarian access within the region, the muzzling of the press, and the "blacklisting" and deportation of human rights activists.[4] Moreover her own website dismissed allegations of security force killings and mass sexual assaults in Northern Rakhine State as "fake news" and "fake rapes" (Global New Light of Myanmar 2016).

Imagining a Myanmar where the Rohingya and other ethnic groups share equal rights with the dominant Buddhist Bamar and live as integrated citizens in a society free from discrimination is certainly idealistic, but it also possible. Realizing that imaginary is far more difficult. The barriers to change appear as impenetrable now as under the military junta, perhaps even more so given the market opportunities and guise of "democracy" that opportunistically seduce foreign governments. But those barriers are not, in truth, impenetrable. If we adopt the definition of state crime as "human rights violations perpetrated by state agents in pursuit of organizational goals" (Green and Ward 2004) then we require a social audience to "name," expose, and challenge those crimes. That audience is best represented by civil society.

This framework, however, poses key problems in the context of Myanmar. The Rohingya have few friends inside their own country. Even Myanmar's large and active human rights community, to whom we might ordinarily look for solidarity and a united struggle, have adopted the regime's stereotype of the Rohingya as "illegal Bengali immigrants."[5] For these activists, encouraged by a deeply racist and Islamophobic national impulse, the Rohingya represent an immigration and security threat, not a human rights issue, and this in turn is used to justify indifference to their suffering at best and complicity with genocide at worst. Rakhine civil society organizations (who at the same time engage in struggles for women's rights and against corporate and military land grabbing) actively promote anti-Muslim hatred.

If we are to reimagine Myanmar as a peaceful, plural, multi-ethnic democracy we must engage that section of civil society who for decades resisted military dictatorship under conditions of brutal repression and endured the junta's squalid prison cells. There can be no democracy for Myanmar while 1.2 million disenfranchised Rohingya face annihilation. Only a united struggle by local, regional and international civil society activists, in which an end to the genocide is understood as a central platform in all human rights struggles, is capable of building a free democratic Myanmar.

Hearteningly, we have seen the small beginnings of this engagement with courageous activists inside Myanmar building alliances in support of their Muslim neighbors. Moreover, Myanmar exiles from a range of political and ethnic communities are beginning to connect in ways not previously envisioned. On March 6th and 7th 2017, under the auspices of the Rome-based Permanent People's Tribunal, the International State Crime Initiative at Queen Mary, University of London hosted the first Tribunal on Myanmar's State Crimes against Rohingya, Kachin and other groups. What was so encouraging and indeed historic was the solidarity shared between the ethnic Kachin and Rohingya diaspora during the tribunal proceedings. And in May 2017 when Aung San Suu Kyi was given the Honorary Freedom of the City of London, Rohingya and Kachin activists stood side by side to protest the award. Both groups had previously pursued entirely separate paths of resistance (and in Myanmar continue to do so). These are very small beginnings, and they are taking place largely outside Myanmar, but they illustrate the possibility and potential of a shared struggle driven by a shared imaginary of a truly democratic Myanmar in which ethnic and oppositional groups overcome historic and state manipulated divisions and hold the state accountable for its myriad crimes.

Notes

1 The study was based on detailed ethnographic research in Rakhine State and Yangon, Myanmar and included 176 interviews with members of Rohingya, Rakhine, Kaman, and Maramagyi communities; international NGOs; government officials; local Rakhine civil society actors, activists; diplomats; journalists; lawyers; monks; imams; business-men and women; photographers; and academics. [The report is available on the International State Crime Initiative website. See: http://statecrime.org/state-crime-research/isci-report-countdown-to-annihilation-genocide-in-myanmar/

2 See Feierstein's stages of genocide (2014).

3 Neither ASSK nor her president, Htin Kyaw, visited Rakhine state during the crisis. Suu Kyi has commented only that investigations will be conducted fairly and according to the rule of law. Her claim that "we have not tried to hide anything on Rakhine" can only be interpreted as denial.

4 On October 31, *Myanmar Times* journalist, Fiona MacGregor, was fired, at the instigation of the Ministry of Information and following Facebook denunciations by the President's Office spokesman, U Zaw Htay, for publishing allegations of the rape of dozens of Rohingya women by Myanmar Army soldiers. The leading English language newspaper was forced to suspend reporting on Rakhine state.

References

Al Jazeera. 2015. "Genocide Agenda." www.aljazeera.com/investigations/genocideagenda.html.

Feierstein, Daniel, and Douglas Andrew Town 2014. *Genocide as social practice: reorganizing society under the Nazis and Argentina's military juntas*. New Brunswick, New Jersey and London: Rutgers University Press.

Funakoshi, Minami. 2016. "Suu Kyi says 'delicate' Myanmar conflict handled by rule of law." *Reuters World News*, November 2, 2016.

Global New Light of Myanmar. 2016. "Clashes continue in the Northern Rakhine, 25 violent attackers dead." November 14, 2016.

Green, Penny, and Tony Ward. 2004. *State Crime: Governments, Violence and Corruption*. London: Pluto Press.

———, Thomas MacManus, and Alicia de la Cour Venning. 2015. *Countdown to Annihilation: Genocide in Myanmar* London: International State Crime Initiative.

Human Rights Watch. 2012. "'The Government Could Have Stopped This': Sectarian Violence and Ensuing Abuses in Burma's Arakan State." July 31, 2012. www.hrw.org/report/2012/07/31/government-could-have-stopped/sectarian-violence-and-ensuing-abuses-burmas-arakan.

———. 2013. "All You Can Do is Pray: Crimes Against Humanity and Ethnic Cleansing of Rohingya Muslims in Myanmar's Arakan State." April 22, 2013. www.hrw.org/report/2013/04/22/all-you-can-do-pray/crimes-against-humanity-and-ethnic-cleansing-rohingya-muslims.

Lindblom, Alina, Elizabeth Marsh, Tasnim Motala, and Katherine Munyan. 2015. "Persecution of the Rohingya Muslims: Is Genocide Occurring in Rakhine State? A Legal Analysis." Allard K. Lowenstein International Human Rights Clinic, Yale Law School: Fortify Rights. www.fortifyrights.org/downloads/Yale_Persecution_of_the_Rohingya_October_2015.pdf.

Zarni, Maung, and Alice Cowley. 2014. "The Slow Burning Genocide of Myanmar's Rohingya." *Pacific Rim Law and Policy Journal* 23 (3): 683.

14

AMBEDKAR AND DU BOIS ON PURSUING RIGHTS PROTECTIONS GLOBALLY

Luis Cabrera

In this era of populism and nativism, when battles for some of the most basic principles of rights and social equality must seemingly be re-fought daily, it may feel as though there is little space left for considerations of *global* justice, much less global institutional development. Yet, some of the most prominent historic champions of those most basic principles of equality and rights have looked beyond the state for support in promoting them within. In so doing, they have indicated an important global institutional imaginary—a multi-level set of political institutions capable of backing individual rights protections domestically, and of giving those facing domestic repression some meaningful place to turn. Such an imaginary is well worth upholding as an alternative vision of political institutions, and it can be of practical use in guiding some current political struggles.

This chapter focuses on institutional alternatives indicated by B.R. Ambedkar and W.E.B. Du Bois. Both are renowned as campaigners for domestic equality, as significant social and political thinkers, and as pathbreakers in their ascribed domestic race and caste categories. Du Bois was the first African-American to earn a PhD at Harvard, in 1895. Ambedkar was the first Dalit (formerly "untouchables") overall to earn a PhD, completing his at Columbia in 1927. Ambedkar became the most prominent champion of Dalits in India, and he ultimately served as chief architect of the country's post-independence 1950 Constitution, which formally barred untouchability practices and established a range of individual rights protections. Du Bois, as a co-founder of and leading figure for decades in the National Association for the Advancement of Colored People (NAACP), similarly challenged the pervasive exclusion and domination of African-Americans. Both demanded a wholesale transformation of their deeply hierarchical societies.

Both also highlighted the potential importance of political institutions beyond the state which would be capable of hearing and addressing challenges to repression within. Du Bois did so in relation to the newly formed United Nations in the mid-1940s, and Ambedkar helped to inspire a current network of Dalit activists to undertake similar UN outreach. Du Bois and the NAACP delivered their "Appeal to the World" to the UN in 1947. It was based in exhaustive documentation of racially motivated discrimination and violence against African-Americans. In drafting the Appeal's introduction, Du Bois highlighted the vast gulf between America's founding ideals of equality and the treatment it had given to African-Americans: "a great nation, which today ought to be in the forefront of the march toward peace and democracy, finds itself continuously making common cause with race hate, prejudiced exploitation and oppression of the common man." He called on the UN and its member countries to pressure the United States to take more decisive action against such discrimination as "a basic problem of humanity."

The effort was strongly resisted by the US government, which had long been suspicious of Du Bois' activities and had put him under surveillance from the early part of the century. The highly visible UN petition in fact gave such foes as the Soviet Union evidence to use in denouncing the US as hypocritical in its global promotion of freedom and rights—something that brought Eleanor Roosevelt to the brink of resigning from the NAACP Board. The Appeal, however, also highlighted an alternative model of political struggle. This was a model where rights claims against a state would not be decided solely by that state. Rather, governments would, in Ambedkar's phrasing, have to answer for their actions "before the bar of the world."

Ambedkar was inspired by Du Bois' efforts and shared his aspirations. He had indicated the alternative model as early as a 1930 speech in which he noted that a right of appeal to the League of Nations had been granted to some vulnerable minorities within central and eastern European countries created after World War I. Such rights of global appeal "would be a very desirable addition to the armoury of the Depressed Classes," he said, though he did not place any strong hope in the possibility that the League or other authorities would actually offer effective aid to those facing repression.

Ambedkar was more hopeful about the United Nations, and he wrote to Du Bois asking for a copy of the NAACP petition. Ambedkar noted some regret later, in his 1951 speech of resignation as India's Law Minister, that he had ultimately decided not to approach the UN himself, but to place his faith in the new Constitution:

> I had prepared a report on the condition of the Scheduled Castes [Dalits] for submission to the United Nations. But I did not submit it. I felt that it would be better to wait until the Constituent Assembly and the future Parliament was given a chance to deal with the matter. … What is the [condition of] Scheduled Castes today? So far as I see, it is the same as before. The same old tyranny, the same old oppression, the same old discrimination which existed before, exists now, and perhaps in a worse form.

Ambedkar died in 1956. Some four decades later, a network of Dalit activists inspired by him both adopted and extended the international outreach blueprint he had indicated. The National Campaign on Dalit Human Rights (NCDHR) was formed to put Dalit rights groups around the country in coalition, and to press the Indian government for action from below and from above. The global outreach has involved lobbying UN human rights bodies as well as the European Parliament, US Congress, and others actors for support in challenging ongoing caste discrimination.

Partly as a result of those outreach efforts, UN bodies have affirmed that caste discrimination is covered by the Convention. Successive Indian governments have resisted such a finding, however, while also resisting international scrutiny of such domestic issues. The current government, led by the Hindu nationalist Bharatiya Janata Party, has effectively barred vital overseas funding for thousands of non-governmental organizations, including numerous ones in the NCDHR network. BJP officials contended in interviews that the Dalit activists are acting primarily as disloyal citizens, airing India's domestic challenges on a global stage. Their claims echo the accusations of disloyal or even treasonous behavior made against both Ambedkar and Du Bois in their time.[1]

Overall, the NCDHR network has succeeded in bringing global attention to caste discrimination, and putting greater pressure on the Indian government. The resistance, scrutiny, and recrimination faced by activists, however, highlights the power states and their governments continue to wield as judges and enforcers in cases involving claims against them. It also highlights some deep, systemic challenges to addressing rights rejections in the current global system.

There is much more to be said about the alternative indicated by Du Bois, Ambedkar and the NCDHR activists, and I have written extensively about it elsewhere (Cabrera 2019). It would be a system in which states, or their ruling governments, would not be the final judges in their own cases when it comes to claims of discrimination, unequal treatment and broader rights rejections. Individuals would have various mechanisms of challenge, and of making domestic repression more visible on the global stage. The current European Union represents a partial model. Or, better, it is a laboratory where struggles over institutional models have been playing out—one where some rights-based challenges can be lodged by individuals, and where state governments continue to try to exert dominant influence.

Ambedkar and Du Bois in some ways imply a more ambitious model, in which fully global institutions would play significant roles in oversight of states' rights records, and in which they would have some substantive powers to address widespread violations. We remain some distance from the latter especially, and there is no suggestion here that a genuinely rights-respecting and rights-protective "world government" is impending or could be realized in the near or medium term. The alternative global imaginary gives important guidance, however, for current efforts. As the American Civil Liberties Union has suggested, in highlighting Du Bois' actions as a model for promoting civil rights, the alternative can direct our attention to existing mechanisms for oversight of states by a neutral global arbiter (NAACP and Du Bois 1947). Those currently engaged in battles to protect very basic rights to equality and against discrimination can make use of UN assessments of states' human rights records in their own struggles, as indeed the Dalit activists have repeatedly done. They have made meaningful use of the features of a global institutional alternative which have emerged, while also affirming broader aspirations for change and helping to make them more prominent as part of a global imaginary—one that embraces a vision of political possibility beyond the state.

Note

1 The author interviewed 26 mid- and senior-level BJP officials and elected representatives, as well as more than 50 NCDHR activists, persons they serve and caste-issue experts in India from 2010–2016.

References

Cabrera, Luis. 2020. "NCDHR's Global Challenge" (Chapter 5) and "The Arrogance of States" (Chapter 6). In *The Humble Cosmopolitan: Rights, Diversity, and Trans-State Democracy*. New York: Oxford University Press.

National Association for the Advancement of Colored People, and W. E. B. Du Bois. 1947. A statement on the denial of human rights to minorities in the case of citizens of Negro descent in the United States of America and an appeal to the United Nations for redress. www.blackpast.org/1947-w-e-b-Du Bois-appeal-world-statement-denial-human-rights-minorities-case-citizens-n.

Bibliography

Ambedkar, B.R. 1943. *Dr. Babasaheb Ambedkar Writings and Speeches : Vol. 9*, edited by Vasant Moon. Bombay: Government of Maharashtra, 389–435. www.mea.gov.in/Images/attach/amb/Volume_09.pdf.

American Civil Liberties Union. "70 Years After W.E.B. Du Bois Appeal to U.N., Groups Press U.S. on Racial Equality." October 23, 2017. www.aclu.org/news/70-years-after-web-du-bois-appeal-un-groups-press-us-racial-equality.

15

WHY SHOULD WE CARE ABOUT CHINESENESS?[1]

Allen Chun

In an opinion piece in *The New York Times* on May 10, 2017, Jill Abramson wrote that

> the Chinese know that one of the best ways to curry favor with any ruler is to shower riches on his family members. There are so many millionaires among the children of its leaders that they have a moniker: the Princelings.

China watchers (sinologists) have made such phenomena staple features of news reporting and social scientific writing on the PRC for decades, so it's perhaps not surprising that the concept of *guanxi* is considered so difficult to render in English that it is often left untranslated, further underscoring its inherent Chineseness.[2] Moreover, the scholarly literature on *guanxi* shows few signs of diminishing. A conference organized by Thomas B. Gold at U.C. Berkeley in March 2015 on "The Field of *Guanxi* Studies" saw presentations and commentaries by two dozen international experts in this ongoing cottage industry. If anything, *guanxi* indexes the rot within a rotten society and system.

However, Abramson's piece was not about China; it was about the Princeling in the West Wing, Jared Kushner. It appeared a day after the "unseemly spectacle" of his sister, Nicole Meyer, hawking golden visas to Chinese investors as a prize for $500,000 investments in the family's real estate projects in Jersey City, which happened just after President Trump signed a renewal of the EB visa program. Never mind the conflict of interests in the Emoluments Clause of the US Constitution: the First Family has set up shop directly in the White House where pay for play is the norm at the top.

If this took place in the PRC, many readers of the *Times* would be crying for regime change. So why is everyone in the United States so complacent? I suppose one can blame unseemly Party politics in Congress or, more generously, respect for the rule of law and the proliferating number of investigations. Yet after criticizing lesser countries for their lack of democratic process, it's ironic that American voters elected a brute con artist who insulted everyone in his path and flaunted his moral indecency.

In defense of himself, Trump has blamed fake news, by others, of course. The blurred lines between reality TV and reality has become the new news. These fictions, inventions, and exaggerations are actually a basic aspect of institutional normalcy. The political sociologist

Philip Abrams once remarked that the state is not the reality that stands behind the mask of political practice but rather the mask that prevents us from seeing political practice as it is. As he put it, the state is "a third-order project, an ideological project. It is first and foremost an exercise in legitimation—what is being legitimated is, we may assume, an unacceptable domination" (Abrams 1988).

This chapter is derived from a recent book on "Chineseness," but it should have ramifications for Americanness (Chun 2017). We tend to view culture as neutral, identity even more so; the fact that we are obliged to have a national identity and that even the definition of a nation is sanctioned at the highest levels of international relations says much about its necessity in the modern era. But as Erik Erikson—who made "identity crisis" a keyword for our time—has astutely noted, identity is literally about "sameness" (*idem*), shared values, or relatedness to group. The fact that the Chinese rendition of identity is *rentong* (assimilation) says much about identification to a group and its values, never mind identity as status. If one also takes into account the content of culture that is inculcated as a product of socialization, then its literal meaning is less important than the fact that people are blind to (take for granted) the subjective values that they are tied to.

My work sought to explicate why Chinese everywhere have different notions of Chineseness that directly shape societal order and interpersonal experience. These differences at a literal level are still the object of ongoing debate, but the point is that they have been produced by entanglements with modernity, coloniality, and nationalism at an underlying level. At the same time, the (discursive) fictions of identity that people construct for themselves as part of their own experience were no less unreal than those we as outsiders have imposed on them through media representations and scholarly "theories." How do we know that East Asian regionalisms, neo-Confucian lineages, or clashes of civilization are any more pertinent as frameworks for explaining the above? We therefore need to deconstruct Orientalisms on *both* ends as a point of departure for unraveling the politicizing processes central to identification in general. I submit that "the native's point of view" is inherently flawed.

I have labeled the Republic of China (ROC) in Taiwan as a "politics of the unreal," but Hong Kong, the PRC, and other societies can be viewed similarly, if viewed literally from "the inside." The evolution of official discourse in postwar Taiwan to this day tends to give the impression that Taiwan has successfully transitioned from its prior claim to the legacy of traditional China and has become a more multicultural Taiwanese nation, which warrants its inevitable separation from the mainland. Interestingly, much of this recent history had been rewritten to reject the Cold War legacy of a prior Nationalist regime and instead emphasize the island's autonomous development since imperial times through its successive waves of colonization by Han settlers, European traders, and Japanese empire long before its return to China.

According to this perspective, the advent of Taiwanese consciousness is a justifiable ethos of self-determination rallied toward the aim of national independence. The reality is on the other hand more complex, even as people at the same time cling to the reality of the Republic of China (ironically, the PRC's rejection of Taiwan's independence efforts is mostly based on its official recognition of the ROC, albeit as a rebel regime). The uneasy, contradictory co-existence of a real Taiwan within an unreal ROC is exacerbated even more by the extent to which all politics is concretely ethnicized, then rooted sacredly to the mythic unity of 2000 years of Chinese civilization. In the heat of the 1996 missile crisis when the PRC was threatening Taiwan's move toward independence with a show of force, I argued sarcastically that, for most Chinese on both sides of the Taiwan Straits, 500 years is not a long time to wait for reunification. One myth familiar to many Chinese is that, after the fall of the Qing dynasty, someone discovered in the attic of a pagoda a placard saying "Restore the Ming (dynasty)!," as if to suggest that it was worth waiting 268 years for this. So when Chinese on both sides contest reunification/independence in terms of such myths, how unreal can politics really get?

Hong Kong identity is a similar fiction that was invented less than 40 years ago. Prior to then, Hong Kongers identified simply as Chinese; its culture was a satellite of Guangdong. Despite its colonial status, the government did not cultivate any connection among the people to Britain, and borders with China were open. The free trade port that eventually galvanized Hong Kong's image to the world in later years was actually the result of the colonial regime's effort to defuse Cold War strife that made the colony a battleground for competing nationalisms. Its cosmopolitan hybrid mass media culture industry that famously created a utilitarian ethos, where lifestyles were commoditized to project the illusion of "apolitical man," was a direct consequence of this policy of depoliticization. But in reality, it created new identities divided by class. Eugene Cooper phrased it best, in arguing that free market development in Hong Kong was "a veritable proving ground for Marxist theory, where enterprising students of Marxist political economy can literally watch chapters of *Capital* unfold before their eyes" (Cooper 1982). Social scientific "theories" that extolled Hong Kong's "administrative absorption of politics" and ethos of "utilitarian familism" were thus post-hoc rationalizations that eventually became taken for granted and mistaken for native "tradition."

The current metamorphosis of the PRC has also seen the emergence of "discourses" too often dismissed as pure propaganda, namely "one country, two systems" and "socialism with Chinese characteristics." However, it has indeed undergone serious transformations that transcend the superficial breakup of Maoist socialism and the open embrace of free market capitalism. Buttressing these developments has been the subtle emergence of a cultural nationalism that has become synonymous with an "unbroken" history of civilization and its collusion with the new politics of state. The fact that Hong Kong's "handover" in 1997 is routinely phrased in Chinese as "return to the motherland" should not be viewed trivially. Similarly, despite the ongoing friction that divides independent minded Taiwan from the PRC, few would disagree that Taiwan had at least two opportunities to claim independence: in 1949, after its retreat from the mainland, and in 1971, after its ouster from the United Nations (one can add the PRC's isolationalist Cultural Revolution era), which cast now distant Cold War mindsets on both sides. I would argue that Taiwan could more easily realize its aim of independence by rewriting history starting from its expulsion from the UN, then flaunt its uprootedness, its eccentricity, a tabula rasa history, i.e. anything but its inherent Taiwaneseness, which ties it inescapably to 2000 years of Chinese civilization.

Chinese everywhere are clouded by their own fog of identity, which is in fact a product of its rootedness to specific historical experiences that have been taken for granted as norm. I think, by way of comparison, this might say much about Americanness as well. The shock of Donald J. Trump's election victory should have been a point of critical introspection. The revenge of a worldview rooted in an era of primordiality *sauvage* ("nativism")[3] has shaken the progressive vision of America and now threatens to reshape reality to new heights of unreality. What would it take for Americans to critically reflect on their own cultural ethos?

Notes

1 This chapter is derived from the author's latest book, *Forget Chineseness: On the Geopolitics of Cultural Identification*. Albany: SUNY Press, 2017.
2 *Guanxi* literally means "relationship," same as in English. Its untranslated glossing has nothing to do with its meaning but rather its prevalence as a phenomenon and its peculiarities of behavior that observers have found *alien*, thus worthy of gazing.
3 Needless to say, Trump's "America First" does not refer to its First Peoples but rather a colonialism made native.

References

Abrams, Philip 1988. "Notes on the Difficulty of Studying the State." *Journal of Historical Sociology* 1 (1): 76.

Chun, Allen 2017. *Forget Chineseness: On the Geopolitics of Cultural Identification*. Albany: State University of New York Press.

Cooper, Eugene 1982. "Karl Marx's Other Island: The Evolution of Peripheral Capitalism in Hong Kong." *Bulletin of Concerned Asian Scholars* 14 (1): 25.

Bibliography

Abramson, Jill. 2017. "The Princeling in the West Wing." *New York Times*, May 10, 2017. www.nytimes.com/2017/05/10/opinion/jill-abramson-the-princeling-in-the-west-wing.html.

PART III

Ecological Imaginations

16

SEEDING THE FUTURE, SEEDING FREEDOM

Vandana Shiva

Humanity Stands at an Evolutionary Crossroads

We will either make peace with the Earth by realizing we are part of her, not her master, owner, conqueror—or the Earth will no longer allow us to exist. We will face extinction as humans even while we push millions of other species to extinction. We will either make peace with our diversity, or destroy the social fabric which diversity weaves, and with it, destroy the social conditions of our continued existence. But we can consciously choose the path of Oneness—of being part of one planet, one humanity, living and celebrating our many diversities, interconnected through bonds of compassion, interdependence, and solidarity. This is the path of the Earth Democracy movement.

We need a new public imagination to address the deep and multiple crises of our times—a public imagination that helps us reclaim our humanity, our freedoms, and our earth citizenship. When we think of the planet and all of humanity in abstractions, taking the path of Oneness seems impossible. But when we think through the real relationships we have with the Earth and each other in the real world, our consciousness expands, and simultaneously the task of making a radical shift becomes simple and possible. The "resurgence of the real" has become a precondition for the continued survival and evolution of our species. Living through illusion is no longer a luxury we can afford. Illusions of separation, atomization, fragmentation make us feel powerless and isolated, while seeing interconnectedness makes silos collapse and turn into bridges. Living in and through non-separability expands our sense of self. Becoming aware of our relationships enlarges our being, and our potential and power. We become aware that rejuvenating the planet and reclaiming humanity are not two different ends, reached through different paths, because the Earth and society are interwoven in one vibrant, indivisible fabric of life in autopoetic freedom.

Both the planet and humanity face the same threat from the same source: the 1% with *one mechanical mind*, which is destroying the intelligence of nature and humanity, running *one money machine* based on violence and war. By appropriating and enclosing the commons, it is promoting poverty, dispossession and disposability. I see the privatization and appropriation of our common wealth as piracy, whether it be the privatization of public lands for drilling and mining, or the privatization of water to sell as a commodity (whether bottled by Coca Cola, Pepsi, and Nestle or as urban water supplied through Suez and Bechtel), or the privatization of seeds, of public health, of education systems. Piracy is the violent appropriation of what is not yours.

The 1% are trying to create *one history* based on hiding their roots in the piracy and colonialism of earlier times and the continued piracy in our times, constructing false identities, false claims to innovation, and false superiority. The illusion of "innovation" has reached its extreme with the claim of patenting life, which is in fact a claim to creation. In every patent on a seed or on a living organism is a loud announcement: "God Move Over." This illusion has real effects in the real world. The will to own and conquer the common wealth of nature and society translates into the will to exterminate. Patents on seeds are pushing species to extinction, pushing farmers to suicide, transforming our daily bread into our daily poison. For people across diverse cultures and diverse beings on the planet, it is truly an end of history.

An unfair, unjust economic system controlled by billionaires creates an undemocratic "democracy." Through the construction of a *delusion of democracy*, representative democracy has become an instrument of corporate power and rule of the 1%, using cultural technologies of divide and rule to create a politics of fear and hate. These structural relations between economies that kill, democracies that are dying, and cultures of fear and hate, demand that we think and act collectively to seed our future and seed our freedoms through Earth Democracy.

In 1999, after we the people stopped the WTO Ministerial Meeting in Seattle, movements got together and launched the World Social Forum in Porto Allegre in Brazil with the vision "Another World is Possible." That is when I first spoke of Earth Democracy as the necessary alternative to destructive corporate globalization. It is an ecological necessity because the worldview of separation combined with an illusion of limitless extraction and exploitation of nature is pushing us to an ecological precipice. It is an economic necessity because a 1% world must render 99% of the population disposable, extinguishing our diverse creativities, potentials and possibilities. It is a democratic necessity because the rule of the 1% is violent dictatorship, destroying our fundamental freedoms and the freedoms of all beings to evolve freely in an interrelated world. It is a social necessity because the world of the 1% must destroy our social being—our communities—through privatization and enclosures of the commons, reducing us to consumers, dividing us on the basis of gender, race, religion. It is a human necessity because participating in a world of limitless greed, profit, violence, and abuse of power robs us of our humanity.

The powerful have divided us, and continue to divide us. Our strength is our Oneness—not a construct, but our very being. We need only to wake up to it. This is where the resurgence of the real begins. The real is the Earth and our oneness with the Earth. The real is our families and friends and communities. The real is the seed that gives rise to seed—not the GMO, patented, toxic non-renewable seed. The real is the food grown with loving, caring hands and mindfulness of the beings in the soil, the sun that blesses the plant, the plant that feeds us—not the fake food that industry manufactures, the toxic chemicals and fossil fuels reaping limitless profits for a few while our health is destroyed. The real is the intelligence pervading life, because life is intelligent. The real is our creativity, the creativity of our bodies and minds, the creativity of our hands—not the "innovation" of tools based on thievery, tools made to control nature and society for extraction and exploitation.

During my 45 years of service to the Earth and my engagement in fostering living economies based on non-violence and real creativity, I have always turned for inspiration to Gandhi's teachings: to act in times of hopelessness, to open spaces when all spaces are shrinking, to cultivate compassion and solidarity in times of greed, fear and hate, to reclaim our power when we are told that power is the monopoly of the few.

The times have changed but the patterns of colonization stay the same. They are based on the violent destruction of people's freedoms and economies, creating supremacy through a strategy of divide and rule. But popular longings for liberation and freedom are perennial, and these desires for freedom shape the path for the resurgence of the real. Three central concepts light this path.

Satyagraha is the deepest practice of democracy: the moral duty to not cooperate with unjust, exploitative and undemocratic processes. This is the first step in breaking free of an enslaving, colonizing system. "Satyagraha"—the force of truth—is Gandhi's word for non-cooperation with systems, structures, laws, paradigms, policies that destroy the Earth and rob us of our humanity and our freedoms, that crush our potential for compassion and sharing. Similarly, Henry David Thoreau coined the term "civil disobedience" in an essay on his refusal to pay taxes to a political system that supported slavery. He argued that higher moral laws compel citizens to disobey lower laws that institutionalize injustice and violence.

Swaraj is self-organization, self-rule, self-governance, autopoesis—it is the basis of real freedom in nature and society, beginning at the smallest scale and emerging over time at higher levels. Resistance by itself does not create freedom from oppression. We also need to sow the seeds of real freedom in our imagination, in our daily lives, and through our diverse and multiple relationships.

Swadeshi is self-making, based on local resources, indigenous knowledge, and community. It allows the expression of our fullest creativity as human beings and as Earth citizens. In Swadeshi we are co-creative with nature's intelligence, creativity, and regenerative potential, as well as the creativity and intelligence of our fellow human beings. Co-creativity with nature combines production with conservation. It is not extractive, polluting, and degrading to the planet and to human communities. It is the foundation of sustainability. It is the core of economic democracy. It is the source of *real wealth*, of well-being and happiness for all.

Real freedom and real wealth creation call for the practice of integrating Satyagraha, Swaraj, and Swadeshi. Resistance alone will not create another world. We must combine it with another imagination, one rooted in the real and combined with constructive action. Sowing the seeds of freedom is not "imaginary." It is a real act, an act in which we become one community with the Earth, one with our hands, hearts, and heads. Oneness is our being, our source of power: our power to resist, nonviolently. It is our power to co-create, nonviolently. This kind of creative public imagination can enable us to live as one humanity on one shared planet, our common home.

17

ECOLOGICAL PUBLICS

Imagining Epistemic Openness

Anna Grear

The contemporary epoch seems heavy with dark imaginings—any quick glance at the daily headlines reveals them day after day: projections, specters and threats, moving like shadow-puppets across the screens of televisions and computers, muttering from radios, from social media sites and newspapers. The threats press in relentlessly, pushing public consciousness ever deeper into a theatre of terrors: the endless 'war on terror'; the looming threat of nuclear catastrophe; the angst generated by rising ethno-nationalisms; the relentless daily struggle of multitudes for survival against poverty, drought, climate change and war; the rise of the robots and the potential threat of mass human unemployment—an entire multiverse of threats that stretch out towards the ultimate dark horizon of the Anthropocene and the threat of irreversible ecological breakdown.

The term 'Anthropocene'—an etymological combination of 'anthropos' ('human'/'man') and 'kainos' ('new'/'current')—is increasingly deployed to communicate the claim that Earth has been capitulated into a new era by humanity as a geological force extensively modifying the Earth System itself, most especially in the form of climate change.[1] In reality, the Anthropocene is the apotheosis of the necrotic, predatory imperatives of Eurocentric petro-capitalism and rampant industrial consumerism as they eat into the living crust of the planet, choke the oceans and pollute the air—it would far better be named the 'Capitalocene' (Haraway 2014; Grear 2015). The Anthropocene/Capitalocene is in many senses an ecological nemesis, and ultimately rests on predatory colonial foundations[2]—those now underpinning the global order of unjust relationships between the states of the global North and those of the global South (Anghie 2005).

The global public imagination remains shaped to an extensive degree by a rationalizing historical discourse of 'civilization'—now taking the form of 'neoliberal economic progress' that both operates and disguises morbidly uneven dynamics of contemporary domination between "imperial and subjected states" (Wood 2005, 12). Indeed, uneven structures and relations are the core characteristic of contemporary globalization, operationalized by the peculiar legal privilege of the transnational corporate form (Gill 1995; Shamir 2005; Ruggie 2018). And just as uneven distribution was (and remains) "a condition for the very existence of modern, fossil-fuel technology" (Malm and Hornborg 2014, 64) deep pathological unevenness[3] remains the hallmark of the appropriative neoliberalism now suffocating the living world in panoptic forms of eco-surveillance and governmentality (Luke 1995; Geisinger 1999).

Against this Anthropocene/Capitalocene horizon, what might it mean, then, to 'recover' public imagination? Where might we start?

I want to start to answer this question by quoting Drucilla Cornell and Stephen D. Seely (Chapter 2) in their contribution to this anthology. Writing on public imagination, and drawing on Spinoza, Cornell and Seely make the important point that the more we open ourselves to being affected by others, the more we allow ourselves to engage in complex situations, the richer our imagination becomes and the more we move away from our own inevitably 'inadequate' ideas towards a rational commons.

Writing in *Octavia's Brood*, Walidah Imarisha argues that "the decolonization of the imagination is the most dangerous and subversive form there is: for it is where all other forms of decolonization are born. Once the imagination is unshackled, liberation is limitless" (Imarisha and Brown 2015, 4).

Nothing, I suggest, could be more urgent than unshackling the human imagination in the age of the Anthropocene/Capitalocene. Nothing could be more pressing than the need to decolonize the public imagination from neoliberalism and its expulsive global grip (Sassen 2014; Näsström and Kalm 2015). Awakening a resistive, fresh imagination is the fulcrum point for global systemic change—and nothing could be more empowering than grasping the radical intimacy between the personal and the global in relation to climate change (the Anthropocene/Capitalocene's most salient marker): If the Anthropocene/Capitalocene horizon insists that 'we'—the all-inclusiveness of this must be challenged, of course—now collectively amount to a geological event of decisive force, then perhaps 'we' (and the meaning of 'we' remains contestable even for progressive narratives[4]) can collectively amount, over time, choice by choice, to a tidal wave of transformation.[5]

Such a prospect, however, mandates a re-imagined politics. For too long, the collective global imagination has been forced into a template supplied by the elitist power structures of the international order, and pushed by neoliberalism's ubiquitous plausibility structures selling the mega-lie that 'there is no alternative.' This lie must be challenged at every level: micro, meso, and macro. It is time to shatter the dominant monoculture of mind ultimately sourced in Eurocentrist colonizing capitalism (Anghie 2005, 4; Chakrabarty 2007).

Cornell and Seely's rational commons arises precisely from encounter with difference and complexity—for, as they suggest, the encounter with diversity provides "the maximal clarification of inadequate ideas." I agree with them that this level and kind of encounter is now fundamental to recovering a non-monolithic, energetic public imagination—as is the affective opening to 'others' lying at the heart of their contribution.

What, though, if we broaden our imagination concerning these 'others'? What if we could embrace new constituencies of meaning-making beyond 'the human'?

The cutting edge of science reveals realities with ethical implications long understood by indigenous populations and by faith-based worldviews—worldviews core to the kind of diversity necessary for a meaningful future commons. New scientific work reveals a world alive with forms of agency that the old dualistic ontology of Eurocentric rationalism foreclosed. It is urgently necessary to include previously excluded human beings and communities in a new public imagination enriched by the diversity of 'others', but against the Anthropocene/Capitalocene horizon it seems dangerously short sighted to continue to believe that the human being is the only actor whose agency counts. Indeed, it seems increasingly out of touch to continue to drag around the carapace of an old necrotic body of Eurocentric thought dulling a different possible sense of the world as it is. If the 'human planet' is increasingly pressed beyond ecological limits, we'd best urgently reimagine both humanity and planet alike.

Of great relevance to this re-imagination is the fact that our best science now insists that the mind/matter split is untenable (Barad 2007): Matter has escaped its imposed (imagined) inertia to announce itself as "materialization[,] a complex, pluralistic, relatively open process"—to step into view as lively materiality—which, once appreciated, relocates all human viewers/knowers "as thoroughly immersed within materiality's productive contingencies" (Coole and Frost 2010, 7). Materiality has its own lively agencies. This insight turns on its head "the conventional sense that agents are exclusively humans who possess cognitive abilities, intentionality and freedom to make autonomous decisions and the corollary presumption that humans have the right or ability to master nature" (Coole and Frost 2010, 10).

Since the conventional sense of Eurocentric human mastery brought us to the Anthropocene/ Capitalocene, what could be more apt than the de-centering of the subject implicit in the terminology itself? What if, instead of seeing ourselves as the isolated selves installed at the heart of the subject-object relations of the international order we could experience ourselves, imaginatively, as we all in reality are: entangled in the complex, lively, nonlinearity and self-emergent properties of materiality itself? What if transits beyond and through skins, leaves, pores, and a range of other breathing portals in bodies ('ours' and 'others') could be rendered visible to human public imagination, enabling politics, law, economics and more to embrace the ceaseless material intra-action of the world as a "spatial and temporal web of interspecies dependencies?" (Haraway 2008, 11). What if 'we' humans developed a completely different view of who is here? What if global public imagination could become so richly ecological[6] that non-human constituencies of meaning-making could become intrinsic to a new reimagined 'public'—even of multiple 'publics'? What if we could really sense, feel and live, day by day, the world as a movement of relations and processes of production that emerge "in a kind of chaotic network of habitual and non-habitual connections, always in flux, always reassembling in different ways?" (Potts 2004). What if such complexity and contingency was something to embrace, rather than to fear? What levels of epistemic openness might then be possible?

The Anthropocene/Capitalocene crisis demands a new ethical responsiveness to materiality—and a new humility. The crisis demands nothing short of a new vision of the human as but one partner in the never-ceasing movement of variegated co-partners entangled as a planetary whole. The crisis demands, in short, a new public imagination—and newly imagined 'publics'—ecological publics full of the freshly appreciated meaning-making capacities of yet-to-be-imagined constituencies. As Imarisha insists, "Once the imagination is unshackled, liberation is limitless."

Notes

1 Crutzen (2002; 2006, 13–18) popularized the term.
2 "The Anthropocene is the outcome of five hundred years of dispossession, capitalist accumulation, and neo/colonial globalization" (Kanngieser and Beuret 2017).
3 For a sustained reflection on unevenness in the contemporary situation, see Radhakrishnan (2003).
4 This is an argument central to the work of Code (2006) on the politics of epistemic location.
5 In this respect, the recent upsurge of protest movement in the 'school strikes for the climate' and the work of *Extinction Rebellion* points to a rising collective sensibility and the emergence of practices of resistance that could potentially build towards a tipping point.
6 In Code's sense, above n. 4.

References

Anghie, Antony. 2005. *Imperialism, Sovereignty and the Making of International Law*. Cambridge: Cambridge University Press.

Barad, Karen Michelle. 2007. *Meeting the Universe Halfway: Quantum Physics and the Entanglement of Matter and Meaning*. Durham: Duke University Press.

Chakrabarty, Dipesh. 2007. *Provincialising Europe: Postcolonial Thought and Historical Difference*. Princeton: Princeton University Press.

Code, Lorraine. 2006. *Ecological Thinking the Politics of Epistemic Location*. Oxford: Oxford University Press.

Coole, Diana H., and Samantha Frost. 2010. *New Materialisms: Ontology, Agency and Politics*. Durham: Duke University Press.

Crutzen, Paul J. 2002. "Geology of Mankind." *Nature* 415(23): doi:10.1038/415023a.

Crutzen, Paul J. 2006. "The Anthropocene." in *Earth System Science in the Anthropocene* edited by Ehlers, Eckart, and Thomas Krafft, 13–18. Berlin and Heidelberg: Springer. doi:10.1007/3-540-26590-2_3.

Geisinger, Alex. 1999. "Sustainable development and the domination of nature: Spreading the seed of the western ideology of nature." *Boston College Environmental Affairs Law Review* 27(1): 43.

Gill, Stephen. 1995. "Globalisation, market civilisation, and disciplinary neoliberalism." *Millennium: Journal of International Studies* 24(3): December: 399–423. doi:10.1177/03058298950240030801.

Grear, Anna. 2015. "Deconstructing anthropos: A critical legal reflection on 'anthropocentric' law and anthropocene 'humanity'." *Law and Critique* 26(3): 225–249. doi:10.1007/s10978-015-9161-0.

Haraway, Donna. 2008. *When Species Meet*. Minneapolis: University of Minnesota Press.

Haraway, Donna. "Anthropocene, capitolocene, chthulucene: Staying with the trouble." Lecture filmed May 9 2014 at University of California, Santa Cruz. Accessed September 18 2015. https://vimeo.com/97663518.

Imarisha, Walidah. 2015. "Introduction." in *Octavia's Brood: Science Fiction Stories from Social Justice Movements*. edited by Imarisha, Walidah, and Adrienne maree Brown Oakland, CA: AK Press and the Institute for Anarchist Studies, pp. 3–6.

Kanngieser, Anja, and Nicholas Beuret. 2017. "Refusing the world: Silence, commoning, and the anthropocene." *South Atlantic Quarterly* 116(2): 363–380. doi:10.1215/00382876-3829456.

Luke, Timothy W. 1995. "On environmentality: Geo-power and eco-knowledge in the discourses of contemporary environmentalism." *Cultural Critique* (31) (Autumn): 57–81. doi:10.2307/1354445.

Malm, Andreas, and Alf Hornborg. 2014. "The geology of mankind? A critique of the anthropocene narrative." *The Anthropocene Review* 1(1): (April): 62–69. doi:10.1177/2053019613516291.

Näsström, Sofia, and Sara Kalm. 2015. "A democratic critique of precarity." *Global Discourse* 5(4): 556–573. doi:10.1080/23269995.2014.992119.

Potts, Annie. 2004. "Deleuze on Viagra (Or, What Can a 'Viagra-Body' Do?) " *Body and Society* 10(1): (March): 19. doi:10.1177/1357034X04041759.

Radhakrishnan, Rajagopalan. 2003. *Theory in an Uneven World*. Malden: Blackwell.

Ruggie, John Gerard. 2018. "Multinationals as global institution: Power, authority and relative autonomy." *Regulation & Governance* 12(3): 317–333. doi:10.1111/rego.12154.

Sassen, Saskia. 2014. *Expulsions: Brutality and Complexity in the Global Economy*. Cambridge: Harvard University Press.

Shamir, Ronen. 2005. "Corporate Social Responsibility: A Case of Hegemony and Counter-Hegemony." in *Law and Globalization from Below: Towards a Cosmopolitan Legality*, edited by Rodríguez-Garavito, César A., and Boaventura de Sousa Santos. Cambridge: Cambridge University Press, pp. 92–117.

Wood, Ellen Meiksins. 2005. *Empire of capital*. London: Verso.

Bibliography

Gonzalez, Carmen. 2015. "Bridging the North-South divide: International environmental law in the anthropocene." *Pace Environmental Law Review* 32(2): 407.

Lewis, Simon L., and Mark A. Maslin. 2015. "Defining the Anthropocene." *Nature* 519(7542): 171–180. doi:10.1038/nature14258.

18

RE-IMAGINING POLITICS THROUGH THE LENS OF THE COMMONS

David Bollier

The rise of so many right-wing nationalist movements around the world—Brexit, Donald Trump, the neo-Nazis in Charlottesville, Virginia, anti-immigrant protests throughout Europe—have their own distinctive origins and contexts, to be sure. But in the aggregate, they are evidence of the dwindling options for credible change that capitalist political cultures are willing to consider. This naturally provokes the question: Why are the more wholesome alternative visions so scarce and scarcely believable?

Political elites and their corporate brethren are running out of ideas for how to reconcile the deep contradictions of "democratic capitalism" as it now exists. Even social democrats and liberals, the traditional foes of free-market dogma, seem locked into an archaic worldview and set of political strategies that makes their advocacy sound tinny. Their familiar progress-narrative—that economic growth, augmented by government interventions and redistribution, can in fact work and make society more stable and fair—is no longer persuasive.

Below, I argue that the commons paradigm offers a refreshing and practical lens for re-imagining politics, governance, and law. The commons, briefly put, is about self-organized social systems for managing shared wealth. Far from a "tragedy,"[1] the commons as a system for mutualizing responsibilities and benefits is highly generative. It can be seen in the successful self-management of forests, farmland, and water, and in open source software communities, open-access scholarly journals, and "cosmo-local" design and manufacturing systems.

The 2008 financial crisis drew back the curtain on many consensus myths that have kept the neoliberal capitalist narrative afloat. It turns out that growth is not something that is widely or equitably shared. A rising tide does *not* raise all boats because the poor, working class, and even the middle class do not share much of the productivity gains, tax breaks, or equity appreciation that the wealthy enjoy. The intensifying concentration of wealth is creating a new global plutocracy, whose members are using their fortunes to dominate and corrupt democratic processes while insulating themselves from the ills afflicting everyone else. No wonder the market/state system and the idea of liberal democracy are experiencing a legitimacy crisis.

Given this general critique, I believe that the most urgent challenge of our times is to develop a new socio-political imaginary that goes beyond those now on offer from the left or right. We need to imagine new sorts of governance and provisioning arrangements that can transform, tame, or replace predatory markets and capitalism. Over the past 50 years, the regulatory state has failed to abate the relentless flood of anti-ecological, anti-consumer, anti-social "externalities" generated by capitalism, largely because the power of capital has eclipsed that of the nation-state and citizen sovereignty. Yet the traditional left continues to believe, mistakenly, that a warmed-over Keynesianism, wealth-redistribution, and social programs are politically achievable and likely to be effective.

The 2008 financial crisis drew back the curtain on many consensus myths that have kept the neoliberal capitalist narrative afloat.

Cultural critic Douglas Rushkoff has said, "I've given up on *fixing* the *economy*. The *economy* is not broken. It's simply unjust." In other words, the economy is working more or less as its capitalist overseers intend it to work. Citizens often despair because struggle for change within conventional democratic politics is often futile—and not just because democratic processes are corrupted. State bureaucracies and even competitive markets are structurally *incapable* of addressing many problems. The limits of what The System can deliver—on climate change, inequality, infrastructure, democratic accountability—are on vivid display every day. As distrust in the state grows, a very pertinent question is where political sovereignty and legitimacy will migrate in the future.

The fundamental problem in developing a new vision, however, is that old ideological debates continue to dominate public discourse. Politics is endlessly rehashing many of the same disagreements, failing to recognize that deep structural change is needed. There is precious little room for new ideas and projects to incubate and grow. New visions must have space to breathe and evolve their own sovereign logic and ethics if they are to escape the dead end of meliorist reformism.

As I explained in a piece in *The Nation* magazine (Bollier 2017), insurgent narratives and projects are actually quite plentiful. Movements focused on climate justice, co-operatives, tradition towns, local food systems, alternative finance, digital currencies, peer production, open design and manufacturing, among others, are pioneering new post-capitalist models of peer governance and provisioning. While fragmented and diverse, these movements tend to emphasize common themes: production and consumption to meet household needs, not profit; bottom-up decision-making; and stewardship of shared wealth for the long term. These values all lie at the heart of the commons.

For now, these movements tend to work on the cultural fringe, more or less ignored by the mainstream media and political parties. But that is precisely what has allowed them to evolve with integrity and substance. Only here, on the periphery, have these movements been able to escape the stodgy prejudices and self-serving institutional priorities of political parties, government agencies, the commercial media, philanthropy, academia, and the entrenched non-profit-industrial complex.

Why is the public imagination for transformation change so stunted? In part because most established institutions are more focused on managing their brand reputations and organizational franchises. Taking risks and developing bold new initiatives and ideas are not what they generally do. Meanwhile, system-change movements are generally dismissed as too small-scale, trivial or apolitical to matter. They also fade into the shadows because they tend to rely on Internet-based networks to build new sorts of power, affordances (structural capacities for individual agency), and moral authority that mainstream players don't understand or respect. Examples include the rise of the peasant farmers' group La Via Campesina, transnational collaboration among indigenous peoples, platform co-operatives that foster sharing alternatives to Uber and Airbnb, and the System for Rice Intensification (a kind of open source agriculture developed by farmers themselves).

Rather than try to manage themselves as hierarchical *organizations* with proprietary franchises, reputations, and overhead to sustain, activists see themselves as part of *social movements* working as flexible players in open, fluid environments. Their network-driven activism enables them to more efficiently self-organize and coordinate activities, attract self-selected participants with talent, and implement fast cycles of creative iteration.

System-change movements tend to eschew the conventional policy and political process, and instead seek change through self-organized *emergence*. In ecological terms, they are using open digital networks to try to create "catchment areas," a landscape in which numerous flows converge (water, vegetation, soil, organisms, etc.) to give rise to an interdependent, self-replenishing zone of lively energy. As two students of complexity theory and social movements, Margaret Wheatley and Deborah Frieze, write:

When separate, local efforts connect with each other as networks, then strengthen as communities of practice, suddenly and surprisingly a new system emerges at a greater level of scale. This system of influence possesses qualities and capacities that were unknown in the individuals. It isn't that they were hidden; they simply don't exist until the system emerges. They are properties of the system, not the individual, but once there, individuals possess them. And the system that emerges always possesses greater power and influence than is possible through planned, incremental change. Emergence is how life creates radical change and takes things to scale (Wheatley and Frieze 2006).

The old guard of electoral politics and standard economics has trouble comprehending the principle of emergence, let alone recognizing the need for innovative policy structures that could leverage and focus that dynamic power. It has consistently underestimated the bottom-up innovation enabled by open source software; the speed and reliability of Wikipedia-style coordination and knowledge aggregation, and the power of social media in catalyzing viral self-organization such as the Occupy movement, the Indignados and Podemos in Spain, the Jasmine Revolution in Tunisia, and Syriza in Greece. Conventional schools of economics, politics and power do not comprehend the generative capacities of decentralized, self-organized networks. They apply obsolete categories of institutional control and political analysis, as if trying to understand the ramifications of automobiles through the language of "horseless carriages."

Instead of clinging to the old left/right spectrum of political ideology—which reflects the centrality of "the market" and "the state" in organizing society—we need to entertain new narratives that allow us to imagine new drivers of governance, production and culture. In my personal work, I see the enormous potential of the commons as farmers and fisherpeople, urban citizens and Internet users, try to reclaim shared resources that have been seized to feed the capitalist machine—and to devise their own governance alternatives. In this, the commons is at once a paradigm, a discourse, a set of social practices, and an ethic.

Over the past five years or more, the commons has served as a kind of overarching meta-narrative for diverse movements to challenge the marketization and transactionalization of everything, the dispossession and privatization of resources, and the corruption of democracy. The commons has also provided a language and ethic for thinking and acting like a commoner—collaborative, socially minded, embedded in nature, concerned with stewardship and long-term, respectful of the pluriverse that makes up our planet.

If we are serious about effecting system change, we need to start by emancipating ourselves from some backward-looking concepts and vocabularies. We need to instigate new post-capitalist ways of talking about the provisioning models and peer governance now emerging. Influencing unfolding realities may be less about electing different leaders and policies than about learning how to change ourselves, orchestrate a new shared intentionality, and hoist up new narratives about the commons.

Note

1 For one critique of Hardin's model, see Angus (2008).

References

Angus, Ian. 2008. "The Myth of the Tragedy of the Commons." *Climate and Capitalism*, August 25, 2008. https://climateandcapitalism.com/2008/08/25/debunking-the-tragedy-of-the-commons/.

Bollier, David. 2017. "To Find Alternatives to Capitalism, Think Small." *The Nation*, August 9, 2017. www.thenation.com/article/to-find-alternatives-to-capitalism-think-small.

Wheatley, Margaret, and Deborah Frieze. 2006. "Using Emergence to Take Social Innovations to Scale." www.margaretwheatley.com/articles/emergence.html.

Bibliography

Hardin, Garret. 1968. "The Tragedy of the Commons." *Science* 162 (3859): 1243–1248. 10.1126/science.162.3859.1243.

PART IV

Rupture and Revolution

19

RUMINATIONS ON DARKNESS AND LIGHT

Elizabeth West

This is an invitation. An invitation to take the hand of imagination—both public and private—from the cerebral, where it loves to dance, and to lead it, spiraling, deep into the most tender and true place in your own heart. Readers of this volume of thoughtful writing on 'public imagination' are undoubtedly masters of the mind. You know how to think, creatively and expansively, and most often, I trust that your thinking is fueled by a foundational passion for justice and dignity on behalf of every living being on the planet.

With this passion at the core of how the world is perceived, we are unlikely to find anyone amongst this readership who is not alarmed by the turn of political events worldwide. Hopeful notes, such as the rise of youth-led resistance to mass ecocide and the outspokenness of a handful of newly minted members of the US Congress, are continually overshadowed by the looming Colossus, steered by a relatively small self-serving cabal which has been sufficiently empowered to do their worst by a populace seemingly gone mad. And of course, it makes sense to investigate the cause of the madness, to do what is possible to open the curtains and let more light into the asylum. Even to unlock the gates and offer the freedom of real facts and new ideas to those incarcerated within.

There are grave dangers threatening large numbers of those of us who live here, on this planet. Trump, his fawning domestic and foreign sycophants, and his fellow authoritarian rulers around the world are knee-deep in the carnage. Terrible suffering is already occurring as a result and more will no doubt follow. Some of us have to counter this race to destruction of all that upholds beauty and decency in human life. Some of us see no choice but to devote ourselves to finding new ways to cut through the deceit and manipulation that has been employed to en-trance and ultimately, enslave so many of our fellow humans.

This is essential work and it requires all the intellectual creativity and rigor that we have at our disposal. It is a time like no other. As many have pointed out, this is not our first go-round with the collapse of goodness in society. But, it is the first time that the collapse is not to any degree contained geographically. If we are to confront the globally rising tide of fear, as well as the fear-mongering which has cynically and deliberately engendered it, and the authoritarian, regressive and repressive reactions to it, we must tap directly into its opposite.

And its opposite—the antipode of fear—is love.

Which, though it can dwell in the mind, arises from the heart.

Too simple? Maybe, but fascination with complexity has historically been a means by which we distance ourselves from reality. From *feeling* reality, from knowing it through experience rather than observation and analysis. Both are legitimate paths to certain kinds of knowledge, but there are times and places where one or the other is more useful in terms of understanding and taking action that meets a designated need. For instance, an objective scientific study of pathogens will lead us toward knowing how to prevent the damage they might do, while a subjective experience of illumination—Maslow's peak experience, if you will—gives us entrance into realms that offer sustenance and confer meaning on the life that has been saved by, say, the antibiotic that halts the previously referenced pathogens.

There is a call to respond to the cruelty both advocated and implemented by totalitarianism around the world from a place of deep love for the light that lives in each and every being on this planet, to respond in a way that fundamentally changes the dialog and upends the underlying assumptions. Fighting for peace is inherently an absurdity. And yet, the willingness of some human beings to disregard all bounds of shared humanity, to deprive others of every right including that of life itself, makes this a particularly difficult challenge.

How does one prevail in a contest where the game is rigged? Where the very nature of the goal itself prevents the actions that seem most likely to achieve it? Many great minds have and will continue to contemplate these conundrums and sometimes, discover ways to slide in sideways, to see the puzzle from a different angle.

Herein lies the tremendous value of cultivating the sphere of public imagination in a time when the rights and lives of all living beings are endangered. The alchemical process of exchanging the inner expanses of personal imaginations in order to spark new thinking is essential if we are to halt, or even slow, the hurtling train of greed, domination, and concomitant widespread—and potentially nuclear—violence.

However, no matter how compelling this call may be, no matter how urgent it is to stand against these forces, there is another, even greater jeopardy which threatens every single one us that we ignore at our peril. In fact, it is likely too late to change the course of environmental avalanche, at least in regard to outcome. The Earth's ability to sustain 7.7 billion homo sapiens (with all our attendant consumptions, constructions and waste products) was always questionable, but when so many of us insist upon living in a manner that is out of balance with the rest of nature, the question becomes one of 'when' and not 'if' a correction will occur. Science is increasingly concluding that the 'when' is not so far off. How large a correction and exactly how distant? No one knows. There really is no precedent. But we all do know—whether we are consciously acknowledging it or not—that the life we live today is not sustainable for the long-term. The mind may rebel, but the heart feels this and it is my belief that it is this inherent knowing that fuels a great deal of the fear we see playing out in the political sphere.

Consider the future of the planet and the species: it is an excruciatingly painful exercise. If we allow ourselves to imagine into the future, there are scenarios that are so impossible, so unbearable to contemplate that the temptation arises powerfully to slam the door and return to crises that we may actually have the ability to ameliorate.

Is there anything to *do?* Absolutely. Things in their thousands. However, it is quite possible that we can but alleviate some of the inevitable suffering. So, here is where the invitation to drop down into your heart becomes an appeal. As human beings, we are gifted with minds that are unequalled, as well as with hearts that truly know no limitation. If our time as a species is finite, which it is beginning to seem credible, then we must give our attention to how we want to live. This is always the case, as our sojourn is short no matter what.

But facing the immanent end of life, or life as we have known it, there is a summons to take stock and make the most of each moment, each breath, each exchange, each dawn and each sunset. To truly *feel* the sorrow of our collective circumstances and to grieve it, to weep, and to rage.

And equally, to rejoice in the beauty and brilliance and unexpected innocence that continues to be so generously offered to us. Simple stuff sometimes: the quiet majesty of a newly unfurled iris, a blue heron standing attentively in the shallows, the unparalleled flavor of tiny spring asparagus, a fleeting instance of communion with another human being, the gentle call of doves nearby. There is no reward, no change in the course of events that is promised by allowing ourselves to be present in our hearts for this life, other than the gift we give ourselves of drinking deeply from the cup we have been given, and using our minds and our hearts *in concert* to partake of the fullness of what it means to be human.

Surely Trump et alii need to be countered; the goodness of human nature longs to be asserted and made manifest. And while we must all find the means forward that reflect our individual inclinations, I want to conclude with a universal benediction that is also an entreaty: whatever we choose to do with the time that remains—no matter how long or how brief—let us embrace the entire range of human expression and experience. Let us reach into the passion and the courage and the particular wisdom that arise uniquely from the human heart-and-mind and allow it to live, fully, as us. Let us not miss out on the extraordinary reality of being all that we were born to be, regardless of the tenebrous times. We can't know if by so doing we will alter anything other than ourselves, but as we live in and from our deepest glory, we cannot help but offer that magnificence as light against the gathering darkness.

20

PUBLIC IMAGINATION AS PROPHETIC LEGACY

Catherine Keller

The public imagination: all too inviting a theme, a question, a possibility! Rather than plunging us one more time into the disheartening immediacy of democratic failure, rather than slamming us yet again into so many closed doors of action, the very thought of the imagination as public suggests unforeseen passageways to the future. The "public" at once leaps beyond its current degradation, while the "imagination," tempted always to private flight, instead swoops and hovers in the interstices of a fresh political assemblage. Suddenly the tedious shadow play of optimism and pessimism is interrupted; real potentiality for a viable earth future winks at us.

Or is this another tempting intellectual chimera, an excuse for more *theoria*—which means after all "seeing," perceiving *images*—and less practice?

Since many of us remain unmotivated by current prescriptions for pure praxis, why not yield experimentally to the temptation to imagine publicly, indeed to imagine a public? The notion of public imagination summons up a proverb that encapsulates an ancient inseparability of theory and practice. In the familiar translation: "Without a vision the people perish."[1] In other words, without a public imagination, the "public" fails. So here we are 2500 years later, with the popular assemblage that in a democracy "the people" signifies, quite possibly in the process of perishing. The *populus* has yielded the new populism that confuses itself with authoritarianism. Resenting its loss of economic dignity, local identity, and common (white) ground, it reacts against "the government" and so undermines its own democratic means of access to needed change. It gets blinded to the actual causes of its discontent. Without a vision, the very idea of "the people" perishes. It has been edged out by what Richard Falk and Victor Faessel call, in the Introduction to this anthology, the "regressive politics" of right-wing populism and nativism, "intensified by disinformation, fake news, and corporatized media." The Foxy barrage of images directing the erstwhile public to blame racial and religious others as well as the politically correct elites "seen" as sponsoring them now fill the space that the public imagination had vacated.

Such images, deforming shared history and selling fake dreams, are what the Hebrew prophets called *idols*. Indeed the more literal translation of the above proverb reads: "Where there is no prophecy, the people cast off restraint."[2] This unrestrained self-indulgence alludes to the moment of regression when the people, in the narrative of exodus, surrender to the nostalgic intensities of idol-worship—the allure of the riches, the golden calf, of Egypt. In other words, the *populus* escaping from slavery turns to embrace the imaginary of its enslavement. Fortunately, if not without great loss, the people of Israel re-collected itself and the liberative imagination persisted, precisely what was then called "prophecy." Prophecy in the Hebrew sense did not signify predictions of the future but its critical envisagement: the public imagination of the future. The discourse of *hope*—not optimism—arises from prophecy, from the anticipation of a "new atmosphere and earth,"[3] when the spirit would "renew the face of the earth."[4] The prophetic hope is conditioned on the public practice of justice: "love justice, practice kindness, walk humbly with your God."[5] Not just among "the people" but, recursively: "love the foreigner, for you were foreigners in Egypt."[6]

My point is not to turn back to the bible for salvation. It is that at least in the West a public imagination of social justice willy nilly echoes the ancient, dissident voices of warning and hope. So scholars of these traditions can help to keep the antecedents exposed, contextual, and diversified. Otherwise we will continue to fall prey to the political theology blustering trumphantly [sic] through the land. In the name of a Christian America it melts its White Christ prosperity gospel cum supernaturalism into the golden calf of consumer bliss and bully power. Thus 45 early delivered a commencement address at the Fallwellian (the Christian analogue to Orwellian?) Liberty University to a huge crowd of ecstatic born-agains, for whom such actual prophetic texts have been buried beneath their biblical literalism. Contradictions—between his secularism and their fundamentalism, between working class self-interest and the current populism—harden into the idol that we hope will not in retrospect be named fascism.

In clearing our eyes now, more recent prophetic utterances are being circulated, notably of Karl Polanyi, warning of a future fascist reaction to the effects of the new capitalism; and Hannah Arendt, who warned of a "new fascist international" that she believed would be provoked *after* WWII by mounting crises of immigration and "white supremacism."[7] And less known: 73 years ago Henry A. Wallace, Franklin Roosevelt's VP, wrote an essay called "The Danger of American Fascists." His grandson recently published an account of it, as describing "a breed of super-nationalist who pursues political power by deceiving Americans and playing to their fears, but is really interested only in protecting his own wealth and privilege" (Wallace 2017). As vice president, Wallace wrote the following: "They demand free enterprise, but are the spokesmen for monopoly and vested interest." They also "claim to be super-patriots, but they would destroy every liberty guaranteed by the Constitution." They posture about putting America first, but it's only a cover. "They use isolationism as a slogan to conceal their own selfish imperialism." They need scapegoats and harbor "an intensity of intolerance toward those of other races, parties, classes, religions, cultures, regions or nations " The citations prove Henry Scott Wallace's point: his grandfather seems to have "predicted President Trump."

Ok, "predicted," but only as long as we don't confuse such prescience with the false notion of omniscient knowledge of the future often projected onto the biblical prophecies (especially of the apocalypse!). But if we are speaking of prophecy as public imagination, it is a strategy to amplify past warnings and past hopes in recognition of their power to open new possibilities: possibilities now, that "flash up," like Walter Benjamin's messianic now-time, precisely as recapitulations of a whole history.

With that politico-theological nicety in mind let me turn to another prophecy from that period, actually by a theologian. Reinhold Niebuhr wrote in 1939:

> the avoidance of social violence depends upon the ability of a wise statesmanship to prevent the lower middle classes and farmers from becoming the political allies of an imperiled capitalistic oligarchy ... Such a political alignment offers the imperiled oligarchy the fascist alternative to capitulation and increases the desperate fury of the

> dispossessed. Unfortunately, the classes which have moral scruples against violence are not always particularly helpful in guiding the political thinking of lower middle-class life away from the deceptions and perils of fascist politics.[8]

Having recently visited a small town in Northeastern Missouri, the image of that sad village haunts me, with three out of four businesses boarded up and agriculture abandoned to the distant profits of agribusiness. Nevertheless the underemployed and overworked locals still cherish their identity as farmers and makers, and they voted predictably.

There is no need for the present international surge of populist authoritarianism to solidify into fascism. The situation is rife with contradictions that threaten the right as well as the left, that indeed shake up the brittle right/left spectrum itself. The very planet is turbulent with climate changes now threatening—as endless environmental protections and promises are cancelled—to become all too predictably apocalyptic. In this ever mounting anthropocene catastrophe, the trumphant denialism of the right meets the disappointed nihilism of the left. It may be helpful, if you hear the apocalypse whispering "too late, too late," to recall that at least in the bible, the concept of "the end of the world" does not exist. Even in the Book of Revelation, where there is indeed great planetary catastrophe environmental and human, there is not an end of the world. There is a New Jerusalem of "clean water for all," of "no more tears" … And it is the most dire of the ancient visions of warning.

In our current imagination, I hope that apocalypse roots down into its etymological significance: *apokalyptein*, to reveal. Not to close down history but to disclose possibility. It can only happen in a great widening of our capacity to coalesce across difference across the democratic spectrum—so as to work mindfully, cannily, maybe even wisely, with all the dispossessed, even those who resent us so middle-fingeringly. We should do this not so that we can all be One, but so that we can foment a new multiplicity, a pluri-singularity, an ecosocial assemblage that works our interdependencies to our mutual advantage. That would mean not social movement but local electoral labor, not just local politics but planetary coalition: collusions between multiple religions, between each religion and its accompanying secularization, so between secular and religious modes of public imagination.

Such a coalition gets fired up not just by human indignations but animal, plant, and elemental precarities. New creation: not a transcendent imposition but a spirited renewal rich with lament for what is and will be lost irretrievably. Such a coalition does not diminish but rather links differences, and so has the chance—the possibility, not the probability—of outmaneuvering the present regime of contradictions. Because we would acknowledge our tensions, deliberately practicing the democratic art of "agonistic respect" rather than mere antagonism (Connolly 2016). In the current shock and outrage at what has happened and what is happening, there is the chance—a bluewaving greengrowing chance—that catastrophe becomes catalyst.

Notes

1 Prov. 29:18 King James Version.
2 New Revised Standard Version.
3 Usually "new heaven and earth," a phrase first used in the Second Isaiah. The heavens, hashamayim, means not a supernatural place but sky, outer atmosphere, visible and invisible.
4 Ps. 104:30.
5 Mic. 6:8.
6 Deut. 10:19, also translated as "stranger," "alien," "immigrant."

7 See William Connolly's timely discussion (2016) of Karl Polanyi's *The Great Transformation*; Arendt (1945).
8 Cited in Pally (2017).

References

Arendt, Hannah. 1945. "The seeds of a fascist international." In *Essays in Understanding*, 140–150. New York: Harcourt Brace.

Connolly, William E. 2016. "Donald Trump and the New Fascism." The Contemporary Condition, August, 2016. http://contemporarycondition.blogspot.com/2016/08/donald-trump-and-new-fascism.html.

Pally, Marcia. 2017. "Apres Macron: Can We Escape from the Neoliberal-Populist Dead End?" ABC Religion & Ethics, May 10, 2017. www.abc.net.au/religion/articles/2017/05/10/4666565.htm.

Wallace, Henry Scott. 2017. "American Fascism, In 1944 and Today." *New York Times*, May 12, 2017. www.nytimes.com/2017/05/12/opinion/american-fascism-trump.html.

21

A NEW AXIAL AGE? OPENING AND DISARRAY

Abdellah Hammoudi

Are we experiencing an axial moment? The "axial age" (Jaspers 2011) has been used by scholars to define the long epoch marking the advent of the three monotheistic religions. As a retrospective concept, it seems unfit for thinking about our present, but the Scriptures and actions attributed to the leaders of those religious movements indicate an awareness of the momentous changes afoot during this era. Similarly, could we think of the current worldwide anguish as generated by the perception of some radical novelty that resists our effort to identify it? I want to consider the possibility that we may be going through something like an "opening," somehow connected to public imagination on a broad scale, and highlight several aspects of it.

First, everyone and everything seems to be on the move and yet we are stuck. Seen from where I come from, North Africa, and many countries south of the Sahara, a sizable proportion of the youth really want to head north. Direction Europe: the wealthiest place on the planet, one that offers the possibility of better living and freedoms not available at "home." Yet, so many are stuck in Northern Africa, to give just one example.[1]

Think of parallels in the Americas, the Levant and the Syrian killing fields, or Australia and elsewhere. We have innumerable accounts from refugee camps of the violence, genocides, ethnic cleansings, droughts, and famines that have put people in motion and yet trapped them in camps where their sense of *being stuck* generally goes unnoticed. Another reality not attended to is that the numerous transit states into which they pass are stuck with them as well.

Second, the ones who do not move resent the ones who succeed in moving back and forth amid the dejection of those left behind, and these resent even more the migratory ease of the global wealthy from North and South. The most important consequence is that states and international organizations still retain power on the frontiers between territories, but they are unable to stop the movement.

Third, change of place is now possible in the virtual world of the internet. Yet, being largely phantasmagoric, it fails to fulfill stringent desires. So, one may experience a full virtual life in Paris or New York but spend one's "real" life in Z'hiliga in Morocco, or Agadez in Niger. Worse, one would interact online with those who physically move about as they please.

The changes we have been witnessing in the West since the late sixties may be pointing to an alteration of consciousness which correlates with an axial moment. May 1968 in France and its aftermath, the movement against the war in Vietnam, and all things New Age in the USA signaled the advent of new modes of change: revolution was not the transformation of a mode of production and the overthrow of the bourgeois classes and powers. It took a novel form: change happened through the erosion of the old bourgeois order. Family, marriage, sex, gender, work, leisure, pleasure, politics, art, war, security, value, capital, inequality, equality … all those familiar figures were still alive, but none worked quite in the same ways as before. The welfare state muddled class issues. Consumption, and consumption of the "sign," became paramount (branding being king).

Historicism ceded its place of honor to an archeology that ceaselessly turned around itself, unearthing geological strata of strange forms and chimera. In the meantime, poets of "advanced" capitalism made the pronouncement of the "end" of History.

What in fact gained ground is an irresistible activity of grand collage production, everywhere generalized by new digital media with often baffling creativity. Collages of styles and times enlarged the market to technologies Marx could never have dreamt of. Thus, about anything could now turn up from any civilization past, contemporary, or virtually future, and at any moment, in this cosmic, sometimes comic, commodity-generating metempsychosis.

This sort of metempsychosis, I suggest, indexes an opening. It discloses the work of agentive forces we are unable to identify properly. It would seem that this is a classic case of a frontier of knowledge. Yet, to say that is not enough, for in this new situation things and voices from different times and places cross paths, often speaking to each other in tongues. These uncanny encounters may well be part of a watershed moment. That is why I use "opening" here coupled with "disarray."

My second contention is that the enduring reality of territorial states running nations more or less in flux is a fact worldwide. But it is crucial to note that those nations are not on the same side of the equation. For example, the breaking and (re-)making of Sudan cannot be lumped analytically with a possible one in Great Britain (involving Ireland and Scotland). Nor can it be lumped with the construction of a transnational Europe. Sudan belongs with the postcolonial weak and poor; Britain with the powerful and wealthy. Sudan was colonized. Britain colonized it. India, Indonesia, or Iran are among the relatively powerful, but not the wealthy, the Gulf States are among the wealthy, not the powerful. China is powerful, but one of a kind. The nuances may extend and proliferate with Brazil, South Africa, and others.

Financial and media centers may still be entrenched in the West, but movement comes from many other centers. Thus another novelty: movement without clear direction doesn't translate as loss of agency, but as the work of myriad agencies. If that is what is happening in between surviving nations, what is happening within them? Anthropologists have rightly insisted that people are now everywhere confronting each other with their differences. These are cultural differences in search of the power to survive.

So what is crucially new here? One answer lies in the unmediated encounters of cultural difference. But this needs a vital qualification. Proponents of "culture" assume that it is a source of orientation for people. They usually discount dis-orientations that may stem from it. Critics posit social embeddedness of "culture." They usually assume a structure hidden from people. Both neglect the enigmatic figures that cultural categories, in current circumstances, may take shape as for both "native" and anthropologist alike. Neither proponents nor critics pay attention to collage and the sort of metempsychosis I consider as major phenomena of our times, unfolding on the most global scale as a source of "opening" that is inseparable from "disarray." Because terms and figures are metempsychosed, the people confronting each other are in fact at a loss as to what their identities should ultimately be about.

The region to which I belong, the majority Arabic speaking one, has had to take the full shock of that opening, with utterly devastating consequences. For it is perhaps the most globalized one in recent memory, at the heart of Western diplomacy and war and the world economy as a whole through the energy market. It is a grand, ghastly field experiment with the lives of its inhabitants. One face of it is the new form of colonialism and apartheid imposed by Israel on the Palestinians. Another is the one conducted by some Arab regimes that employ systemic violence, torture, and glaring forms of discriminations and inequality. A most telling experiment is the form of violence currently going on in the "Caliphate's" dominions, a reign of terror that follows in the wake of the American experiment with a "New Middle East." The region is but one experimental field, if perhaps a most gruesome one.

Thus, our historical moment of "opening and disarray" is a global reality of confounding reversals in politics and identity. How are we to understand, say, the sudden passages from Catholic to jihadist? And what about from secular to radically pious, or the back and forth between radical and quietist Islam? Nothing here is specific to Islam or religion. But how it works depends on which side of the opening a person resides. In the West one is confronted with seemingly infinite lifestyle "choices" available in a fast moving market. Elsewhere, it may live with the burdensome reality of being physically stuck while virtually on the move or geographically contained while living the life of a restless refugee.

Today confrontation often occurs in enigmatic collages of cultural and linguistic expression. Actions may be taken or policies executed without much translation or mediation. But on the ground accommodations may happen regardless. This is not to say that we could dispense with understanding. Rather, it is to say that we need more of it. Because of the current overwhelming collage of cultural practices, it is often hard to envision grounds for commensurability. Perhaps only some leaps of creativity, similar to ones which seem to have occurred in an "axial age," may bring some new directions to our times of extreme volatility. Originating in, and responding to, the predicament of "opening and disarray," they may bring together the very diverse crisscrossing lives which are not on the same side of the global.

It is our distinct responsibility to hold on to another meaning of "opening"—which is "promise."

Note

1 Mhani Alaoui, in her recent dissertation at Princeton University, provides a good description of the forced stasis in Morocco, for people who are obsessed by the desire to leave.

References

Jaspers, Karl 2011. *The Origin and Goal of History*. Hoboken, NJ: Routledge. Reprints.

Bibliography

Alaoui, Mhani. 2009. "Migratory Trajectories: Moroccan Borderlands and Translocal Imaginaries." PhD diss., Princeton University.

22

REVOLUTIONARY POLITICS AND PUBLIC IMAGINATION

Behrooz Ghamari-Tabrizi

Revolutionary moments, *like a thunderbolt from the blue*, tear open the world of possibilities—possibilities that are articulated, albeit in ambiguous terms, in public imaginations of the good life. Revolutionary moments, from the time of the French revolution to the recent Arab uprisings, have also been stifled by institutional restrictions and the demands of the postrevolutionary *Realpolitik*. Such demands often compel revolutionary subjects to abandon their essential desire for *possible* realities and instead become content, as Robert Musil lamented in *The Man Without Qualities,* with a pragmatic sensibility of *real* possibilities. Where do we stand today? Are we losing the ability to imagine that *another world is possible*? Are we losing the ability to imagine what that other world might look like? Are we witnessing today the realization of what Rousseau feared in the mid-eighteenth century about the emergence of a particular form of authority that penetrates mankind's innermost thoughts and desires?

Much has been written about the paradoxical core of the Enlightenment: its substantive emancipatory outlook and its instrumental oppressive practice. Enlightenment thought advocated a secular eschatology that promoted the pursuit of worldly happiness against the Christian submission to Divine providence. It fostered the desire for earthly riches against the hope for heavenly salvation. Yet revolutions around the globe, most significantly the Haitian Revolution that inaugurated the nineteenth century, most profoundly expressed a public imagination that rested upon a commitment to the world of possibilities.

The twentieth century witnessed a repeated perversion of public imagination. Utopia and utopian thinking increasingly became associated with terror and totalitarianism, rather than with hope and emancipation. From a highbrow philosophical assertion, the end of history turned into an everyday reality that colonized the very essence of imagination. The ability to transcend present and to think of the world anew appeared to be a story the end of which we already knew, so we told ourselves, as the first act was unfolding. Despite restoring faith in the possibility of change, every revolution that once stood at the threshold of a novelty, failed to realize the kind of imaginations and desires that had given rise to them. In every instance, the *Realpolitik* of existing possibilities colonized the imaginative spirit through which the demands for change were articulated.

Revolutions express a public desire to *make* history, rather than reproducing it along the same prescribed futures. Revolutions open moments of possibilities to enact historical transformations without predetermined goals. But since the dawn of the age of revolutions, they have always been understood as "that transitory phase" that bridges one stage of history to another. Even Marx, *the* theorist of revolution, and his successors believed that revolution was a moment of transition, thus limiting the significance of politics to the *realization* of a predestined future. The evolutionary core of this radical ideology rendered public imagination as mere utopianism, thus confining politics in the prison house of a historical telos.

The Islamic Revolution in Iran in 1979 puzzled western pundits and intellectuals who understood revolutionary movements only with reference to the European experiences. They were confounded by the religious character of a historical movement that was hitherto understood as the most secular expression of social change. European political philosophers who understood revolutions to be the ultimate manifestation of the incessant expansion of the secular realm saw in Iran only a counter-revolution, a momentary pause in the otherwise progressive March of History.

Iranians were dreaming, as Michel Foucault wrote in an essay during his visit to Iran in 1978. It was true, he observed, that there were economic difficulties, political repression, and corrupt administrations. It was also true that they knew that they needed to change the whole country, its economic order, and political system. But, above all, they told themselves that *we have to change ourselves.* "Our way of being, out relationship with others, with things, with eternity, with God, etc., must be changed, and there will only be a true revolution if this radical change in our experience takes place" (Foucault 2005). Foucault's Parisian friends and foes found his enthusiasm for the revolution in its religious expression hilarious. They ridiculed the transformative power of a political spirituality that he identified in the Iranian revolutionary movement.

In Iran, the revolution spread as a phenomenon of history and, at the same time, as a phenomenon that defied it. With all the ambiguities associated with their political discourse and religious expressions, Iranians intended to think of their future anew and refused to turn themselves into subjects of the discursive authority of a world that is perpetuated in tired conceptions of "History." The Iranian revolution unfolded without closing the window of possibilities, without subjecting the revolutionary movement to the logic of historical inevitabilities.

More recently, the Arab uprisings that began in Tunisia in 2010 and spread throughout North Africa and the Middle East reminded us of the perils of the failure to recognize the significance of public imagination. Unlike the Iranian Revolution thirty years earlier the Arab uprisings not only overtook the streets of major cities and squares but also dominated the global mediascape. The media operated paradoxically both as an instrument of the effective dissemination of revolutionary action and, at the same time, as a means of its discursive restraint. Although by and large the masses on the streets identified their movement as a call for human dignity *(kerāma)* and an end to social injustice and corruption *(kefāya),* only a few weeks after their emergence the news reports and scholarly analyses identified the moment as the "Arab Spring." In order to make the uprisings legible, a great majority of observers in the West situated it in a recognizable assembly of points of references. By naming it the "Arab Spring," the uprisings entered a conceptual and discursive universe with a written past and a known future direction.

The "Arab Spring" was a discourse, in the making for five years, constructed to close the window of possibilities and subject the uprisings to historical inevitabilities. After the massive rallies to condemn the assassination of the former Lebanese Prime Minister, Rafik Hariri, in February 2005, conservative as well as a number of liberal and Left columnists began to ponder the wisdom of George W. Bush's Middle East project. They considered the mass protests against the Syrian influence in Lebanon, the "Cedar Revolution," an "Arab Spring" that heralded the fruition of the Bush policy of exporting democracy to the land of unfriendly tyrants. A series of editorial columns in *Le Monde, the Independent, Der Spiegel,* and *Foreign Policy* debated whether the "Cedar Revolution" of 2005 invokes the "Spring Time of Nations" in Europe of 1848, Prague Spring of 1968, or Eastern Europe of 1989.

The Arab Spring of 2005 did not materialize the way the pundits predicted. But the uprisings of 2010–11 turned into a full bloom "Spring," albeit a short-lived one. The dominant explanations of the uprisings interpreted this *spring*, whether it was a reference to Prague of 1968, or Europe of 1848, as a triumph of liberalism and the discovery of Enlightenment in the Arab world. According to these interpretations, what the uprisings of North Africa and the Middle East expressed was what might be called, in Alain Badiou's word, "*a desire for the West*" (Badiou 2012, 48). Not only did this view conflate competing interests of the uprising in single reductionist desire for the West, but more significantly, it subjected the public imagination of those who rose up to *make* history to the slavish unfolding of its inherent logic.

The narrative of "Arab Spring" denied the 2010–11 uprisings the *singularity* with which they could be comprehended and advanced outside the recognized patterns of revolutionary transformation. The discourse of "Arab Spring" devoured the Egyptian liberals and revolutionaries alike and denied them the impetus to articulate the significance of the uprising in its own terms. They considered any deviation from the conventional narratives of revolution to be failure and inauthentic to their movement. The election of Mohamed Morsi of the Muslim Brotherhood invariably and quickly became the case in point. Even before the Morsi Administration showed its incompetence and autocratic tendencies, liberals and many actors on the Left regarded a Muslim Brother president as the epitome of *one step forward, two steps back,* thus their Orwellian jubilance over the July 2013 military coup to save democracy.

Instances abound when historians, political actors, intellectuals, and all those who give voice to public imagination render them as demands that are only legible with reference to the inherent logic of linear historical progress. Public imagination is the space of engagement with politics in its creative and uncertain terms, a space that allows thinking about possible realities without the inhibiting constraints of real possibilities.

Bibliography

Badiou, Alain. 2012. *The Rebirth of History: Times of Riots and Uprisings*. London: Verso.

Bloch, Ernst. 1986. *The Principle of Hope*. Cambridge: MIT Press.

Foucault, Michel. 2005. "Iran: The Spirit of a World without Spirit: Foucault's Conversation with Claire Brière and Pierre Blanchet." In *Foucault and the Iranian Revolution: Gender and the Seductions of Islamism*, eds Janet Afary and Kevin Anderson, 250–260. Chicago, IL: University of Chicago Press.

Musil, Robert. 1996. *The Man Without Qualities*. Translated by S. Wilkins and B. Pike. New York: Vintage.

23

THE GREAT GRAMSCI

Imagining an Alt-Left Project

Dayan Jayatilleka

In the construction of a new public imagination, as in every other form of human endeavor, you are caught between two realities: you have to go back to where you got it wrong, but you can't go back home again.

Today's political crisis involves responses to the realities of our time, the current world order in both its political and economic dimensions, which some Marxists might define as neoliberal imperialism. "Our time" here refers to the history of the world after the fall of global socialism. On the left or progressive center-left, there is an absence of global public imagination. Or rather, it is no longer "global." What we have are competing blocs of opinion, each of which contains legitimate and justifiable elements. But these competing and internally contradictory blocs of opinion collide and collude, forming unprecedentedly complex, heterodox, and fluid patterns.

Meanwhile, as the century and the millennium turned, progressivism was being identified with liberalism, and liberalism with the neoliberal status quo. What we didn't know from the outside was that, devoid of a viable progressive alternative, the neoliberal world order was spawning a new fundamentalism within what Jose Marti called "the belly of the beast." A strange mutation occurred in which stances that were once antithetical began to meld. Those of us who lived in either the Third world or the Second saw a merger of human rights and military interventionism, resulting in the devastation of states and societies. The political options that we supported in the West, those of Clinton and Blair, became a grotesque nightmare. And soon we were caught between *two* nightmares: western (neo)liberal interventionism on the one hand, and on the other the Frankenstein it spawned, namely radical Islamist terrorism—a religious version of Pol Pot's Khmer Rouge, which likewise had mutated into a radically evil force in the wake of misguided interventionism from the West.

If both sides of this state of affairs, both the right and the left, have some elements of legitimacy, is it possible to pull them together? Perhaps, but somewhere along the line, perhaps in reaction to class reductionism, the leftwing political movements in the West forgot about class and substituted identity and gender instead. The right picked it up. The left also forgot about nation and patriotism—and the right picked them up as well. Meanwhile, if you were in the Third or Second worlds, the radical religious right picked them up.

We on the left were accustomed to Democratic New Mandarins—the "best and the brightest" who took us into Vietnam—and we had lived through Republican administrations that made diplomatic breakthroughs to Russia and China. Thus, we've witnessed unexpected political turns, but

I never thought I'd see Russophobia as a marker of the liberal left in the US. By comparison, in the Third and Second worlds, many leftists understand the logic of recent Russian assertiveness. We had witnessed the expansion of NATO to Russia's borders, the Ukrainian coup, and the attempt to do in Syria what had been done in Iraq and Libya, and we were glad that Putin was pushing back, restoring some sense of a global balance against rampant unipolar impunity. Could one imagine that the American left would accuse a rightwing administration of being "soft" on Russia and Syria?

With all the talk of fascism that's going round, perhaps we should revisit the phenomenon in context. German fascism was able to prevail not only because of the well-known split in the left, but also because the pusillanimous Weimar republic failed to address the national pride that had been wounded by the inequities of the Versailles Treaty. There was something wrong with the world order of that day, just as there is with the liberal world order of our time. While this does not justify the Nazi option, it does not mean that every right-wing challenge to the liberal world order is fascist. Nor does it mean that the liberal world order should not be challenged. It is the failure of contemporary progressives and liberals in the West to challenge it that opened the space for Brexit and then for Trump.

This was the first great recent failure of the left: the absence of a sense of crisis—of the reality of the crisis. Something is desperately awry when the leadership of the left is unable to relate to the *angst* of working people, the directly productive working classes. There was a Third world within the First and they weren't only people of color, many were poor and white as well. The liberal left in the US was far too enamored of the need to defend the Obama "revolution," yet the mistakes began at the very outset of his presidency with the bailout of the banks instead of a Rooseveltian New Deal, and ended with the folding of the Obama legacy back into the Clintonian heritage and candidacy. The progressives were too far from Bobby Kennedy of the '68 campaign, too much in tune with Hillary and too little with Bruce Springsteen's blue collar blues.

The second greatest failure of contemporary progressives and the left, which must be addressed in order to construct a new public imagination, are the unavoidable issues of the nation, nationalism, and patriotism. Suffering in a fascist jail, Antonio Gramsci wrestled with what had gone wrong in his time and what needed to be done to put it right. Our left contemporaries learned from much of what he wrote on hegemony and culture but missed one of his most important themes, that of the nation, nation building and state building. He understood that the left had abandoned those tasks and argued that picking up where Machiavelli left off was a task of the left, by which he meant wrestling with the tasks of nation and state building. Indisputably an internationalist, he notably criticized "cosmopolitanism" as a doctrine that hampered the task of nation building.

It is not entirely illegitimate that in many parts of the world, for the right and left, Putin is a hero, and almost a role model, just as De Gaulle and Gaullism were at an earlier time. In Asia, Duterte is intriguing and fitfully admired, as is Erdogan in his own land. All round the compass, nationalist populism, even when it doesn't enjoy an arithmetical majority, seems to embody the Rousseauvian general will. This is a symptom that cannot be ignored.

The contemporary left abandoned Gramsci and instead embraced cosmopolitanism—and has paid the price. As with every serious revolutionary from Mao and Ho Chi Minh to Fidel Castro and Amilcar Cabral, Gramsci combined class, mass and nation into a bloc, and it was a "majoritarian" bloc in the best sense of the word, not a collocation of minorities.

A *neo-progressive project* needs to grapple with the crisis of neoliberalism, learning from the Latin American left to reject hegemonic liberal-"humanitarian" interventionism which destroys national/state sovereignty in the global South, while nevertheless fighting against terrorism as well as the conditions that create it, and eschewing right-wing nationalism while refusing to concede the nation and patriotism to the right. This project must turn to Gramsci so as to rediscover and re-appropriate the nation, reimagine a "people-nation" and build a "national popular" bloc. Intellectuals such as Eric Hobsbawm and Stuart Hall diligently deployed Antonio Gramsci's thinking to unpack Margaret Thatcher's authoritarian populism and its reworking of nationalism. They prescribed the application of Gramsci's concept of the "national popular." Meanwhile, in the USA, a witting or unwitting "neo-Gramsci Lite" helped shift the Democratic Party to its winning Clintonian culture in the 1990s. While its strength was that it outlined a new strategy, its weakness was that it did not outline a new public imagination.

A neo-progressive public imagination must be based on a moral and the ethical perspective. An ethics of violence—that is, its correct use (Jayatilleka 2007)—is a central component. It must acknowledge that whenever violence is wittingly used against the innocent, against unarmed civilians, be it by states or movements, it is terrorism and is therefore wrong and must be opposed. Terrorism cannot be deployed, condoned or ignored even when it is directed against an entity we are inimical towards. But progressive morality has a more general application. If someone reveals a truth, says what is right, causing no harm to the innocent, he or she must be applauded and defended on that occasion—be it Assange, Snowden … or Trump ("you think our country is so innocent?"[1]). This is the only way by which the moral, ethical and intellectual hegemony that Gramsci spoke of can be accumulated by the progressive cause.

Thus the neo-progressives must seek to occupy the "moral Sierra Maestra" (as I have dubbed it elsewhere), the moral high ground, while always grasping the realities of politics and power. This is a difficult dialectic, but for those of us in the global South, Fidel Castro showed how the Nietzschean synthesis of "Caesar with the soul of Christ" could be even remotely approximated.

Note

1 Donald Trump comment in an interview with Bill O'Reilly of Fox News, broadcast on February 5, 2017.

References

Jayatilleka, Dayan 2007. *Fidel's Ethics of Violence: The Moral Dimension of the Political Thought of Fidel Castro.* London: Pluto Press and University of Chicago Press.

24

A DIALECTIC OF UTOPIA/DYSTOPIA IN THE PUBLIC IMAGINATION OF THE 21ST CENTURY

Stephen Gill

An avenue for characterizing one aspect of the public imagination of today's world—apparently configured by what has been widely characterized as a rising populism across both the left and particularly the reactionary right—is with reference to a recent upsurge of interest in utopian/dystopian thinking. Since Donald Trump was elected President of the United States, Aldous Huxley's *Brave New World* and George Orwell's *1984* have resumed prominence in the concerned public imagination and are again top of the bestseller lists. Both discuss how repressive autocratic/totalitarian elements place subject populations under regimes of total surveillance and propagate "Orwellian" versions of the truth,[1] while citizens are palliated by the happy drugs of a somatic culture.[2] These dystopian perspectives are contrasted in the conclusion to this piece with my political hypothesis of the "post-modern Prince" with its "feasible utopias" reflected in the imaginaries and collective action of diverse progressive forces.

Utopias have tended to emerge in response to wars, crises, and significant periods of dislocation: in the context of the Peloponnesian Wars, Plato's *The Republic* (ca. 380 BC) was premised on creating a good society led by wise elite Guardians. Utopian thought has typically been concerned with concepts of justice, order, the good society, and radical change, often based on common ownership of land/property. Indeed, utopias—and their dialectical other, dystopias—are "ways to interpret the present with an eye to an (imaginary yet positive) future." A dystopia may be taken as a utopia "that malfunctions" or "only functions for a particular segment of society." Dystopias "resemble actual societies historically encountered—planned but not planned well enough to be just" (Gordin et al. 2010).

These insights seem to capture very well aspects of current imaginaries in US, European, and in some respects world politics.

Important elements of the population who are dissatisfied with the dystopian conditions of growing inequality in the United States (and with it, the end of the American Dream) are separated into increasingly distinct left and right components. On one side, a majority of young educated Americans, particularly those between the age of 18 and 35 with college degrees, actually supports "socialism"—a word that used to be taboo in American political culture. On the other hand, many so-called white Americans, who continue to work but whose conditions of material existence have been undermined considerably over the last 25 years as real wages have stagnated and employment has become more precarious, have tended to gravitate towards the political right. Many of these people voted for a plutocratic billionaire president who is avowedly misogynist, racist, and who delights in scapegoating immigrants and "Others," claiming that by doing so he can lead a revival in American fortunes. US decline is caused, so the Trumpists argue, by the academic "pointy heads" and Washington élites with their pathetic liberal internationalism. Now Hercules has been chosen by the people to clean the Augean stables—to "drain the swamp."[3]

The USA is caught at an impasse amidst a concatenation of global crises, requiring urgent solutions that cannot be addressed simply by a combination of rabid nationalism and the free play of market forces. What seems imperative is a restoration of public goods not just in the United States but also on a worldwide basis. President Trump and his key advisers deny the reality of climate change and various other threats to the biosphere and insist on extending and intensifying a fossil fuel based, energy intensive, and consumerist market civilization while arming America to the teeth so that anyone who might oppose this agenda can be forcibly denied a hearing. Trumpism regards them as enemies of the people. With significant components of the population in a state of denial, public imagination in the United States is in dire shape.

Some observers have called this development a reflection of growing populism. In many respects, however, it closely resembles the extreme inequalities, governing strategies, and reactionary rhetoric that submerged liberalism and democracy in the 1930s.

As noted, this seems to reflect the contradictory and regressive condition of public imagination in the United States. It does not fully correspond with developments in the rest of the world. Despite the rise of President Trump and the vocal intensities of his xenophobic allies such as Madame Le Pen in France, Nigel Farage in the United Kingdom, and Islamophobes and immigrant-haters such as Dutch politician Geert Wilders, in the European Union—at least so far—the center has been able to hold. Paradoxically, Trump's espousal of a particular form of realpolitik and his links, both political and business, to President Putin and to autocrats and dictators throughout the world has tended to produce a renewed political impetus towards European integration and support for its welfare systems, at precisely the moment when centrifugal tendencies such as Brexit had been threatening to splinter the E.U. apart.

Furthermore, my sense is that establishment and popular media organs, many owned and controlled by reactionary plutocrats such as Rupert Murdoch, ignore or dismiss the progressive and imaginative elements at work in the world. These alternative visions are rarely and not fully reflected in official versions of an increasingly monopolized mediated "truth." Even the edited versions of establishment media "truths" are now repudiated by President Trump and his entourage of plutocrats and right wing political advisers who believe, as did Dr. Goebbels, that it is preferable to employ ultra-propagandandistic narratives endorsing hatred and racialist discourse to discredit opponents, foster discontent, and confuse and inflame the minds of the citizenry.

Nonetheless, we should remember that there are and always will be alternatives—and many of these uphold ethical principles associated with egalitarianism, solidarity, social justice, and constraints on the arbitrary use of violence.[4] Progressive imaginaries seek to protect the sanctity of life on the planet in a quest for the "development of sustainability"—a regenerative and reconstructive concept that stands in stark contrast to the oxymoron of 'sustainable development" advanced by giant corporations, ritually included in the business plans and advocacy work of companies that exploit nonrenewable resources and call for business as usual. This is why organizations such as the World Social Forum and other forms of activism give rise to a certain kind of optimism of the will—alternative utopias or political myths of human possibility that envision the possibility of global cooperation across civilizations in ways that are sustainable and regenerative for the biosphere and that are socially just—in ways that deploy knowledge and innovations that can help to reinvigorate the peoples and politics of the planet.

In sum, assessing the public imagination must relate not simply to disorientation, to conditions of bare life or to the narrow economism of mainstream debates over Brexit and budget deficits. It also involves a dialectic of utopia/dystopia. One element in this thinking is what I call a "feasible utopia" of the "post-modern Prince." It builds upon Gramsci's concept of the *Modern Prince* (1929–35), which was his response to the dystopias of the 1930s and an effort to think through the possibility for the emergence of a new democratic communism. Gramsci had drawn upon Machiavelli's *The Prince* (c.1532), a work that sought to discern the contours and possibilities of an ethical state amid the crises associated with the external domination of Italian principalities by major European powers during the Renaissance. Both works consider the internal and external determinants of the possibilities of political transformation.

The "post-modern Prince"[5] is a political hypothesis or political myth of possibility that seeks to relate new forms of political agency to the conditions, crises and contradictions of our times. It reflects plural, progressive forces in collective action, with the goal of recreating work and society and their relations to nature and the biosphere in a fruitful, forward looking and socially just manner that is welcoming to the dispossessed, the refugees, and the outcasts of the planet. The concept is an attempt to capture new imaginaries, many from the creative ranks of indigenous peoples, landless workers, women's groups,[6] concerned scientists, public workers, progressive trades unions, environmentalists, and peoples young and old seeking to forge new political alternatives, both real and imagined. Here I should emphasize that much of the most forward-oriented political thinking of the post-modern Prince, encompassing new imaginaries and epistemologies, rises from among indigenous peoples and is articulated by collective leadership involving both men and women; indeed, the post-modern Prince is simultaneously the post-modern Princess!

What is at issue here is the idea of an alternative type of society—a feasible political myth or utopia—appropriate to the post-modern conditions of the 21st century and its potential future. As Gramsci once put it, the Modern Prince—the myth-Prince—cannot be a real person, it must be a set of political forces that are actually asserting and recreating themselves, engaging in the making of history. One of the principles of the post-modern Prince—understood in the plural—is epistemological, namely that knowledge should not be treated as a commodity, but as part of the global commons as it is built from the broad intellectual and cultural heritage of humankind. Other key principles of the post-modern Prince are associated with human dignity and equality, democracy, social justice, political accountability, public healthcare, and the development of an ethic of caring and regenerative sustainability. The praxis of the post-modern Prince/Princess invokes a radical politics of redistribution, recognition, and emancipation.

Of course, this set of democratic and radical potentials has to be assessed in relation to the dominant reactionary and regressive alternatives now being posed as either challenges to, or that seek to reassert the supremacy of, market-based disciplinary neoliberalism. Institutionalized over the past 30 years, its resilience should not be underestimated.

A key question in this context concerns the political fate of the middle classes in both North and South and how far they will orient themselves politically towards more progressive or reactionary futures.[7] Such preferences are forged in the context of a citizenry among whom many are disoriented by the stresses, dislocations, and dystopias associated with a hypercompetitive and historically myopic/somatic market civilization. This vortex of social forces indicates that rather than history ending, a new phase of global struggle has begun. We may be at an historical crossroads.[8]

Notes

1 It is also important to reflect upon wider issues of surveillance (Big Brother) in relation to projects of *global* governance that seek to create a US controlled "global panopticon," a post-modern dystopia

that seeks to put everyone and everything under constant 24/7 monitoring by the Pentagon and NSA. This project is intended to inscribe the disciplinary gaze of its imperial power on everyday life, facilitated by the social technologies and the compliant accumulation strategies of firms like Facebook, Apple and Microsoft. President Trump promises to intensify such surveillance. For an earlier attempt to theorize this aspect of global politics see Gill (1995).

2 In the US today, according to Nicholas Eberstadt (author of "Men Without Work: America's Invisible Crisis"), a socially inert residue of the somatic culture includes possibly as much as one in eight of the US male population aged between 25 and 54. These are people who do not work for income, nor indeed do any kind of work, including housework. They are not registered as unemployed since they are not seeking work. They spend their days watching television, or surfing the Internet under the influence of antidepressant drugs. For more detail see NPR transcript (2017).

3 When I reviewed this piece for publication in this collection on 31 May 2019 I checked the *New York Times* Best Seller list and the top raked non-fiction work (with 5 weeks on the list) was: *The Mueller Report,* with related materials by *The Washington Post*: Redacted findings from the special counsel's investigation into Russian interference in the 2016 presidential election and potential obstruction of justice by the president. President Trump consistently claims that news media such as the Washington Post are purveyors of "fake news."

4 For example, drone strikes against so-called adversaries causing casualties amongst innocent people carried out under the instructions of President Obama.

5 For extended discussions of the post-modern Prince and the idea of a feasible utopia, see Gill (2008).

6 Witness the large-scale marches and demonstrations in hundreds of cities world-wide in early 2017 and in 2018 and 2019 world-wide marches and demonstrations to try to force political focus on dealing with climate change and related ecological problems, and the ways that they unequally impact societies and locations. The growing salience of such issues was reflected in the May 2019 election results for the European parliament where Green parties made sweeping gains.

7 One dimension of this question concerns whether they will favor the extension of the public goods and the social commons noted above, as well as preferences for greater social inclusion, improved provisions for social reproduction and stewardship of the biosphere, and more generally the socialization of risk on behalf of the majority. By contrast, many middle-class people associated with self-employment and small businesses, for example, may well favor further marketization of social and economic life, more gated communities, and the repression and othering of strangers and the marginalized.

8 On a range of issues relating to the crossroads of history see Gill (2015).

References

Gill, Stephen 1995. "The global panopticon? The neoliberal state, economic life, and democratic surveillance." *Alternatives: Global, Local, Political*, 20 (1): 1–49. https://doi.org/10.1177/030437549502000101.

———. 2008. *Power and Resistance in the New World Order*, 237–269. London: Palgrave Macmillan UK.

———. 2015. *Critical Perspectives on the Crisis of Global Governance: Reimagining the Future*, 181–199. Basingstoke: Palgrave Macmillan.

Gordin, Michael, Helen Tilley, and Gyan Prakash 2010. *Utopia/dystopia: conditions of historical possibility*, 1–2. Princeton, N.J.: Princeton University Press.

Bibliography

Eberstadt, Nicholas. 2017. "An Economist On The 'Miserable 21st Century." Interview by Scott Simon. Weekend Edition Saturday, NPR, February 25, 2017. Audio. www.npr.org/2017/02/25/517181348/an-economist-on-the-miserable-21st-century.

———. 2016. *Men Without Work: America's Invisible Crisis*. West Conshohocken: Templeton Foundation Press.

PART V

Across the Border

25

THE FUTURE OF NATIONAL AND GLOBAL (DIS)ORDER

Exclusive Populism versus Inclusive Global Governance[1]

Ahmet Davutoğlu

The demise of the Cold War system promised to engender a new global order. Yet this didn't happen. Instead, the world has grappled with many monumental crises, turning points, and transformative events without drawing the right lessons from them, resulting in reactive and conjectural formulas that have aggravated the problems. The international system has consequently accumulated a plethora of issues, problems and crises, each built upon the remnants of previous unresolved or frozen crises. Therefore, when we speak of the current crises we should beware of the dangers of conjecturalism, short-termism, and particularism in analyzing them. Unfortunately, the responses and reactions to the present election cycles in the West—which generously rewarded populist, xenophobic, and neo-nationalist groups—have led to some soul-searching among the political and intellectual class, as well as concerned citizens in the West and elsewhere, yet few have shown a willingness to investigate the root cause of this trend by situating it in a historical context. Recent developments aren't occurring in an evolutionary way, and as I have suggested elsewhere, we can best respond to our current cycles of change if we understand the ensemble of earthquakes that are shaping our world.

Earthquakes in World Politics

The global system was first shaken by a geopolitical earthquake following the end of the Cold War. During this period, the map of Eurasia was redrawn, Cold War geopolitics came to an end, and new states emerged. With the breakdown of the authoritarian political structure of the Communist bloc, a new wave of democratization came to the fore in Eastern and Central Europe as well as new regional initiatives, such as the European Union. Then, just over a decade later, the global system witnessed a security earthquake with September 11, 2001. While values such as freedom and democracy were at the center of the geopolitical earthquake, the basic conceptual framework after 9/11 has revolved around the issue of security, creating an atmosphere of animosity, anxiety and distrust in the international sphere. The third major earthquake, which has been even more deeply felt, struck the financial systems, first in the United States in 2008, followed by the Euro-crisis in 2010, and an unfolding global financial crisis. The fourth major earthquake emerged in the Arab World from 2010 onwards and was sociopolitical/economic in nature. Until and unless this earthquake fulfills its initial promise to deliver dignity, freedom, democracy, and economic advancement to Arab peoples, it will continue to shake the whole region to its very foundations.

Short-termism and conjectural policies were primarily employed to deal with these earthquakes, leaving them unresolved and paving the way for what is now taking place: a systemic earthquake characterized by a rising tide of extremism that ranges from the terrorist activities of groups like DAESH to the populist surge in recent elections in Europe and the United States. One of the more worrying consequences of these earthquakes has been a rise in populist autocracies, exclusivity, unilateralism, the selfish pursuit of narrowly defined national interests at the expense of common values and goods.

On a more personal note, Turkey has been at the center of all these earthquakes. As an academic who has spent a significant amount of his intellectual and academic life examining the root causes of these earthquakes, and later as foreign minister and prime minister of Turkey who had to formulate policy responses to these seismic events, I came to recognize a pattern of short-termist and reactive national, regional, and international responses that fail to address broader questions of global governance and systemic order.

Challenges and Shortcomings of the Current 'Order'

Post-truth, post-order, post-fact and similar concepts have been abundantly utilized to describe what the world is going through. For instance, while the term 'post-truth' is employed to account for the context—the factors that have paved the way for what we are now experiencing—the term 'post-order' is used to describe the global system, or lack thereof. If not viewed with some skepticism and distance, these concepts invite a lack of intellectual or analytical rigor, serving the unintended purpose of relieving agents of their responsibility for what is happening. Fresh thinking not held hostage by newly popularized concepts should be combined with the understanding that the traditional usage of once explanatory concepts, such as right and left, is significantly limited in accounting for the current phenomenon.

The present international 'order' sustained largely by the American power—supposedly underpinned by values such as democracy, rule of law, free markets, and by institutions such as UN, G20, IMF, WB, WTO—is facing severe challenges. First, the Trump administration with its declared policy of 'America first' seems to be turning away from the system, the most topical of the crises today. Arguably, its impact could be mitigated through either the US establishment's commitment to world order, or a more collective ownership of it. Secondly, the declared value system of the prevalent order has either been selectively applied or not applied at all in many contexts. For instance, during the fourth earthquake engendered by the uprisings across the Arab World, international actors largely adopted short-termist and self-defeating policies instead of standing by the order's declared values such as democracy. This has left people with the unpalatable choice of terrorism versus police states, which in turn has significantly diminished the legitimacy of the international order for large segments of the world population. Third, the institutions of the prevalent international order are in dire need of reform and updating. Take the example of the UN: it is an institution largely devoid of success stories, and hence credibility. Moreover, the governance structure of these institutions isn't inclusive, so they act like exclusive clubs primarily designed to serve the interests of the powerful at the expense of the weak. As long as international institutions are regarded this way, their legitimacy will always remain doubtful.

The recent debates on the future of the international 'order' have been triggered by Brexit and the election of Trump. Yet the heated nature of the present shouldn't inform our responses to this deep crisis. Some concepts, issues and 'facts' should come under serious scrutiny. The ideas of change and order, as well as the agent of change and order, should be thoroughly examined before we can offer any sustainable, inclusive and just response to the current systemic crisis.

The Necessity of the Change and Modalities of Order

Given the present systemic earthquake, the political and intellectual classes should begin by recognizing that change is both necessary and inevitable. Once this is established, the next questions are about what must change, and how. One of the defining shortcomings of the current international 'order' has been its overreliance on technocracy. It is unrepresentative, with a democratic deficit at its core, which has led to the progressive dwindling of social ownership of the system. This in turn has created a vicious circle: the more the social basis of the current order has diminished, the more it has relied on globalist technocracy for its survival, yet the more it has relied on this technocracy, the further people have become alienated from the system. A large proportion of societies across the world regard this system as a tutelary imposition on a global scale. This grievance plays right into the hands of populist autocrats. Therefore, the tension between the technocratic nature of the system and the rising demand that it be more representative needs to be tackled head on.

Once this is settled, then proponents of maintaining a reformed version of the present 'order' should counter the more regressive and exclusionist demands for change advanced by the populists with a much more progressive and inclusive idea of change. This means that any international order that isn't rule and value-based and isn't in principle reflective of a large segment of humanity's values and interests will be bound to fail. Easier said than done, obviously. Still, there are two main approaches.

The first option is to agree on a set of principles and values and build the order based on them. That way, the value foundation of the order is clear to everyone. We would have a set of rules and a playbook that are applicable to everyone. Moreover, this approach also provides the criteria and benchmarks with which to judge performance and detect any malfunctioning of the system. Such a value-based and inclusive order would give it further legitimacy and a broad social basis worldwide.

The second approach is to try to build some kind of order based on conjecture and pragmatism. This form of order will be on shaky ground and from day one it will be questioned. It will face a cycle of crises engendered by zero-sum competition and rivalries. As such, rule-based inclusivity and principle-driven fairness should form part and parcel of any order—and the current order should at least strive to update itself with these factors in mind. While the present system should already in theory reflect the first approach, its applications in practice show it to be closer to the second.

Who has responsibility to establish or maintain the order? At the national level we have two candidates: the establishment or the populist leaders of the new anti-systemic waves. The trouble is that the establishment doesn't possess the necessary legitimacy to build a new or dramatically update the old order. But the new populists have neither the intention nor the know-how to establish a new order or significantly revise the incumbent one. The interaction, the struggle between them will shape the national order, which in turn will shape the international order. At the international level, the UN should have functioned as the primary platform for discussion on a reformed or new order, yet its track record doesn't encourage high hopes.

The Need for a More Inclusive Global Governance

All in all, the rising populist tide and systemic crises have clearly illustrated that the current international 'order' is in the process of delegitimation on two levels. First, it is rejected as a source of injustice, unfairness and imposition, a symptom of the decay of the global elite and its indifference to or detachment from people's grievances in societies across the world. Second, the current 'order' is questioned by large groups of states, particularly the rising powers including Turkey, who rightly regard it as unrepresentative, as almost exclusively reflecting the projections and priorities of the victorious Western powers of World War II. The system's inability to fairly accommodate and represent them not only reduces its legitimacy, but undermines its functioning. The combined impact of these two factors generates the contemporary crisis of legitimacy. At this stage, the crucial question is whether this delegitimation will lead to the complete disintegration of the system. In other words, it is yet to be seen whether this systemic earthquake will culminate in the dissolution of the present order, or in its refinement. To avoid disintegration, major reforms need to be undertaken to re-establish legitimacy, which is the only way that the current order will survive this systemic earthquake.

Otherwise, present trends are worrisome and resemble 19th century politics or the pre-World War II period. An ongoing economic crisis, an increase in isolationist tendencies among major powers, an uptick in populist policies and autocracies, unilateralism, a perception of politics and international interactions as zero-sum games, and similar features represent frightening trends that can, however, be reversed. The choices are clear. The world will either once again head towards the mutually destructive 'balance of power system' or strive to establish a mutually-rewarding, more benevolent, inclusive, fair, and humanitarian global governance structure. While narrowly-defined interests and self-defeating unilateralism form the main character of the former system, shared values and rules, and a mutually-rewarding multilateralism, will define the general contours of the latter option.

The unfulfilled hope since the 1990s has been to realize a future shaped by global governance. The difference between global governance and international order is that international implies that nation-states are main units and the order is formed as a result of the relations and dialogue between nations. Global governance is more interactive, more dialogue—based, and more transnational. In that sense, it is not only dialogue among nation-states but among human beings, with an interactive, interconnected system creating an international order. Therefore, humanity at this stage needs rule- and value-based, multilateral, consensual, fair and inclusive form global governance.

Note

1 The extended version of this chapter will be published as a book in 2020 (Davutoğlu, Forthcoming).

References

Davutoğlu, Ahmet. Forthcoming. *Systemic Earthquake*. Cambridge, UK: Cambridge University Press.

26

THE INDISPENSABILITY OF UTOPIAS

A Note on Davutoğlu's Vision of Global (Dis)order

Celso Amorim

I spent a good part of my professional life as a diplomat or government minister, working on multilateral issues in the areas of trade, peace and security, environment and health, among others. I had many disappointments and a few achievements. Most significant among the latter was the effort made jointly by Brazil and Turkey to help in finding a solution to the "problem" posed by the Iranian Nuclear Program. Together with my friend, then Turkey's Foreign Minister, Ahmet Davutoğlu, I strived to find a way forward for this vexing issue. Although the Tehran Declaration of May 17th 2010[1] was eventually refused by the P-5, led by the United States, and new sanctions were imposed on the Islamic Republic,[2] it served as an inspiration (if not in the precise content, at least in spirit) to the Joint Comprehensive Program of Action spearheaded by President Obama some years later. I base this claim on an article by Anne Marie Slaughter, a former head of the planning staff of Secretary of State Hillary Clinton, published in November 2011 at a moment when tensions between Tehran and Washington were escalating, to a large extent due to the obsessive fear of an "existential threat" on the part of the latter's main ally in the Middle East. In her piece, entitled "Diplomacy is the Least Damaging Option with Iran," Slaughter (2011) summarizes the Tehran Declaration and says that the US and its allies should "turn back to Brazil and Turkey."

It was therefore with great interest and intellectual respect that I read Ahmet Davutoğlu's essay on "The Future of National and Global (Dis)order." I followed attentively his analysis on the several "earthquakes" that shook the so-called world order in the post-Cold War period, resulting in a "systemic earthquake" that forces us to re-think many of the concepts used to define international politics. I agree with his criticisms on overreliance on technocracy and on the democratic deficit in international relations as well as with his plea for an inclusive, value based, global governance. Davutoğlu's strong case for a "humanitarian global order" and "collective ownership" has my full sympathy. Like others who commented on his article, I also think that incremental reforms are not sufficient and that the "root causes" of these "earthquakes" should be confronted. Perhaps most pressing is the issue of inclusiveness. I do not underestimate the importance of a United Nations reform that makes it more democratic and responsive to the present world realities. Updating the composition of the Security Council (especially in relation to the permanent members) would be not only a matter of realism and fairness. More than likely it would also help in finding solutions to apparently intractable questions. A more consistent presence of some major developing countries in the UNSC might work as a bridge between the positions of Western Powers, on the one hand, and Russia and China, on the other. Countries like India, Brazil and South Africa[3] cherish many of the values that Washington, London and Paris claim to champion, such as human rights and representative democracy. At the same time, these nations are very sensitive to principles like non-intervention and respect for national sovereignty, which are very much at the core of "negative" attitudes assumed by Moscow and Beijing, allegedly causing the "paralysis" of the Council. My experience in dealing with the Iraq question when Brazil occupied the presidency of the Security Council in January 1999, reinforced my conviction that developing countries—if they summon the will—have an important role to play in matters of peace and security, apart from their obvious relevance for negotiations relating to trade, sustainable development, climate change, etc.[4]

Similarly, strengthening bodies like the Peace Building Commission and ECOSOC (UN Economic and Social Council) and giving more power to organs that deal with sustainable development and human rights would be welcome changes. Even evolutionary steps in relation to informal groups such as the G-20—designated by U.S. President Barack Obama as the main forum for coordination of economic policies—may have positive effect on decisions that affect the whole world. Arguably, with some adjustments, such as a better representation of African nations, the G-20 might have its agenda expanded to subjects other than financial ones. None of these reforms, however, would in and by themselves avoid the threats posed by narrow self-centered attitudes. There would be no guarantee that, even with improved governance structures, questions of transcending importance such as total nuclear disarmament (the only way, in my opinion, to ensure sustainable non-proliferation) or combatting climate change, which are posed in Richard Falk's "Response" (2017) would receive the treatment they deserve by changes, however positive, in the structure and composition of international bodies. No "structural reform" would have the magical power of pre-empting the rise of conservative nationalist ideologies of the kind represented by Donald Trump or Marine Le Pen.

In his essay, Ahmet Davutoğlu mentions "the selfish pursuit of narrowly defined national interests at the expense of common values and goods." Overcoming this kind of mindset requires great efforts that go beyond systemic changes if the latter relate to structural and operational aspects of global governance. In my opinion, the prevalence of this mindset is one of the main obstacles to obtaining the kind of systemic change proposed by Davutoğlu. On this point (and many others), I tend to agree with the emphasis placed by Robert Johansen (2017) on *political education*. Although I accept that it is not the role of policy makers to address the "manifestly undiminished imperfections of the individual human being" as Louis René Beres suggests, (2017) I do believe there is room for trying to convey the notion that 'my well-being depends on the well-being of my fellow humans." Or, to put the same thought in the frame of international relations: "the well-being of my country depends on the well-being of other countries." How to separate such an "enlightened" approach from interventionist doctrines—including ones allegedly based on humanitarian considerations—is not a simple task. The disastrous situation that followed the intervention in Libya, whose main justification was based on the "right to protect" (R2P), is a case in point. But it is a task we must face.

During my years as foreign minister, both president Lula[5] and I stressed the importance of *solidarity*, starting with our own neighbors but also extending to other countries of the Global South. To rebut the criticism of this initiative from most of the Brazilian media and a large portion of our ruling elite, I argued that "generosity" (a term that normally has no place in realist analyses and which, I concede, is often misused or manipulated) consists in looking at one's own interest in the long run. Without this kind of perception, I do not see how we can get rid of the *short-termism* and the *pursuit of narrow interest* denounced by Davutoğlu. Political education—or appropriate public information—is a task that requires bold actions, and not very popular ones, at the national as well as the international levels. Davutoğlu's insistence on broader participation of individuals and groups of individuals over and above the nation states may be an important way of encouraging the development of the kind of solidarity and long-term perspective that the world needs.

Here is a final thought: Earthquakes being by their very nature unpredictable (at least at the present stage of scientific knowledge), I am not naive enough to claim that even with the best advocacy, we will be able to avoid them. But, at least, some more reasonable responses, based on more solid reasoning, may be found, to the benefit of our grandchildren and to the continuous evolution of mankind. If I may be allowed some self-indulgence, I would quote the last three or four lines of my book on Brazilian foreign policy, with which I tried to summarize our approach: "... if politics is not to be limited to the raw pursuit of narrow self-interest, utopias are indispensable. Without them we are inevitably consigned to the role of mere spectators, watching the unfolding of history without ever helping to write it."

Notes

1 Details on the process which led to the Tehran Declaration, signed by Turkey, Iran and Brazil, as well as on its aftermath, can be found in Amorim (2015).
2 Sanctions in addition to those already in place were imposed on Iran by the Security Council on June 9th, barely three weeks after Iran agreed to all the substantive points contained in the so-called Swap Agreement proposed by the US and its allies (which in this case included the four other Permanent Members as well as Germany).
3 A similar case may be made for other countries, like Indonesia and Turkey. But it is not my purpose here to discuss the merits or de-merits of individual countries.
4 At that time, three panels were established to deal with different aspects of Iraq's problem: disarmament, humanitarian issues, and Kuwait's prisoners and property. The main consequence of the panels was the replacement of the existing Commission tasked to verify Iraq's disarmament (UNSCOM) by a new one with somewhat modified targets and procedures (UNMOVIC). For a critique of the progress and limitations of UNMOVIC see Blix (2004).
5 Luiz Inacio Lula da Silva was president of Brazil from 2003 to 2010.

References

Amorim, Celso. 2015. *Acting Globally: Memoirs of Brazil's Assertive Foreign Policy*. Lanham, Maryland: Hamilton Books.

Beres, Louis René. 2017. "Fixing the Microcosm: Global Governance and World Order." *global-e* 10, no. 51.

Blix, Hans. 2004. *Disarming Iraq*. 1st ed. New York: Pantheon Books.

Davutoğlu, Ahmet. "The Future of National and Global (Dis)order."

Falk, Richard. 2017. "Exclusive Populism versus Inclusive Global Governance: A Response to Ahmet Davutoğlu." *global-e* 10, no. 33.

Johansen, Robert. 2017. "Solve Global Problems? Build Global Governance." *global-e* 10, no. 37.

Slaughter, Anne-Marie. 2011. "Diplomacy is the Least Damaging Option with Iran." *Financial Times*, November 9, 2011.

27

IMAGINING THE RIGHT TO PEACE

Marjorie Cohn

In 1945, after two horrific wars claimed nearly 100 million lives across the globe, the countries of the world came together and created the United Nations system "to save succeeding generations from the scourge of war." By adopting these words as the lynchpin of the U.N. Charter, the member states imagined that peace was possible. But the adoption of the Charter and the U.N. system did not put an end to war. Indeed, the resort to military force has become the default method of resolving—yet also, repeatedly creating—international disputes.

It is time to rekindle what the drafters of the Charter imagined. That requires instilling in the public imagination the notion that peace is possible. Is there a human right to peace? There is indeed, and much needs to be done to make that right a reality.

Legal Codification of the Right to Peace

Peace is not simply the absence of war. Peace requires that all states refrain from interfering in the internal affairs of other states, settle their disputes peacefully, and create conditions necessary to eliminate the causes of international conflict, including an end to the arms race. The right to peace is inherent in the very fabric of the U.N. Charter. Through the Charter and subsequent U.N. resolutions, the human right to peace is ripening into a norm of international law.

Article 2(3) of the Charter requires that member states "shall settle their international disputes by peaceful means in such a manner that international peace and security, and justice, are not endangered." Moreover: "All members shall refrain in their international relations from the threat or use of force against the territorial integrity or political independence of any state," according to Article 2(4). Under Article 51, member states are only permitted to use military force in self-defense after an armed attack by another state or with the approval of the Security Council. In 1970, the U.N. General Assembly (GA) adopted Resolution 2625, which defines the non-intervention mandate as "an essential condition to ensure that nations live together in peace with one another."

GA Resolution 33/73, promulgated in 1978, states, "Every nation and every human being, regardless of race, conscience, language or sex, has the inherent right to live in peace.' And in 1984, during the Cold War when the danger of nuclear war was ubiquitous, the GA adopted Resolution 39/11, which "solemnly proclaims … a sacred right to peace" whose realization constitutes "a fundamental obligation of each state." To ensure the right to peace, state policies must "be directed towards the elimination of the threat of war, particularly nuclear war," Resolution 39/11 provides.

Recent Violations of the Right to Peace

Shortly after the September 11, 2001 terrorist attacks, George W. Bush invaded Afghanistan, even though it had not attacked the U.S. The terrorists—nineteen men, including 15 from Saudi Arabia—committed a crime against humanity, but it was not an Afghan military operation. Bush's invasion therefore did not constitute lawful self-defense and the Security Council did not approve it. Yet what is now the U.S.'s longest war continues to claim lives. In 2003, before he invaded Iraq and changed its regime, Bush tried to secure the imprimatur of the Council for his intervention. The Council refused. Bush then cobbled together prior Council resolutions from the first Gulf War in an unsuccessful attempt to legitimize his illegitimate war, which was not conducted in self-defense. Bush's war on Iraq was a disaster that keeps on giving. It has resulted in hundreds of thousands of deaths, led to the rise of ISIS, and dangerously destabilized the region.

John Bolton, Bush's temporary U.N. ambassador and now Donald Trump's national security adviser, infamously declared,

> There is no United Nations. There is an international community that occasionally can be led by the only real power left in the world, and that is the United States, when it suits our interest, and when we can get others to go along.

Bolton added, "When the United States leads, the United Nations will follow. When it suits our interest to do so, we will do so" (NPR 2005).

Democratic presidents have not fared much better in making the promise of the United Nations a reality. Bill Clinton could have helped prevent the genocide in Rwanda. Instead, he stopped the U.N from acting to halt the killing of 800,000 people there. Clinton's secretary of state, Madeleine Albright, called the U.N. "a tool of American foreign policy" (Deen 2005).

The pattern of law-breaking continued during the Obama administration. Its program of targeted killing with drones and manned bombers violated the Charter and the Geneva Conventions. Obama's forcible regime change in Libya violated the International Covenant on Civil and Political Rights and created another vacuum that ISIS filled. Now Trump's administration is violating the Charter and the Geneva Conventions by targeting civilians in Syria and Iraq, and launching 59 Tomahawk missiles in Syria. These actions constitute war crimes.

Why Isn't the Right to Peace a Reality?

Why hasn't the right to peace become a reality? Because the only international forum for peacekeeping is failing to live by its stated principles, and instead is continuing to serve largely as an instrument of U.S. foreign policy.

The Trump administration has, like its predecessors, thwarted the United Nations in other ways. Nikki Haley, Trump's former U.N. ambassador, endeavored to suppress a U.N. report in which independent experts concluded "beyond a reasonable doubt" that Israel's treatment of the Palestinians constitutes "the crime of Apartheid." Pressured by Haley, the U.N. secretary general removed the report from the U.N. website. The chairperson of the U.N. agency that published the report resigned in protest against the removal.

In April, 2017, all 100 U.S. senators signed a letter to the U.N. secretary general decrying "the U.N.'s anti-Israel bias" and "continued targeting of Israel by the U.N. Human Rights Council (HRC) and other U.N. entities." Israel's Ministry of Foreign Affairs had called the HRC biased because it issued the 2009 Goldstone Report, prepared under the direction of noted Judge Richard Goldstone. The report found Israel guilty of international law violations in its December 2008-January 2009 war on Gaza, which killed 1,400 Palestinians and 13 Israelis.

In 2016, under pressure from the Israel lobby, Obama approved a record $38 billion in military aid for Israel over the next 10 years. But as his presidency came to an end, Obama finally stood up to Israel. When the Security Council voted to condemn Israel for building illegal settlements in occupied Palestinian territories, Obama's administration abstained instead of issuing a veto, which allowed the resolution to pass. Resolution 2334 says the settlements have "no legal validity," calls them "a flagrant violation under international law," and demands Israel "immediately and completely cease all settlement activities." The newly elected, but not yet inaugurated, President Trump intervened unsuccessfully to prevent Resolution 2334 from coming to the Council floor.

In order to prevent the International Criminal Court (ICC) from investigating and prosecuting Israel, the United States opposed Palestine becoming a party to the Rome Statute. Palestine, recognized as a non-member observer state by the GA, acceded to the Statute in 2015 and asked the ICC to investigate Israel for building illegal settlements and committing war crimes in Gaza. The ICC prosecutor opened a preliminary examination, which is currently pending.

The U.S. government continues to resist accountability for its own violations of the law by refusing to ratify the Rome Statute, which provides for prosecution of individual leaders for war crimes, genocide, crimes against humanity, and the crime of aggression. Obama declared, "I don't believe that anybody is above the law. On the other hand, I also have a belief that we need to look forward as opposed to looking backwards" (Koppelman 2009). Those responsible for committing war crimes during the Bush administration were never brought to justice during Obama's presidency, which signaled to Trump he could commit war crimes with impunity.

How Do We Enforce the Right to Peace?

We cannot count on the U.S. government to enforce the right to peace. Each successive administration has used military force in violation of the U.N. Charter. Clinton bombed Kosovo and Iraq. Bush invaded Afghanistan and Iraq. Obama continued Bush's wars and used drones in seven countries. And Trump continues the wars and drone bombings and has escalated by bombing Syria.

Since his inauguration, Trump's attacks on workers, immigrants, the poor, women, LGBTQ people and the environment have propelled hundreds of thousands of people into the streets, their congresspersons' offices, and town hall meetings. But there are not large numbers of people protesting Trump's military interventions. There is almost no pushback in Congress, even among Democrats. The corporate media parrots the administration's line on the need to bomb Syria and conduct regime change in Venezuela (Cohn 2019a) and Iran (Cohn 2019b), which would be illegal. Most people in the U.S. are unaware that Trump's foreign policy not only violates U.S. and international laws but also makes us less safe. When people elsewhere see their loved ones cut down by U.S. bombs, they seek to do us harm.

We must organize mass protests to demand that Washington comply with the Charter by refraining from attacking other countries and joining with Russia, Turkey, Iran and Syrian president Bashar al-Assad to pursue a diplomatic solution to the war in Syria. We must work toward nuclear disarmament in accordance with our legal obligations under the Nuclear Non-Proliferation Treaty.

Trump's provocation of North Korea creates a risk of nuclear conflagration. Astoundingly, he has indicated a willingness to use nuclear weapons as a tool of foreign policy. But if one steps back from the drama surrounding the Trump administrations' ties with Russia, the benefits of closer relations with Russia come into focus. Stoking the flames of a new Cold War between the two most heavily armed nuclear powers imperils the right to peace.

There is little awareness in the United States about the human right to peace. It is critical that we educate people about our legal obligations, by writing, speaking out and widely circulating articles about the right to peace. The first step toward making peace a reality is to imagine that peace is possible.

References

Cohn, Marjorie. 2019a. "US Takes Illegal, Dangerous Actions Toward Regime Change in Venezuela." *Truthout*, April 17, 2019. https://truthout.org/articles/us-takes-illegal-dangerous-actions-toward-regime-change-in-venezuela/.

———. 2019b. "An Attack on Iran Would Violate US and International Law." *Truthout*, May 23, 2019. https://truthout.org/articles/an-attack-on-iran-would-violate-us-and-international-law/.

Deen, Thalif. 2005. "UN Faces New Political Threats From US." *Global Policy Forum*, November 23, 2005. www.globalpolicy.org/component/content/article/157/27018.html.

Koppelman, Alex. 2009. "Obama: 'We need to look forward.'" *Salon*, January 12, 2009. www.salon.com/2009/01/12/obama_prosecutor/.

NPR. 2005. "Background: John Bolton's Nomination to the U.N." NPR, June 3, 2005. www.npr.org/templates/story/story.php?storyId=4648850.

28

PUBLIC IMAGINATION ABOUT PUBLIC AFFAIRS

Johan Galtung

A key slogan during the student revolt in Paris May 1968 was: Imagination au pouvoir! Bring imagination to power!

France is now suffering from more imagination deficit than ever. But to call Le Pen-Front National "extreme right" when the issue is for or against the EU is not helpful; left–right was a 20th century dichotomy. And why not think bigger, beyond the EU: for or against EUR-ASIA? Russia and China are ready and so is trade, as indicated by the growing number of trains plying the rails between London and Beijing. Today is about the West-East axis, not only the old colonial obsession with North–South (neo)colonialism. And how about both, EURASIAFRICA? After all, they do hang together geographically!

Another word is for imagination is creativity, like the spirit of the engineer with matter, the architect with space, the artist with form, the scientist with connections, humans with relations. We have tried to make creativity a trademark of the Transcend approach—transcend meaning "go beyond," go beyond fixed positions of any kind. How it works is very simple, grounded in the assumption that underlying violence and the threat thereof are unsolved conflicts. Identify them, have dialogues with all parties to identify the goals in their visions for the future—of Afghanistan, of West Asia (not that London-made "Middle East"), of a good marriage, whatever. Where creativity enters is here: what might a new social reality look like that would make such goals compatible? Examples are to be found.

Out of the Cold War came a UN security commission for Europe, building on the economic commission to become, via energetic diplomacy in Helsinki, the Organization for Security and Cooperation in Europe. Next up: West, Central, Northeast Asia? South Asia already has SAARC, and Southeast Asia ASEAN. More recently, up came antagonistic states once fighting over a contested area, now considering joint ownership instead, like a *zona bi-estatal* in the Andes between Ecuador and Peru or the relaxation of Philippine fishing access in disputed areas of in South China Sea. There are many more examples (see our Track Record),[1] some realized, some not (yet).

There is something static, almost dead really, about the state systems, particularly in how states relate to each other. As if states have found a final form, and as if their relations will always remain anarchic. The concern for security—no violence within and without—is indeed legitimate, but dominant answers in terms of police and military, using violence and the threat thereof, dominate what might otherwise be possible. They often involve knee-jerk reflexes, devoid of imagination, not even of reflection. Even more seriously, as if the agenda for inter-state relations had only one point: "security" of a kind that often seems to entail scanning the world guided by what is also known as paranoia.

But states cooperate when trading, across gaps of distrust, even paranoia. They do, and often very creatively, for mutual and equal benefit, greatly helped by price mechanisms defining what is "equal." Both are better off with a good business deal, but they do not want the other side to be much better off. They watch each other, knowing that the survival of the other party may be a condition for their own survival; but if not, then as winners gripped by the fear of being losers.

However, cooperation through exchange for mutual and equal benefit can be expanded beyond economic goods supplied and demanded. The theory and practice of negative and positive peace may be helpful concepts for explaining this. Negative peace points to non-provocative security, defensive defense, including guarding well what should be defended (rather than hunting for terrorists everywhere). No violence, no exchange of bad for bad, including psychologically bad in the form of threats.

Positive peace goes significantly beyond that into exchanging good for good, as in trade, and we would put our finger on skills as a key element. "You seem to do well something I am not good at, but on the other hand, I am quite good at X." At the personal level we may think of cooperation between the bright student with no skills in sport and the sporty but somewhat dumb one, lifting each other up. What about following a similar logic at the inter-state level?

Using an Octagon map of our present multi-polar world, with Russia-India-China-Islam emerging, USA-EU declining, and Latin America Caribbean-Africa as the old "third world," we get 8x7/1x2 = 28 bilateral relations. All these poles have bad but also good aspects, and it is entirely legitimate to be on guard against the bad and entirely illegitimate not to be open to the good aspects, like skills.

Examples abound.[2] Take two giants, nos. 1 and 2 in population (not smaller Western states), China and India. China is good at lifting the bottom up (even if they still have a long way to go) while India is not, ridden by caste; India is good at accommodating cultural diversity with its linguistic federalism (even if not in Assam), China less so. How about meeting, comparing notes in an open-ended dialogue, itself an instrument of mutual and equal benefit? And preferably, not doing so behind closed doors because others may also have much to learn, not least from the willingness simply to have problems openly discussed.

Take the old super-powers, USA and Russia, one good on individual freedom to innovate and practice, the other on divesting itself of an empire almost without violence—both very weak where the other is strong. Of course, it takes some courage for them, as also for China and India, to admit shortcomings, but it is not beyond the realm of possibility. The entire world would benefit from a skills market where good could meet with good, not only bad meeting with bad via traditional modes of competition, conflict, and deterrence.

There is a major problem, however. We have been drilled with endless repetition of the "developed vs. developing" dichotomy so that many of us believe the former have no problems whereas the latter do. Much better would be a yin-yang perspective on both: that something is missing in all, something is accomplished by all. The limitation lies in our limited public imagination. Expand it, and new world visions open up in our minds, shared with others in new speech, enacted by new acts. We can if we will. We will if we imagine.

Notes

1 See Galtung (2017).
2 They are spelled out in Galtung (2012).

References

Galtung, Johan. 2012. *A Theory of Peace: Building Direct Structural-Cultural Peace*. Grenzach-Whylen/Germany: Transcend University Press.

Galtung, Johan 2017. "The Transcend Track Record." In *The Art of Peace*. Grenzach-Whylen/Germany: Transcend University Press. Online version (2016) available at: www.galtung-institut.de/wp-content/uploads/2016/08/GALTUNG-MEDIATION-TRACKRECORD-.pdf.

29

IMAGINING GLOBAL GOVERNANCE

Alternatives to Trump, Brexit, and New Wars

Mary Kaldor

Human beings imagine their own futures, to paraphrase Marx, but they do so in circumstances transmitted from the past (Marx 1852). Our political and social institutions were designed for a different era—the era of mass production, cheap oil, automobiles and aircraft, roads and suburbia, radio and television, mass consumption and high military spending. That era, the American dominated model of development, began to falter already in the 1970's when the United States experienced its first trade deficit and its defeat in Vietnam. The response to decreasing rates of profit was neo-liberalism and privatization—what has become known as market fundamentalism or sometimes globalization. The deregulation of global flows of capital allowed for the spread of new technologies, particularly information and communication, and the rise of new economic centers (most notably China and India), but also grotesque inequalities, the disproportionate growth of finance capital, and the increasing co-optation of states—especially the United States and the United Kingdom—by corporate power.

There is an evident parallel with the 1920's and 30's when the British dominated model of development, which relied on heavy industry, railways and ships, newspapers and telegraph, coal, and empire was coming to an end, as well as strong similarities between the crash of 1929 and the crash of 2008. Like now, that crash heralded a rightward, not a leftward shift in politics. Whether we are talking about fascism in the 1930s or the Trump and Brexit phenomena today we can interpret this rightwards tendency as a failure of the political imagination. It was the inability of the dominant political classes to tell a story that made sense of our present and offered a plausible imagined future, their tendency to repeat a tired rhetoric that contradicted everyday lived experience, that made possible a negative backward-looking alternative story. In both the 1930s and today, it was a failure of the left—the belief by the representatives of the left that they needed to compromise with market fundamentalism in order to capture power—that created a gaping hole in the collective imagination. So it was that the new, claiming to be old, scions of the right were able to manipulate nostalgia for a time when our institutions seemed to work and to attribute blame for the breakdown of our institutions on the so-called newcomer, 'the other' who has spoiled our golden past. In the 1930s, this kind of thinking led to the rise of fascism and culminated in a war.

So are contemporary developments likely to lead to war? In my view this is highly likely, but, rather than an inter-state war like the wars of the twentieth century, we confront instead what I call a 'new war' on a global basis. A 'new war' (Kaldor 2012) is a mixture of crime, sectarian conflict, and massive violations of human rights as in the former Yugoslavia or in Libya, Yemen, and Syria today. A new war is a product of backward-looking blame games—the Serbs, for example, who mobilized popular sentiment through an appeal to an imaginary heroic history where pure orthodox Serbs win or lose battles against the evil Turks and genocidal Albanians, or the Salafists who recruit rootless young men with the claim that the corruption of Western capitalism could be solved through a return to literal interpretations of the Koran, or ethnicized Russians who counter the democratic multi-ethnic Ukrainian movement with sectarian narratives. In this type of war, conventional battles are rare and most violence is directed towards civilians—the 'other' of this twisted form of political imagination.

The Russians call this type of war 'non-linear war'. The Russian Chief of Staff, Valeri Gerassimov, explained that (Galeotti 2014) frontal assaults are a thing of the past and that nowadays it is possible to destabilize countries through support for domestic opposition, special forces, information warfare, and what the Russians call 'political technology' (seen at work in the UK Brexit referendum and the 2016 US presidential election). Indeed, old-fashioned military power has been shown in recent wars to be extraordinarily ineffective, in the classic sense of 'compellence'. The Iraq and Afghan wars have left both countries with greater instability than before the invasions. Russia razed Grozny to the ground twice yet it is still characterized by criminality and terrorism. The battle against ISIS in Iraq and Syria is producing more casualties than inflicted by ISIS, yet ISIS is already reappearing in liberated areas. Today's rightwing populism is not primarily directed against other states but against groups (Muslims, immigrants, Mexicans, Jews, blacks …) and against internationalism, especially the United Nations and the European Union. While the Korean crisis is alarming, a different sort of 'new war' violence seems more likely. Trump's behavior is eerily reminiscent of Milosevic, and it is increasingly pervasive violence of the sort already experienced in the former Yugoslavia, Africa, and the Middle East that could easily come to characterize the US (especially given the availability of guns) and maybe Britain too.

The hugely destructive and tragic wars of the twentieth century involved the entire population and profoundly restructured societies; victory was achieved through mobilization around a new narrative based on mass participation that had the potential to shape the new model of development. In contrast, a global new war will be decentralized and fragmented and is likely to increase inequalities, to benefit a few obscenely rich groups, and to entrench backward-looking exclusive ideologies. Casualties are unlikely to be as high as earlier wars but mass forced displacement and widespread environmental degradation has already become normal. Such wars as we have discovered elsewhere tend to spread through extremist ideas, transnational crime, and trauma. They are also very persistent and very difficult to end.

So is there an alternative to a global new war? Can we tell a new story that would enable us to imagine new or reformed institutions that could counter rather than win wars? Such a story would need to be relevant for a global, resource saving, socially just model of development based on information and communications technologies. Writing in 1939, the historian E.H. Carr drew a distinction between utopia and realism in International Relations (Carr 2016). Utopians propose various international schemes for world peace. Realists analyze the world in terms of states and the military and economic power they possess. Carr argued that the Utopians of the inter-war period had failed to take realism into account even though the realists often found it necessary to clothe their power in utopian language in order to exert power. I think the opposite is the case today. Utopianism, the construction of effective global institutions, is the only realistic option. Putin and Trump clothe their actions in the language of traditional realism (statism and sovereignty) and this can only lead to war and violence. The only way to address the problems that we face today is through a new or reformed set of institutions at international or global and local levels. It is absurd to argue that welfare is no longer affordable when the world has become far richer than ever before. Welfare and income distribution require a reduction in the overall share of finance capital and the regulation of global financial flows so as to protect policy making at local levels. Rich individuals and companies no longer pay taxes. Therefore, safe havens have to be closed down and a new family of taxes (on finance, on multinationals, on carbon) need to be raised to redistribute income and pay for global public services like resource-saving infrastructure, peace and human security, and global health initiatives. In new wars, it is at local levels that resistance is most effective, especially among women, allowing some cities and towns to keep out of the violence. At present, cities like London, Seattle, or New York are leading the resistance to right-wing populism; they need to make common cause with each other and with global institutions.

Currently, the dominant narratives are polarized between a right-wing nationalist populism and global neo-liberalism. The left is divided between the old nationalist left and those, like Clinton and Blair, who compromised with neo-liberalism. What we need is a new global emancipatory narrative that is global, green, socially just, and realistic, another way of seeing the world not through the national prism but through the prism of lived cosmopolitanism and realistic engagement with the problems we face. It has to resonate with everyday experience and can only be constructed through campaigns and struggles as well as practical implementation. The seeds of this narrative already exist in local initiatives or movements like the global Women's March on the day of Trump's inaugural. What is lacking is an imagined institutional framework.

President Barak Obama recently made the point (Wintour 2017) that "this generation is the most sophisticated, the most tech-savvy, the most entrepreneurial, but they do not have much faith in existing institutions." Is it possible for the political imagination to encompass new sorts of institutions and models of global governance that do not replace the state but restrain its worst aspects—war and fascism—and overcome its limitations in addressing contemporary global issues like climate change or financial speculation? One consequence of Brexit is that a new generation, which had taken the existence of the European Union for granted, is now discovering its European identity, how much it values freedom to work, study, and play across the European Union and how important the existence of the Union is in upholding political, social, and environmental rights. This has produced new movements, debates, proposals, and discussions about how to democratize and reform the European Union. Could something similar happen, for example, in relation to the United Nations as a consequence of UN votes on Jerusalem, Iran, or North Korea? In other words, could global governance come to be viewed not as an abstract technical preoccupation of a global elite, but as something that can capture the popular imagination of a new generation—a new realistic utopia?

References

Carr, Edward Hallett. 2016. *The Twenty Years' Crisis, 1919-1939*. London: Palgrave Macmillan.

Galeotti, Mark. 2014. "The 'Gerasimov Doctrine' and Russian Non-Linear War." In Moscow's Shadows, July 6, 2014. http://inmoscowsshadows.wordpress.com/2014/07/06/the-gerasimov-doctrine-and-russian-non-linear-war/.

Kaldor, Mary. 2012. *Old and New Wars: Organized Violence in a Global Era*, 3rd ed. Cambridge: Polity.

Marx, Karl. 1852. "Feb. 1848 to Dec. 1851." In *The Eighteenth Brumaire of Louis Bonaparte*. Translated by Saul K. Padover. Marx/Engels Internet Archive. www.marxists.org/archive/marx/works/1852/18th-brumaire/ch01.htm.

Wintour, Patrick. 2017. "The Prophet of Dystopia." *The Guardian*, December 27, 2017. www.theguardian.com/us-news/2017/dec/27/barack-obama-tells-prince-harry-leaders-must-stop-corroding-civil-discourse.

30

POLITICS OF COMPASSION IN AN AGE OF RUTHLESS POWER

Kevin P. Clements

The world is confronted by many challenges that cannot be resolved within states alone. Climate change, negative globalization, economic vulnerability, social and environmental precarity, war, refugees, political corruption, and high levels of alienation from political processes and institutions are driving state dysfunction and rising levels of political extremism all around the world.

The challenges of our time are not North-South problems anymore. They are global, and they are having a profoundly pathological impact on state systems and democratic politics everywhere. In the first instance, they reflect and are producing deeply divided societies. For example, there have been few clear winners in many recent elections (e.g the United Kingdom, the United States, Germany, New Zealand, Austria were all largely divided down the middle). Second, there has been a deliberate cultivation of existential fear and anxiety by opportunistic leaders and their media allies. This has been used to justify the expansion of dominatory[1] and authoritarian politics. Third, against the social democratic trends of the late 20th century a permissive environment has been created for the promotion of a politics of inequality and greed. The richest one percent of the world's population, for example has seen its share of global wealth increase from 44 percent in 2009 to 48 percent in 2014 and more than 50 percent in 2016.[2] Fourth, the protection of this global wealth has resulted in an expanded use of coercive diplomacy and military intervention with disastrous consequences for all the countries concerned.

While these trends are eliciting some resistance, so far it has been reactive rather than proactive and not well rooted in dynamics capable of challenging arbitrary and authoritarian rule. It is therefore vital to formulate new socio-political imaginaries that can inspire creative resistance as well as political actors motivated by serving the common good rather than sectional interests. Because Left-Right politics have lost their traction since the end of the cold war, many democracies have been caught in the politics of a paralyzing present. This is why it is critical to articulate social and communitarian spaces to generate forms of public imagination that are progressive, emancipatory, and effective against ruthless power and dominatory politics.

To do this effectively requires an embrace of diversity, ambiguity, and some degree of disorder. Progressive political actors have to be willing to live with questions that have no simple solutions while providing a strong and effective counterpoint to the simplistic solutions of autocratic populists. This is a critical antithesis to the authoritarian imagination that prioritizes political order and hierarchy in vain attempts to control a chaotic world. Authoritarian regimes are incapable of resolving complex transnational problems in an interdependent world because their intent is domination. We need a fundamental paradigm shift.

The first step in this process is to develop a rationale for ensuring that political imaginaries focus attention on how states, societies, and communities might move from dominatory to collaborative power. If we are to generate a genuine paradigm shift from a notion of sovereignty based on "power over" others to one based on "power with" others, it is critical that we embrace value and normative systems capable of sustaining egalitarian, relatively non-coercive, and integrative sensibilities. This means concentrating more attention on social rather than political sources of continuity, change, predictability, and order.

States like to argue that social systems are dependent on their coercive capacity, without which anarchy would reign. It is important to reverse the optics on these assumptions. Social and economic relationships are arguably more critical to effective, capable, and legitimate governance than coercive capacity. When states reveal the iron fist behind the velvet glove of enlightened governance it is normally because their policies (economic, social, or political) have failed and large numbers of citizens no longer believe that the state is acting in their interest. Most political theory and politicians with authoritarian inclinations therefore concentrate on the state as the principle ordering agent, with coercive agency as its major weapon. It is time to focus attention on more fundamental social dynamics if we are to develop paradigms capable of doing justice to diversity and to inclusive, resilient, and democratic polities.

The second step, therefore, is to focus attention on what currently delivers unity, stability, and harmony. The most fundamental social dynamic governing most relationships and the DNA for peacefulness is the norm of reciprocity. It has been systematically isolated and marginalized from the realm of the political by those who want to argue the primacy of the state, yet it is the norm of reciprocity that holds most communities and societies together through time. Without it states would have to depend almost completely on their monopoly of force. Predictable social relationships are much more important than "imposed" political order. Reciprocity is the glue that governs the millions of social exchanges that take place every day, most of which have nothing to do with the realm of politics. The norm of reciprocity generates altruism among kin and non-kin groups; it limits selfishness and challenges freeloaders and dominators; it creates the sociological and social psychological basis for equality, integration, and harmony, and is capable of providing a critical frame for anti-authoritarian resistive politics. To do this effectively, however, means linking this fundamental social rule to what I call the politics of compassion.

For me, therefore, new political imaginaries must be deeply rooted in basic norms of sociation and exchange accompanied by altruistic political programs aimed at serving the common good rather than narrow state interests. The politics of compassion, therefore, is the opposite of dominatory, fear driven, xenophobic politics based on a monopoly of force and coercion. I think that it has the capacity to be a new political paradigm for an interdependent world. It starts with compassionate citizens, who elect compassionate politicians capable of utilizing political mechanisms toward more compassionate societies. Its radicalism hinges on insisting that social (rather than economic and political) criteria be the major foci of political decision making (for example, by asking how economic, political, and military decisions will impact social well-being and community. The New Zealand Labour, Green, NZ First government, for example, has just released its 2019 budget. They labelled it a "Wellbeing" budget and it uses metrics aimed at promoting cultural identities, civic engagement and responsive governance, social connections, mental health, and so on. This is a good example of directions that progressive politics need to move in). The politics of compassion, therefore, is inclusive rather than exclusive, egalitarian rather than hierarchical, and it rests on sociation and relationships instead of domination. It aims at resolving problems non-violently, collaboratively, empathetically, and altruistically.

For this idea to take hold, however, it is vital that leaders interested in promoting a politics of compassion build transparent and open communications and incentives to reward fair, equal, reciprocal, and resilient exchanges between peoples. In this process, more attention should be directed to enhancing the power of unifiers in communities and diminishing the power of dividers. The challenge, however, is understanding and combating all the dynamics which threaten to undermine these values—possessive individualism, neo-liberalism, and elite-driven politics.

Compassionate citizens do not occur by accident. They need to be nurtured and rewarded. In the first instance this suggests paying more attention to emotional intelligence. Compassionate citizens should be encouraged to lead by example rather than direction and to focus on positive rather than negative sanctions in relation to social order. The promotion of compassionate politics should reinforce positive relationships, decrease the prevalence of toxic negative emotions and behavior, increase optimism and hope, build resilience and energy levels, and counter fear-based politics. Compassionate politics is loving kindness in action. It pays particular attention to health, education, and welfare—key to life and societal happiness, and critical reinforcers of reciprocity. This is why welfare states have been so successful on most well-being indicators, even though these systems are not immune to authoritarian impulses if subject to the politics of fear.

For a new, socially driven imaginary to succeed it must first, however, analyze and negate politics and practices of domination everywhere. This means analyzing relationships of domination and subordination at the personal and social as well as formal political levels. The #metoo movement is a wonderful example of women challenging patriarchal entitlement, harassment, and dominant relationships in workplaces and in homes. It is around these kinds of movements that political respect is forged and compassionate politics become possible.

Second, there can be no compassionate politics that does not place equality and inclusion at its heart. This means a radical critique of the ways in which our social processes produce and reproduce patterns of hierarchy, power, and privilege. But it also means giving priority to the weakest and poorest and, as mentioned above, an identification and reinforcement of individuals and groups who are willing to sustain the social fabric in the face of economic and political subversion.

Third, it means focusing on inclusive participatory processes capable of doing justice to the concrete experiences of those who are victims of domination, violence, marginalization, and humiliation. This new paradigm rests on personal transformation and a willingness to live courageous, hopeful, and loving lives. These are critical ingredients for speaking "truth" to power, for challenging dominatory power, force, and coercion.

Finally, promoting the politics of compassion demands a few practical steps.[3] People should learn the capacity to reach out to those they fear. Second, we should strive to transcend simplistic dualistic thinking so that we might touch the heart of complexity, develop more empathetic consciousness, and eliminate the unproductive naming and blaming of others for our own mistakes. A third step is imagining beyond what is seen—a quality at the heart of what this essay series has been investigating. How do we (whoever the we is) develop new imaginaries suitable for the 21st century? Finally, as John Paul Lederach suggests, we might want to risk vulnerability one step at a time. To do this means quietly replacing the old paradigms with something new, and ensuring that the risks we take will be transformative rather than ineffective. If we wish to enhance the dignity of every single human being on the planet, it is critical that we focus on emancipatory relationships—fully aware of their risks, but emboldened by the mandate for a radical alternative to a destructive, inhumane status quo.

Notes

1 Dominatory politics/processes refer to all those exchanges that result in the intentional or unintentional subordination of others and the development of persistent hierarchies based on age, race, gender or class.
2 Members of this global elite had an average wealth of $2.9 million per adult in 2016. (Oxfam 2016).
3 Derived from Lederach (2010).

References

210 Oxfam Briefing Paper. "An Economy for the 1%." Oxfam, January 18, 2016. www.cdn.oxfam.org/s3fs-public/file_attachments/bp210-economy-one-percent-tax-havens-180116-en_0.pdf.

Lederach, John Paul. 2010. *The moral imagination: the art and soul of building peace*. Oxford: Oxford University Press.

Bibliography

Sidanius, Jim, and Felicia Pratto. 1999. *Social Dominance: An Intergroup Theory of Social Hierarchy and Oppression*. Cambridge: Cambridge University Press.

CODA

Victor Faessel

This volume has its origins in a thought piece that I shared some years ago with Richard Falk on the contemporary public life of myths. Not specifically the myths of pantheons and their celestial inhabitants. Nor the mythology of early 20th-century psychologists, their drives, complexes, and archetypes, nor their 19th and 20th century counterparts among classicists, anthropologists, political philosophers, semioticians, historians, literary canon keepers (and bashers). Nor again 'myths' as equated nowadays with public ignorance or popular delusions, political obfuscations, historical fabrications, fake news, pop culture heroism (and heroics), and their like. Rather, my reflections were about each and every one of these things. This is because all of them contribute something to the background of what it means today to think in a global setting about the public relevance of certain kinds of *stories*—salient, valorized, significance-bearing conduits of imagination that stir and channel the passions of individuals, groups, nations, whole civilizations. I was thinking here as well in terms of 'discursive traditions' that are also about critique and proposal, the stretching of the boundaries of the possible. About identifying that uncertain terrain where utopian imaginings impart both wisdom and restraint. For their diverse audiences, such narratives are part of what shape cultural identity, often playing a significant and at times powerfully affective role in displays of civic political imagination.

It had been my starting point that the one thing most urgently needful of attention in everything that counts as 'mythology' since the middle of the 20th century must be the public, political force of myth and myths, their relationship to social action—for better and for worse. If the 20th and early 21st centuries teach us anything at all, it is that such stories—whether revered ones of the (supposedly) timeless or distant past, the modern (Enlightenment) ones erected against them, or the new/old/mashed up 'counter-'narratives that now proliferate effusively in the latter group's wake—retain potentials of emotive salience that can translate into considerable social energy. This gives them a force that impacts not just the private and public lives of peoples everywhere, but the very biotic conditions of human existence. Today, entering a bio-ethical crisis of our own making that imperils not just 'sovereign' human political constructs but the natural foundation of human and non-human species, we are called upon to cast, recast, and embrace narratives that capture a sense of the origins and destiny of all earthly life, prior to its division into 'kingdoms'.

The Introduction to this volume is what evolved from the generous comments Richard offered to my reflections on myth and politics. Unsurprisingly, and characteristically, his reading broadened and elevated the scope of my original paragraphs in crucial ways that impart much of the shape of the collection, because the essay that grew from our exchange, helpfully critiqued and extended by Michael Curtin, became the nucleus around which to invite responses from a wide array of contributors. To be sure, they were not solicited with explicit reference to my mythic nexus of concerns. Their chapters speak more often indirectly to the narrative, story-mediated dimensions of public imagination. But it seems fair to say that the historical and contemporary problem of and prospects for precisely these dimensions of group, national, 'civilizational' public imagination lie close to the heart of each essay. This is because, wherever one looks, whatever policy or political philosophy or prognostication, whatever social vision or historical remembrance, whatever religious, spiritual, and cosmological conviction, or prejudice, or polemic, or conspiracy theory, all are mediated by narratives. All are objects of imaginative play—but also of conscious rhetorical construction, and of intentional discursive deployment.

What seems clear in our time is that, worldwide, more people than ever are waking up to the failure of a dominant economistic narrative and its underlying "anthropology" (i.e., basic vision and "logos" of the human being) whose material day-to-day upshot creates wealth for the few, injustice for the many, conflict and now obvious ecological crisis for all. There is a palpable sense that the lid is being held down, sat on, more and more desperately, by obscene wealth and its political servant class at the helm of corroded and too often democratically neglected institutions of government. Our era's heightened awareness of injustice is manipulated with dependable, yet socially poisonous tropes of 'invading' and/or 'immoral' others—little *myths* that work well in challenging or transitional times to distract segments of the population needful of, or receptive only to, the simplest explanations. Their social cost, as all can see, is extremism and polarization.

But, as many of the chapters collected here suggest, potentials for engaged, enlivened, humane, and ecologically sensitive publics are present and do flourish today. They just have a hard time getting across in the fragmented cultural maelstrom of partisan politics, ubiquitous advertising, and social media that mostly benumb and trivialize imagination. But it is important to remember that humane imaginaries have never ceased to flourish, that social and economic betterment, the rule of law, the right to vote, the right to equality and justice and self-determination are the hard-won victories of the ceaseless, restless imagination of human dignity, realized by people struggling for a better future for themselves and others—often at times when such aspirations seemed, at best, utopian.

In order for visions of a better future to gain traction, however, individual consciousness en masse has to be propelled beyond styles of *being political* in which affect (that which moves us prior to conscious filtering) remains isolated, solitary, reactive, and projective. Political engagement is too often now 'socially' expressed though online sharing, trolling, hating in virtual 'public spaces' become theaters of caustic and violent outburst, narrowing what ought to be multisided political debate to ceaseless tension between tribes that are civically disconnected and imagine themselves in a state of war against their opponents. Whatever the emergent narrative of hope and transformation toward a just, sustainable and shareable human future, it will have to stimulate more people to adopt informed and interpersonal (i.e., public) modes of participation. At stake is the danger of abandoning public spaces—*civic* spaces—and surrendering them to gangs, mobs, unscrupulous agitators, rage killers, and militias (self-styled or state sanctioned). Where today it is possible to speak of an increasingly assertive 'virtual demos' that has outward, tangible public effects, it seems vitally important to sustain old-fashioned arguments for something at least close to a modern civic demos that is at once radically more inclusive but also more systematically and collaboratively devoted to rendering naked the agents of cynical power, of civic fragmentation, and of ecological collapse.

As for the role of imagination in a revitalized public sphere, it needs to urge us beyond the usual binary agonies—of cosmopolitan versus tribal (national); frugal and generous versus greedy and rapacious; generally thriving commonweal versus egoistic and exclusive competition—towards a collective dedication to an ethos that is *creaturely*, one that extends like filial attachment toward animals and the biological foundations of life, transcending andro- and anthro-centrism. In short, we need to envision a humane ecological consciousness that allows both the most immediate and the most remote to flourish within the same mental habitat, that embraces transcendent and cosmic vision while honoring myriad neighborhoods of immediacy.

Public Imagination

The two words in juxtaposition make for a rather unstable plank. There is something at first nonsensical about the term. Does it mean, expressions of private individual imagination that spill into the public realm (for better or worse)? Or, the imagination of a public, should such a thing be possible? (Many would deny it.) And if we agree that publics exist, what are they? Whose are they? What about the differences between Western and non-Western publics, which vary widely, for example, on issues of individual vs. collective rights and responsibilities? And what about the private sphere? Do we mean to deny, denigrate, devalue it? Indeed, the more one mulls the words "public imagination," the sense of a certain kind of threat or challenge seems to creep in.

To our way of thinking this would be a very good thing. For if public imagination in an age of authoritarian and populist politics, of recrudescent nativism, racism, and revanchism, and of ecological calamity's arrival should mean anything, it should be about unsettling any sought-after quiescence of secure isolation, safety in walled-off communities of the like-minded. The social facts of justice, equality, tolerance, freedom—to the extent that they actually exist where one happens to live—are only 'facts' in this sense because they have been and continue to be fought for by *coalitions* of conscience and commitment. In our time, the forces (these are people, not abstractions) who would deny or restrict or even abolish those hard-won gains would like for us to believe that they and their friends are taking over public space. News and media—including much 'social' media—that have forfeited all allegiance to social good for the pursuit of profit wherever and however it can be squeezed out, would have us believe the same. But those facts of 'civilized' life that even haters and racists and militiamen take for granted were wrested from fear and benightedness by an imagination not just for private individual good, but also in and for the general, public good. As a form of political passion, this sensibility needs to catch on.

Asking about the private sphere points to questions only adumbrated within the pages of this collection. Of course, it goes without saying that imagination, in the end, feels like a very private thing. But where its forms, preoccupations, and stirrings become matters of discussion, shared affective facts having as their object the quality and structure of group concerns, then imagination is a very public matter indeed. It will always become so, if given access to public space. It is ridiculous, it would be nonsensical, to think that a small collection like this could ever aspire to say all there is to say on the matter. The hope, the point of this set of reflections is to stimulate dialogue, debate, and conversation—ideally, of the kinds that spark small fires of intersubjective community imagination with wildfire potential. Minds and souls in numbers, fired up, not just launching but coordinating movements, medleys of cooperative ethical passion become concrete acts toward a future no one can wait for any longer. A future whose imperatives the old, tired, exclusive myths will never deliver.

APPENDIX

Sara Lafia

Visualizing public imagination reveals latent patterns throughout the volume. To discover major topics, I modeled the text of each chapter using a statistical technique called latent Dirichlet allocation (LDA). The resulting topics were then visualized in 62 "topic bubbles" that provide a semantic overview and enable comparisons.

As expected, "public" is a prevalent topic throughout the volume, but its usage is also situated in specific political and cultural contexts, with populism and authoritarianism emerging as bridges. Less prominent topics, ranging from media to torture, are interspersed.

While cross-cutting notions of law, rights, and religion are central as well, contrasting ideas are visible on the periphery. Topics about peace and war, national and global, religious and secular, minority and majority reflect a diversity of perspectives. Overall, the visualization points to major, minor, central, and peripheral ideas, providing a complement to the book's introduction, table of contents, and index.

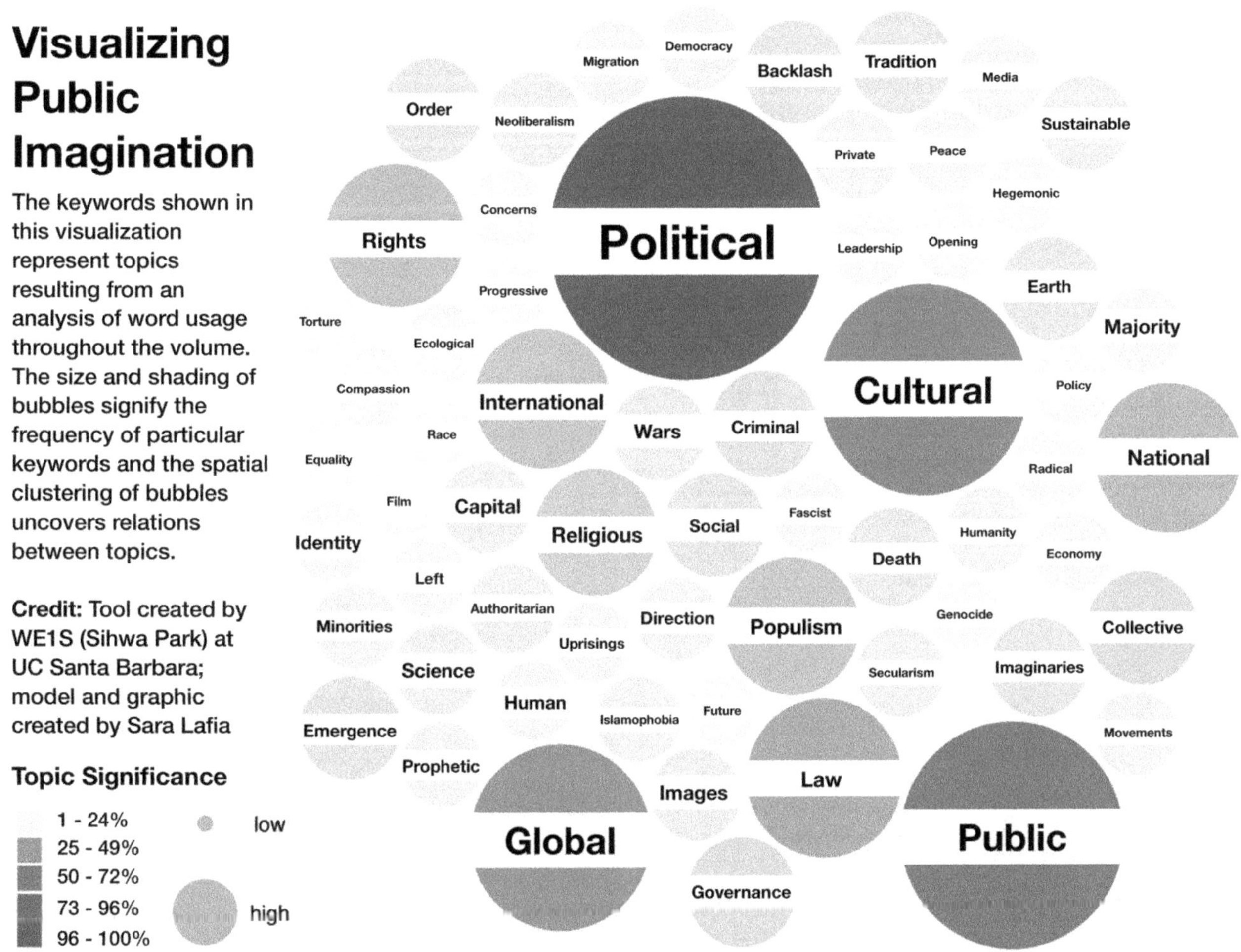

Figure A.1 Visualization of Key Concepts, their Frequency of Appearance and Relations.

INDEX